T0207264

Lecture Notes in Computer Science   14092

Founding Editors

Gerhard Goos
Juris Hartmanis

Editorial Board Members

Elisa Bertino, *Purdue University, West Lafayette, IN, USA*
Wen Gao, *Peking University, Beijing, China*
Bernhard Steffen ⑩, *TU Dortmund University, Dortmund, Germany*
Moti Yung ⑩, *Columbia University, New York, NY, USA*

The series Lecture Notes in Computer Science (LNCS), including its subseries Lecture Notes in Artificial Intelligence (LNAI) and Lecture Notes in Bioinformatics (LNBI), has established itself as a medium for the publication of new developments in computer science and information technology research, teaching, and education.

LNCS enjoys close cooperation with the computer science R & D community, the series counts many renowned academics among its volume editors and paper authors, and collaborates with prestigious societies. Its mission is to serve this international community by providing an invaluable service, mainly focused on the publication of conference and workshop proceedings and postproceedings. LNCS commenced publication in 1973.

Spyridon Bakas · Alessandro Crimi ·
Ujjwal Baid · Sylwia Malec · Monika Pytlarz ·
Bhakti Baheti · Maximilian Zenk ·
Reuben Dorent
Editors

Brainlesion:
Glioma, Multiple Sclerosis, Stroke and Traumatic Brain Injuries

8th International Workshop, BrainLes 2022
Held in Conjunction with MICCAI 2022
Singapore, September 18, 2022
Revised Selected Papers, Part II

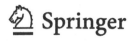 Springer

Editors
Spyridon Bakas ⓘ
University of Pennsylvania
Philadelphia, PA, USA

Ujjwal Baid ⓘ
University of Pennsylvania
Philadelphia, PA, USA

Monika Pytlarz ⓘ
Sano, Center for Computational Personalised
Medicine
Kraków, Poland

Maximilian Zenk ⓘ
German Cancer Research Center
Heidelberg, Germany

Alessandro Crimi ⓘ
Sano, Center for Computational Personalised
Medicine
Kraków, Poland

Sylwia Malec ⓘ
Sano, Center for Computational Personalised
Medicine
Kraków, Poland

Bhakti Baheti ⓘ
University of Pennsylvania
Philadelphia, PA, USA

Reuben Dorent ⓘ
Harvard Medical School
Boston, MA, USA

ISSN 0302-9743   ISSN 1611-3349 (electronic)
Lecture Notes in Computer Science
ISBN 978-3-031-44152-3   ISBN 978-3-031-44153-0 (eBook)
https://doi.org/10.1007/978-3-031-44153-0

This Springer imprint is published by the registered company Springer Nature Switzerland AG
The registered company address is: Gewerbestrasse 11, 6330 Cham, Switzerland

Paper in this product is recyclable.

Preface

This volume contains articles from the Brain Lesion workshop (BrainLes), as well as the Brain Tumor Segmentation (BraTS) Challenge, the Brain Tumor Sequence Registration (BraTS-Reg) Challenge, the Cross-Modality Domain Adaptation (CrossMoDA) Challenge, and the Federated Tumor Segmentation (FeTS) Challenge. All these events were held in conjunction with the Medical Image Computing and Computer Assisted Intervention (MICCAI) conference on the 18th–22nd of September 2022 in Singapore.

The submissions for each conference were reviewed through a rigorous double-blind peer-review process. The review process involved the evaluation of the submitted papers by at least three independent reviewers, ensuring high quality and reliability of the accepted papers. The average number of papers reviewed by each reviewer was two, which helped to maintain the consistency and fairness of the review process.

The presented manuscripts describe the research of computational scientists and clinical researchers working on brain lesions, and specifically glioma, multiple sclerosis, cerebral stroke, traumatic brain injuries, vestibular schwannoma, and white matter hyper-intensities of presumed vascular origin. This compilation does not claim to provide a comprehensive understanding from all points of view; however, the authors present their latest advances in segmentation, registration, federated learning, disease prognosis, and other applications to the clinical context.

The volume is divided into five chapters: The first chapter comprises the accepted paper submissions to the BrainLes workshop, and the second through the fifth chapters contain a selection of papers regarding methods presented at the BraTS, BraTS-Reg, CrossMoDA, and FeTS challenges, respectively.

The aim of the **first chapter**, focusing on the accepted **BrainLes workshop submissions**, is to provide an overview of new advances of medical image analysis in all the aforementioned brain pathologies. It brings together researchers from the medical image analysis domain, neurologists, and radiologists working on at least one of these diseases. The aim is to consider neuroimaging biomarkers used for one disease applied to the other diseases. This session did not have a specific dataset to be used. BrainLes workshop received 15 submissions, out of which 10 papers were accepted.

The **second chapter** focuses on a selection of papers from the **BraTS 2022** challenge participants. BraTS 2022 had a two-fold intention: a) to report a snapshot of the state-of-the-art developments in the continuous evaluation schema of the RSNA-ASNR-MICCAI BraTS challenge, which made publicly available the largest ever manually annotated dataset of baseline pre-operative brain glioma scans from 20 international institutions, and b) to quantify the generalizability performance of these algorithms on out-of-sample independent multi-institutional sources covering underrepresented Sub-Saharan African adult patient populations of brain diffuse glioma and from a pediatric population of diffuse intrinsic pontine glioma (DIPG) patients. All challenge data were routine clinically acquired, multi-institutional, skull-stripped multi-parametric magnetic resonance imaging (mpMRI) scans of brain tumor patients (provided in NIfTI file format). Total number of manuscript sent to review in BraTS were 16, from which 9 were accepted.

The **third chapter** contains a selection of papers from the **BraTS-Reg 2022** challenge participants. BraTS-Reg 2022 intended to establish a benchmark environment for deformable registration algorithms, focusing on estimating correspondences between baseline pre-operative and follow-up scans of the same patient diagnosed with a brain glioma. The challenge data comprise de-identified multi-institutional mpMRI scans, curated for each scan's size and resolution, according to a canonical anatomical template (similarly to BraTS). The unique difficulty here comes from the induced tumor mass effect that harshly shifts brain tissue in unknown directions. Extensive landmarks points annotations within the scans were provided by the clinical experts of the organizing committee. Among 13 papers submitted in BraTS-Reg challenge, 9 were accepted.

The **fourth chapter** contains a selection of papers from the **CrossMoDA 2022** challenge participants. CrossMoDA 2022 was the continuation of the first large and multi-class benchmark for unsupervised cross-modality domain adaptation for medical image segmentation. Compared to the previous CrossMoDA instance, which used single-institution data and featured a single segmentation task, the 2022 edition extended the segmentation task by including multi-institutional data and introduced a new classification task. The segmentation task aims to segment two key brain structures involved in the follow-up and treatment planning of vestibular schwannoma (VS): the VS tumour and the cochleas. The goal of the classification challenge is to automatically classify T2 images with VS according to the Koos grade. The training dataset provides annotated T1 scans (N=210) and unpaired non-annotated T2 scans (N=210). CrossMoDA received 8 submissions, from which 7 were accepted.

The **fifth chapter** contains a selection of papers from the **FeTS 2022** challenge participants. This was the continuation of the first computational challenge focussing on federated learning, and ample multi-institutional routine clinically acquired pre-operative baseline multi-parametric MRI scans of radiographically appearing glioblastoma (from the RSNA-ASNR-MICCAI BraTS challenge) were provided to the participants, along with splits on the basis of the site of acquisition. The goal of the challenge was two-fold: i) identify the best way to aggregate the knowledge coming from segmentation models trained on the individual institutions, and ii) find the best algorithm that produces robust and accurate brain tumor segmentations across different medical institutions, MRI scanners, image acquisition parameters, and populations. Interestingly, the second task was performed by actually circulating the containerized algorithms across different institutions, leveraging the collaborators of the largest to-date real-world federation (https://www.fets.ai) and in partnership with the largest open community effort for ML, namely MLCommons. FeTS challenge received a total of 13 submissions, out of which 11 papers were accepted.

We heartily hope that this volume will promote further exciting computational research on brain-related pathologies.

The BrainLes organizers,

Ujjwal Baid
Spyridon Bakas
Alessandro Crimi
Sylwia Malec
Monika Pytlarz

Organization

Main BrainLes Organizing Committee

Ujjwal Baid	University of Pennsylvania, USA
Spyridon Bakas	University of Pennsylvania, USA
Alessandro Crimi	Sano Science, Poland
Sylwia Malec	Sano Science, Poland
Monika Pytlarz	Sano Science, Poland

BrainLes Program Committee

Maruf Adewole	University of Lagos, Nigeria
Bhakti Baheti	University of Pennsylvania, USA
Ujjwal Baid	University of Pennsylvania, USA
Florian Kofler	Technical University of Munich, Germany
Hugo Kuijf	University Medical School of Utrecht, The Netherlands
Andreas Mang	University of Houston, USA
Zahra Riahi Samani	University of Pennsylvania, USA
Maciej Szymkowski	Sano Science, Poland
Siddhesh Thakur	University of Pennsylvania, USA
Benedikt Wiestler	Technical University of Munich, Germany

Challenges Organizing Committee

Brain Tumor Segmentation (BraTS) Challenge

Ujjwal Baid	University of Pennsylvania, USA
Spyridon Bakas (Lead Organizer)	University of Pennsylvania, USA
Evan Calabrese*	University of California San Francisco, USA
Christopher Carr*	Radiological Society of North America (RSNA), USA
Errol Colak*	Unity Health Toronto, Canada
Keyvan Farahani	National Institutes of Health (NIH), USA
Adam E. Flanders*	Thomas Jefferson University Hospital, USA
Anahita Fathi Kazerooni	University of Pennsylvania, USA

x   Organization

Felipe C Kitamura*	Diagnósticos da América SA (Dasa) and Universidade Federal de São Paulo, Brazil
Marius George Linguraru	Children's National Hospital, USA
Bjoern Menze	University of Zurich, Switzerland
Luciano Prevedello*	Ohio State University, USA
Jeffrey Rudie*	University of California San Francisco, USA
Russell Taki Shinohara	University of Pennsylvania, USA

* These organizers were involved in the BraTS 2021 Challenge, the data of which were used here, but were not directly involved in the BraTS 2022 Continuous Challenge.

The Brain Tumor Sequence Registration (BraTS-Reg) Challenge

Hamed Akbari	University of Pennsylvania, USA
Bhakti Baheti	University of Pennsylvania, USA
Spyridon Bakas	University of Pennsylvania, USA
Satrajit Chakrabarty	Washington University in St. Louis, USA
Bjoern Menze	University of Zurich, Switzerland
Aristeidis Sotiras	Washington University in St. Louis, USA
Diana Waldmannstetter	University of Zurich, Switzerland

Cross-Modality Domain Adaptation (CrossMoDA) Challenge

Spyridon Bakas	University of Pennsylvania, USA
Stefan Cornelissen	Elisabeth-TweeSteden Hospital, The Netherlands
Reuben Dorent (Lead Organizer)	King's College London, UK
Ben Glocker	Imperial College London, UK
Samuel Joutard	King's College London, UK
Aaron Kujawa	King's College London, UK
Patrick Langenhuizen	Elisabeth-TweeSteden Hospital, The Netherlands
Nicola Rieke	NVIDIA, Germany
Jonathan Shapey	King's College London, UK
Tom Vercauteren	King's College London, UK

Federated Tumor Segmentation (FeTS) Challenge

Ujjwal Baid	University of Pennsylvania, USA
Spyridon Bakas (Task 1 Lead Organizer)	University of Pennsylvania, USA
Timothy Bergquist	Sage Bionetworks, USA
Yong Chen	University of Pennsylvania, USA
Verena Chung	Sage Bionetworks, USA

James Eddy	Sage Bionetworks, USA
Brandon Edwards	Intel, USA
Ralf Floca	German Cancer Research Center (DKFZ), Germany
Patrick Foley	Intel, USA
Fabian Isensee	DKFZ, Germany
Alexandros Karargyris	IHU Strasbourg, France
Klaus Maier-Hein	DKFZ, Germany
Lena Maier-Hein	DKFZ, Germany
Jason Martin	Intel, USA
Peter Mattson	Google, USA
Bjoern Menze	University of Zurich, Switzerland
Sarthak Pati	University of Pennsylvania, USA
Annika Reinke	DKFZ, Germany
Prashant Shah	Intel, USA
Micah J Sheller	Intel, USA
Russell Taki Shinohara	University of Pennsylvania, USA
Maximilian Zenk (Task 2 Lead Organizer)	DKFZ, Germany
David Zimmerer	DKFZ, Germany

Contents – Part II

BraTS-Reg

Applying Quadratic Penalty Method for Intensity-Based Deformable
Image Registration on BraTS-Reg Challenge 2022 3
   Kewei Yan and Yonghong Yan

WSSAMNet: Weakly Supervised Semantic Attentive Medical Image
Registration Network 15
   Sahar Almahfouz Nasser, Nikhil Cherian Kurian, Mohit Meena,
   Saqib Shamsi, and Amit Sethi

Self-supervised iRegNet for the Registration of Longitudinal Brain MRI
of Diffuse Glioma Patients 25
   Ramy A. Zeineldin, Mohamed E. Karar, Franziska Mathis-Ullrich,
   and Oliver Burgert

3D Inception-Based TransMorph: Pre- and Post-operative Multi-contrast
MRI Registration in Brain Tumors 35
   Javid Abderezaei, Aymeric Pionteck, Agamdeep Chopra,
   and Mehmet Kurt

CrossMoDa

Unsupervised Cross-Modality Domain Adaptation for Vestibular
Schwannoma Segmentation and Koos Grade Prediction Based
on Semi-supervised Contrastive Learning 49
   Luyi Han, Yunzhi Huang, Tao Tan, and Ritse Mann

Koos Classification of Vestibular Schwannoma via Image
Translation-Based Unsupervised Cross-Modality Domain Adaptation 59
   Tao Yang and Lisheng Wang

MS-MT: Multi-scale Mean Teacher with Contrastive Unpaired Translation
for Cross-Modality Vestibular Schwannoma and Cochlea Segmentation 68
   Ziyuan Zhao, Kaixin Xu, Huai Zhe Yeo, Xulei Yang, and Cuntai Guan

An Unpaired Cross-Modality Segmentation Framework Using Data
Augmentation and Hybrid Convolutional Networks for Segmenting
Vestibular Schwannoma and Cochlea 79
　　Yuzhou Zhuang, Hong Liu, Enmin Song, Coskun Cetinkaya,
　　and Chih-Cheng Hung

Weakly Unsupervised Domain Adaptation for Vestibular Schwannoma
Segmentation 90
　　Shahad Hardan, Hussain Alasmawi, Xiangjian Hou,
　　and Mohammad Yaqub

Multi-view Cross-Modality MR Image Translation for Vestibular
Schwannoma and Cochlea Segmentation 100
　　Bogyeong Kang, Hyeonyeong Nam, Ji-Wung Han, Keun-Soo Heo,
　　and Tae-Eui Kam

Enhancing Data Diversity for Self-training Based Unsupervised
Cross-Modality Vestibular Schwannoma and Cochlea Segmentation 109
　　Han Liu, Yubo Fan, Ipek Oguz, and Benoit M. Dawant

FeTS

Regularized Weight Aggregation in Networked Federated Learning
for Glioblastoma Segmentation 121
　　Muhammad Irfan Khan, Mohammad Ayyaz Azeem, Esa Alhoniemi,
　　Elina Kontio, Suleiman A. Khan, and Mojtaba Jafaritadi

A Local Score Strategy for Weight Aggregation in Federated Learning 133
　　Gaurav Singh

Ensemble Outperforms Single Models in Brain Tumor Segmentation 142
　　Jianxun Ren, Wei Zhang, Ning An, Qingyu Hu, Youjia Zhang,
　　and Ying Zhou

FeTS Challenge 2022 Task 1: Implementing FedMGDA + and a New
Partitioning 154
　　Vasilis Siomos, Giacomo Tarroni, and Jonathan Passerrat-Palmbach

Efficient Federated Tumor Segmentation via Parameter Distance Weighted
Aggregation and Client Pruning 161
　　Meirui Jiang, Hongzheng Yang, Xiaofan Zhang, Shaoting Zhang,
　　and Qi Dou

Hybrid Window Attention Based Transformer Architecture for Brain
Tumor Segmentation 173
    Himashi Peiris, Munawar Hayat, Zhaolin Chen, Gary Egan,
    and Mehrtash Harandi

Robust Learning Protocol for Federated Tumor Segmentation Challenge 183
    Ambrish Rawat, Giulio Zizzo, Swanand Kadhe, Jonathan P. Epperlein,
    and Stefano Braghin

Model Aggregation for Federated Learning Considering Non-IID
and Imbalanced Data Distribution 196
    Yuan Wang, Renuga Kanagavelu, Qingsong Wei, Yechao Yang,
    and Yong Liu

FedPIDAvg: A PID Controller Inspired Aggregation Method for Federated
Learning 209
    Leon Mächler, Ivan Ezhov, Suprosanna Shit, and Johannes C. Paetzold

Federated Evaluation of nnU-Nets Enhanced with Domain Knowledge
for Brain Tumor Segmentation 218
    Krzysztof Kotowski, Szymon Adamski, Bartosz Machura,
    Wojciech Malara, Lukasz Zarudzki, and Jakub Nalepa

Experimenting FedML and NVFLARE for Federated Tumor Segmentation
Challenge 228
    Yaying Shi, Hongjian Gao, Salman Avestimehr, and Yonghong Yan

Author Index 241

Contents – Part I

BrainLes

Deep Quality Estimation: Creating Surrogate Models for Human Quality
Ratings 3
    Florian Kofler, Ivan Ezhov, Lucas Fidon, Izabela Horvath,
    Ezequiel de la Rosa, John LaMaster, Hongwei Li, Tom Finck,
    Suprosanna Shit, Johannes Paetzold, Spyridon Bakas, Marie Piraud,
    Jan Kirschke, Tom Vercauteren, Claus Zimmer, Benedikt Wiestler,
    and Bjoern Menze

Unsupervised Anomaly Localization with Structural Feature-Autoencoders 14
    Felix Meissen, Johannes Paetzold, Georgios Kaissis, and Daniel Rueckert

Transformer Based Models for Unsupervised Anomaly Segmentation
in Brain MR Images 25
    Ahmed Ghorbel, Ahmed Aldahdooh, Shadi Albarqouni,
    and Wassim Hamidouche

Weighting Schemes for Federated Learning in Heterogeneous
and Imbalanced Segmentation Datasets 45
    Sebastian Otálora, Jonathan Rafael-Patiño, Antoine Madrona,
    Elda Fischi-Gomez, Veronica Ravano, Tobias Kober,
    Søren Christensen, Arsany Hakim, Roland Wiest, Jonas Richiardi,
    and Richard McKinley

Temporally Adjustable Longitudinal Fluid-Attenuated Inversion Recovery
MRI Estimation / Synthesis for Multiple Sclerosis 57
    Jueqi Wang, Derek Berger, Erin Mazerolle, Othman Soufan,
    and Jacob Levman

Leveraging 2D Deep Learning ImageNet-trained Models for Native 3D
Medical Image Analysis 68
    Bhakti Baheti, Sarthak Pati, Bjoern Menze, and Spyridon Bakas

Probabilistic Tissue Mapping for Tumor Segmentation and Infiltration
Detection of Glioma 80
    Selene De Sutter, Wietse Geens, Matías Bossa, Anne-Marie Vanbinst,
    Johnny Duerinck, and Jef Vandemeulebroucke

Robustifying Automatic Assessment of Brain Tumor Progression from MRI ...   90
  Krzysztof Kotowski, Bartosz Machura, and Jakub Nalepa

MidFusNet: Mid-dense Fusion Network for Multi-modal Brain MRI
Segmentation 102
  Wenting Duan, Lei Zhang, Jordan Colman, Giosue Gulli, and Xujiong Ye

Semi-supervised Intracranial Aneurysm Segmentation with Selected
Unlabeled Data 115
  Shiyu Lu, Hao Wang, and Chuyang Ye

BraTS

Multimodal CNN Networks for Brain Tumor Segmentation in MRI:
A BraTS 2022 Challenge Solution 127
  *Ramy A. Zeineldin, Mohamed E. Karar, Oliver Burgert,
  and Franziska Mathis-Ullrich*

Multi-modal Transformer for Brain Tumor Segmentation 138
  Jihoon Cho and Jinah Park

An Efficient Cascade of U-Net-Like Convolutional Neural Networks
Devoted to Brain Tumor Segmentation 149
  *Philippe Bouchet, Jean-Baptiste Deloges, Hugo Canton-Bacara,
  Gaëtan Pusel, Lucas Pinot, Othman Elbaz, and Nicolas Boutry*

Tuning U-Net for Brain Tumor Segmentation 162
  Michał Futrega, Michał Marcinkiewicz, and Pablo Ribalta

Diffraction Block in Extended nn-UNet for Brain Tumor Segmentation 174
  Qingfan Hou, Zhuofei Wang, Jiao Wang, Jian Jiang, and Yanjun Peng

Infusing Domain Knowledge into nnU-Nets for Segmenting Brain Tumors
in MRI 186
  *Krzysztof Kotowski, Szymon Adamski, Bartosz Machura,
  Lukasz Zarudzki, and Jakub Nalepa*

Multi-modal Brain Tumour Segmentation Using Transformer with Optimal
Patch Size 195
  Ramtin Mojtahedi, Mohammad Hamghalam, and Amber L. Simpson

Brain Tumor Segmentation Using Neural Ordinary Differential Equations
with UNet-Context Encoding Network 205
  *M. S. Sadique, M. M. Rahman, W. Farzana, A. Temtam,
  and K. M. Iftekharuddin*

An UNet-Based Brain Tumor Segmentation Framework via Optimal Mass
Transportation Pre-processing   216
    Jia-Wei Liao, Tsung-Ming Huang, Tiexiang Li, Wen-Wei Lin,
    Han Wang, and Shing-Tung Yau

BraTS-Reg

Robust Image Registration with Absent Correspondences in Pre-operative
and Follow-Up Brain MRI Scans of Diffuse Glioma Patients   231
    Tony C. W. Mok and Albert C. S. Chung

Unsupervised Method for Intra-patient Registration of Brain Magnetic
Resonance Images Based on Objective Function Weighting by Inverse
Consistency: Contribution to the BraTS-Reg Challenge   241
    Marek Wodzinski, Artur Jurgas, Niccolò Marini, Manfredo Atzori,
    and Henning Müller

Employing ConvexAdam for BraTS-Reg   252
    Christoph Großbröhmer, Hanna Siebert, Lasse Hansen,
    and Mattias P. Heinrich

Iterative Method to Register Longitudinal MRI Acquisitions
in Neurosurgical Context   262
    Luca Canalini, Jan Klein, Annika Gerken, Stefan Heldmann,
    Alessa Hering, and Horst K. Hahn

Brain Tumor Sequence Registration with Non-iterative Coarse-To-Fine
Networks and Dual Deep Supervision   273
    Mingyuan Meng, Lei Bi, Dagan Feng, and Jinman Kim

Author Index   283

BraTS-Reg

Applying Quadratic Penalty Method for Intensity-Based Deformable Image Registration on BraTS-Reg Challenge 2022

Kewei Yan[✉] and Yonghong Yan

University of North Carolina at Charlotte, Charlotte, NC 28223, USA
{kyan2,yyan7}@uncc.edu

Abstract. Registration of Magnetic Resonance Imaging (MRI) scans containing pathologies is challenging due to tissue appearance changes, and still an unsolved problem. In this paper, we present our implementation of the *Quadratic Penalty Deformable Image Registration (QPDIR)* algorithm for the Brain Tumor Sequence Registration (BraTS-Reg) Challenge 2022. The QPDIR algorithm is an intensity-based algorithm which turns computation of deformation field to an optimization problem of minimizing terms of image dissimilarity and regularization. The terms are computed based on processing exhaustive search among image blocks and the optimization is performed using a gradient-free quadratic penalty method. The whole optimization problem is decomposed to several sub-problems and each of them can be solved by straightforward block coordinate decent iteration. The data set of the BraTS-Reg Challenge 2022 has 160 cases. For each case, pre-operative images and follow-up images of 4 different modalities including t1, t1ce, flair and t2 are provided. For each case, we apply QPDIR to register image pairs of each modality to produce the deformation field, and then add the deformation field to landmarks, and merge the predict landmarks of each modality together to compute the final predict landmarks of the case. During the validation phrase, our method produces the average median absolute error(MAE) of 4.425, the average Robustness of 0.734 and the average negative numbers of Jacobi Determinant of 87960.95. The testing phase rank of our method is at 7. Detailed study of case ID 142 are shown in the paper.

Keywords: BrasTS-Reg Challenge 2022 · Deformable Image Registration · Block Matching · Quadratic Penalty

1 Introduction

Image registration is a fundamental image processing task that match multiple images together to overcome the image translation issues such as rotations and scales. Medical image registration is a clinical application of image registration

S. Bakas et al. (Eds.): BrainLes 2022, LNCS 14092, pp. 3–14, 2023.
https://doi.org/10.1007/978-3-031-44153-0_1

and can be widely applied into radiation therapy tasks. As a early stage for treatment planning or delivery, the goal for medical image registration is to establish a transformation between medical image pairs thus to build the mapping of shared features such as anatomical points.

The model of medical image registration are usually iterative-based [18]. The model receives moving image and fixed image then outputs the transformation, which is represented by a deformation field. The objective function, which can also be regarded as a measurement of similarity of images, are computed based on moving image and fixed image. The optimizer tries to update the parameters of the model for maximizing/minimizing the objective function. The transformation generated by optimized model is then applied to moving image to get the predict image. The predict image works as moving image for the next iteration until the criteria is met.

The early age image registration is limited in cases of rigid registration. One of the most popular methods could be curving [10] or 3D-SIFT [19], which, applying matrix as the transformation. Demons [21,23] is also regarded as a good solution to diffeomorphic image registration. However, Demons is not good at large motion deformable registration. Along with better understanding of image registration tasks, the transformation of deformable registration cases is regarded as a flow thus velocity field is used as the transformation between moving image and fixed image. Large Diffeomorphism Deformation Metric Mappings(LDDMM) [5] and region-specific diffeomorphic metric mapping (RDMM) [20] are the most representative ones among the algorithms using such idea. With the development of machine learning/deep learning(ML/DL) methods, medical image registration is also trying to utilize ML/DL to get better spacial accuracy, including CNN [9], GAN [15], RNN [8] and transformer [7]. With ML/DL methods, it is straightforward to build an end-to-end model, that is, the transformation can be estimated directly by feeding the model with image pairs. In these cases, displacement field is a popular choice.

For the task of BraTS-Reg Challenge, we use QPDIR, which is presented by Castillo [6], to process medical image registration to all 4 modalities and merge the results of each modality together to generate the final result of each case. The advantages of using QPDIR algorithm to process medical image registration can be concluded as: 1) This algorithm is less likely to be constrained by data volume since there is no pre-training at all. 2) Using gradient-free method is not sacrificing information richness of images. 3) The quadratic penalty method breaks the whole optimization problem down and make the code to benefit higher level of parallelism.

In the following several sections, related work, algorithm, results, and conclusion are presented, respectively.

2   Related Work

For large motion deformable registration, Beg et al. [5] shows a diffeomorphic metric mapping methods named Large Diffeomorphism Deformation Metric Mappings (LDDMM). Both moving image and fixed image are regarded as fluid, then the process of registration is the process of moving image continuously flowing towards fixed image. Shen et al. [20] extend this methods to region-specific diffeomorphic metric mapping (RDMM). In this case, the regularization of $L(\mathbf{x}, t)$ turns to a function of time t. Thus, LDDMM turns to an instance of RDMM. Avants et al. [1] presents symmetric image normalization (SyN) method for diffeomorphic image registration. Comparing with Beg et al. [5], the registration start from the time stamp 0.5 according to Diffeomorphism. Later, Avants et al. extend SyN to ANTs [2] toolbox to enable customized medical image registration, such as, update objective function from sole regularization to the sum of regularization and similarity including intensity differences, MI, and landmark guidance.

Besides 'traditional' methods, ML/DL based methods are applied to medical image registration as well. Convolution Neural Network (CNN) has proved itself with good performance on image processing tasks such as classification and segmentation. Based on its capability of extracting feature maps, the convolutional layer is further applied to other network frameworks including generative adversarial network (GAN) U-net and transformer.

Fan et al. [9] presents a fully convolutional network (FCN) to predict the transformation field. This is a standard format of end-to-end model which is wildly used in machine learning based methods: images pairs are received as inputs and transformation field are predicted as output. Convolutional layers are applied to extract features and provide hierarchical loss to compute objective function. Besides, ground truth is introduced for getting higher accuracy.

Convolution layers can also be applied to different framework constructions. Mahapatra et al. [16] applies GAN to generate deformation image and the deformation field based on moving image, then applying the discriminator network to check if the is generated image is close enough to the fixed image. The loss function is defined by sum of NMI (correlation), SSIM (correlation) and VGG (distance) between fixed image and predicted image. Unet is another popular framework using convolutional layers. Balakrishnan et al. [4] presents Voxel-Morph a learning framework for deformable medical image registration. For this frame work, it has two settings. The unsupervised setting is composed with Unet-based network, and the optional setting is composed with image segmentation module. The objective function is given according to the intensities of the inputs and When a new pair of the inputs are fed, the network computes a deformation field by evaluating the function directly.

The transformer/self-attention based models are originally designed for Natural Language Processing (NLP) [22]. Inspired by recurrent neural network (RNN), including long-short memory [11] and gated RNN [8], these models adapt the encoder-decoder network structure and enhance the power of RNN-based long-sequencing models. Unlike RNN's concentrating on symbol positions and modeling dependency based on the symbol distance in input and output, transformers/self-attention mechanism just free the constrain on distance-based dependency modeling [12] and make it possible to get short paths forward and backward signals in the network and launch multi-tasks among symbols and subsequences thus processing longer sequence with better parallelism comparing with RNN's.

Chen et al. [7] presents TransMorph, which is a transformer for unsupervised deformable medical image registration. There are three settings for the Trans-Morph, one unsupervised setting composed with a transformer encoder and a CNN decoder and two optional settings, including affine network for a raw image matching, and labeled images to improve the registration result. A detailed evaluation with the accuracy of TransMorph and other algorithms is also presented in this publication. With the same test dataset of brain CT and in terms of DSC, numbers of methods including we mentioned before such as SyN, LDDMM, and VoxelMorph are tested and evaluated.

For machine learning based methods, the interpretability is one of the main concern given that for most of the cases neural network is regarded as a black box. Lipton et al. [14] claims that the property of interpretable models falls in two categories: transparency and post-hoc interpretability. Thus in our approach, we use an iterative optimization method with mathematics algorithm for much better explainability.

3   The Quadratic Penalty Deformable Image Registration (QPDIR) Algorithm

The QPDIR algorithm is an intensity-based algorithm presented by Castillo [6]. The objective function F can be written like,

$$\Sigma_{i=1}^{N} F(d_1^{(i)}, d_2^{(i)}, d_3^{(i)}; x_i, R, T) + \frac{1}{2\alpha} \Sigma_{j=1}^{3} ||Ad_j||^2$$

The input image pairs are denoted as R and T for moving and fixed image, respectively. The total number of blocks is N. The displacement field is denoted as d of size of $3 \times N$. The matrix A is of size of $N \times N$.

The F part is for similarity and the A part is for regularity, i.e. the measurement for smoothness of the displacement field d. In this objective, $d_j^{(i)}$ is notation of mapping $d_j(x_i)$, which means the mapped coordinates of certain points x_i of certain dimension x, y, or z according to $j = 1, 2, 3$. d_j stands for the vector of $d_j^{(i)}$, $d_j = [d_j^{(1)} d_j^{(2)} ... d_j^{(N)}]^T$, taking care for the mapping of the whole dimension of x, y, or z. According to Castillo [6], the pattern of the loss function is well suited for the Quadratic Penalty Function Optimization method [17], then, this problem can be divided into several sub-problems formatted as,

$$\Sigma_{i=1}^{N} F(d_1^{(i)}, d_2^{(i)}, d_3^{(i)}; x_i, R, T) + \frac{1}{2\alpha} \Sigma_{j=1}^{3} ||Az_j||^2 + \frac{1}{2\mu} \Sigma_{j=1}^{3} ||z_j - d_j||^2$$

with introduction of auxiliary variable z.

Also, since this is a intensity-based method, there is no need to apply gradients to smooth the images thus avoiding to causing either extra computation efforts or information loss.

3.1 Displacement Field

Displacement field is one of the most popular type of transformation used in image registration. It can be used for handling both rigid and deformable cases, and is usually used in deformable cases of ML/DL methods, for its straight-forward representation of transformation filed with no need for smoothing on images. Like other transformation fields, displacement field is a collection of vector from moving images pointing to fixed images. For displacement field d and image feature $\mathbf{x}$, the corresponding feature of predicted image $\phi(\mathbf{x})$ can be presented by,

$$\phi(\mathbf{x}) = \mathbf{x} + d(\mathbf{x})$$

3.2 Block Matching

The block matching methods used in this work as is shown in Fig. 1 is the exhausted search method plus quadratic penalty algorithm, that is, along with certain size of block dimensions and search window dimensions, a block coordinate descent algorithm is processed. The algorithm can be described in Algorithm 1.

The block matching algorithm is guided by a mask image. The mask image is generated by image segmentation. We firstly apply a standardization to make the pixel value of the images fall into the range of 0 to 255. Thus, we use threshold of 100 to transfer non-zero values to 1 and 2: if the standardized pixel value is non-zero and less than or equal to 100, it will be turned to 1; if the standardized pixel value is greater than 100, it will be turned to 2. Since the zeros are untouched, as the outputs of image segmentation, the mask images are partitioned by indices from 0 to 2. Thus, a "dart throw" algorithm is developed to sample the blocks covering partitioned areas. Then, with a certain dimensions of blocks and search windows, an exhausted search is processed to compute corresponding parts of the displacement field.

Algorithm 1 Block Coordinate Descent Algorithm

Give a initial displacement estimates z_1, z_2, z_3

   Step 1: Update d_1, d_2, d_3 for i = 1, 2, 3, ..., N to get minimum value of

$$F(d_1(x_i), d_2(x_i), d_3(x_i); R, T) + \frac{1}{2\mu}\Sigma_{j=1}^{3}(d_j(x_i) - z_j(x_i))^2$$

   Step 2: Update z_j^* for j = 1, 2, 3 to get minimum value of

$$\frac{1}{2\alpha}||Az_j(\mathbf{x})||^2 + \frac{1}{2\mu}(z_j(\mathbf{x}) - d_j(\mathbf{x}))^2$$

   Step 3: If $\Sigma_{j=1}^{3}||z_j - z_j^*||_\infty$ is 0 for j = 1, 2, 3, then, stop iteration with solution z_j^*, otherwise, set $z_j = z_j^*$, for j = 1, 2, 3, and go back to Step 1

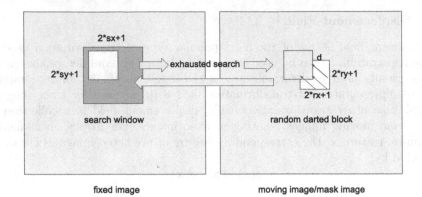

Fig. 1. An illustration for block matching algorithm. Without loss of generality, the algorithm is shown in pattern of 2D. rx, ry are the radius of block, and sx, sy are the radius of searching window. d is part of the (corresponding part of) displacement field.

Based on the Block Coordinate Descent algorithm, the QPDIR method can be described in Algorithm 2. To add more detail to Algorithm 1, the computation of $n \times N$ matrix A for regularity can be described as,

$$A = I_N - [a(x_1; X - x_1)H^{(1)}...a(x_N; X - x_N)H^{(N)}]^T$$

The matrix I_N is identity matrix of dimension N. Matrix H is obtained by removing i^{th} row of I_N, corresponding to $X - x_i$. In this equation, $a(x; X)y$ is a moving least square(MLS) [13] operator. Plus, the penalty parameter μ is of dynamic value along with the radius of search window to scan moving image with different scales, and according to Castillo [6], μ is given by computing l as the radius of search window,

$$l = \sqrt{2\mu}$$

4   Results

In this section, a case study of ID 142 and results of our team on validation phrase are presented. According to BraTS-Reg Challenge 2022 data set [3] , there are 20 cases for validation and the case ID ranges from 141 to 160. For each case, pre-operative images and follow-up images of 4 modalities including t1, t1ce, flair and t2 are provided. The dimensions of the images are 240, 240 and 155 for height, width and depth. The resolution of the images is 1 mm^3. Besides the images, landmarks which are the height, width and depth coordinates of region of interests(ROI) are provided for evaluation. The corresponding predict landmarks on fixed image of registration can be generated by applying the deformation field to the landmarks and the similarity between the predict landmarks and ground truth, which is the collection of landmarks on fixed image marked by experts, are evaluated.

Algorithm 2 QPDIR Algorithm

Give a set of voxel location $X = x_i$ for i = 1, 2, 3, ... N and corresponding initial displacement estimates z_1, z_2, z_3, regularization parameter α, and initial value of penalty parameter μ.

    Step 1: Update z_j^* and initialize z_j for j = 1, 2, 3 as is described in Algorithm 1
    Step 2: If μ is less than 0.5 for j = 1, 2, 3, then, stop iteration with solution z_j^*, otherwise, set $z_j = z_j^*$, for j = 1, 2, 3, $\mu = \mu \times 0.5$ and go back to step 1
    Step 3: Apply MLS to compute the full displacement field.

The experiment is set in this way: For each validation case, we group the image pairs by modalities. For each group, we apply registration to the image pair to generate the deformation field, which is a displacement field, and we apply the generated displacement field to the landmarks to compute the predict landmarks. Then, we average every single predict landmark of all 4 groups to get the predict landmarks of the case. At last, these predict landmarks are evaluated along with ground truth provided in validation phrase. The results are shown in Table 1.

A case study of ID 142 is presented for visualization and data analysis. As for the visualization, we show images of case ID 147 (Fig. 2) and cases ID 142 (Fig. 3) to illustrate the input/output of the registration: the fixed and moving image pairs are the inputs while mask and predict images are the outputs. The images are slices sharing the same depth index and are grouped by modalities. For each modality, fixed image, moving image, mask image and predict image are presented in order. As for the data analysis, we show the statistics, including means (Table 2) and standard errors (Table 3) of predict landmarks of case ID 142 to show the robustness of our experiment setup. For each table, X,Y, and Z stands for the index of height, width and depth. The elements in Table 2 will be rounded and thus be used as the predict landmarks of case ID 142 for evaluation.

According to Fig. 2, there are three inputs received by the algorithm: fixed image, moving image, and mask image. In this figure, given that the whole image is a stack of images, slices of images of case 147 are shown for illustration. The fixed image (target image) is the pre-operative image before treatment. The moving image is follow-up image after treatment and the mask image is the segmentation result for moving image for guiding the registration. The predict image is the out put, which is generated by applying the displacement field on the moving image.

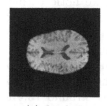 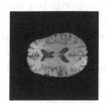 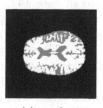 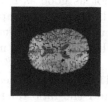

   (a) fixed t1   (b) moving t1   (c) mask t1   (d) predict t1

Fig. 2. Case ID 147 visualization

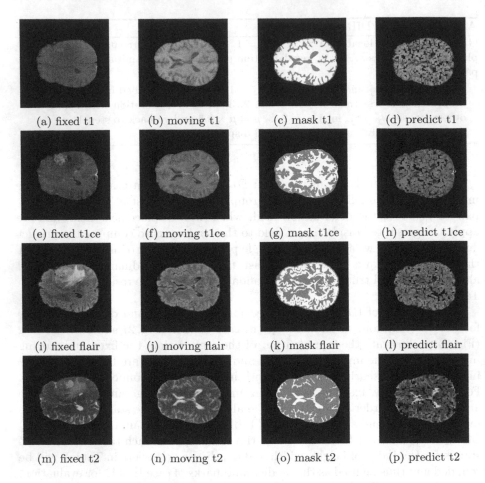

Fig. 3. Case ID 142 visualization

According to Fig. 3, the images are label in the format of "image modality". For instance, image(a) is the fixed image of registration of modality t1 of case ID 142. In the slice of fixed image, the frontal horn of lateral ventricle and occipital horn of lateral ventricle are pushed by the mass effect of tumor. As is shown in the predict image, the change is roughly captured by the displacement field, however, in this case, the horn structures do almost vanish, then the result is not as good as is shown in case 147. In the predicted image, we noticed that there are some gaps, which indicates pixel misses. This is caused by the block overlapping: blocks can overlap each other after applying displacement field to them, then, since no new pixels are created, there will be some gaps.

According to Table 1, the median absolute error(MAE) ranges from 1 to 11.5, getting a mean value of 4.425. The Robustness is measured by the ratio and the ratio ranges from 0.333 to 1.0. That means in average around 73.4%

Table 1. Evaluation on validation data set. There are in total 20 validation cases, and for each case there are 4 pairs of fixed and moving images corresponding to 4 modalities. The three columns for evaluation are: MAE, median absolute error; Robustness, ratio of that predict coordinates improving MAE; JD. TC30 neg., number of negative elements in Jacobian Determinant.

Case Id	MAE	Robustness	JD. TC30 neg.
141	10.5	0.5	113847
142	5	0.875	222224
143	11.5	0.75	114525
144	8.5	1.0	127442
145	11	0.875	240649
146	10	0.875	19860
147	2	0.35	14421
148	2.5	0.8	23888
149	2	1.0	38480
150	2	0.579	42844
151	1	0.7	109671
152	2	0.895	22700
153	2	0.333	4029
154	2	0.4	63360
155	2	0.421	122252
156	3	1.0	95170
157	3.5	0.9	132886
158	1	0.9	76109
159	5	0.727	85721
160	2	0.8	89141
mean	4.425	0.734	87960.95

of the predict landmark are getting MAE improved. Also, the mean number of negative elements of Jacobi Determinate is 87960.95, takes in average around 16.9% of the total elements.

According to Tables 2 and 3, comparing with the table of the mean value, the std ranges from 0 to 2.63, which is relatively small. It supports that the experiment setup is robust.

Table 2. Case ID 142 data analysis: mean value of predict landmarks of modalities of t1, t1ce, flair and t2.

Landmarks	X	Y	Z
1	115.5	86.64433757	86.76933757
2	87	65.45412415	65.70412415
3	96.5	72.39433757	72.51933757
4	121.25	90.875	90.9375
5	102.25	76.875	76.6875
6	156.5	117.4330127	117.3080127
7	179.5	134.8943376	135.0193376
8	137.75	103.375	103.5625

Table 3. Case ID 142 data analysis: standard error value of predict landmarks of modalities of t1, t1ce, flair and t2.

Landmarks	X	Y	Z
1	0.5773502692	0.9574271078	0.2687549099
2	0.8164965809	0.5773502692	0.1691019787
3	0.5773502692	1	0.2988584907
4	0.5	0.5	0
5	0.5	1.290994449	0.5593175386
6	1.732050808	1.258305739	0.3349883504
7	0.5773502692	0.5773502692	0
8	0.5	2.62995564	1.506106076

5   Conclusion

In this work, we apply QPDIR algorithm to the image registration task on BraTS-Reg Challenge 2022. This algorithm is featured with gradient-free quadratic penalty method, and the method makes it possible to decompose the optimization problem to sub-problems which can be solved by straightforward block coordinate decent iteration. For evaluation, we apply QPDIR to each case to register the pairs of pre-operative image and follow-up image of all 4 modalities. We compute the mean values of predict landmarks across all the modalities to generate result of predict landmarks of each case. The results are evaluated by median absolute error(MAE), ratio of that predicted coordinates improving MAE(Robustness) and number of negative elements in Jacobian Determinant. We also show the visualization and data analysis of certain case ID to illustrate the input/output of the algorithm and to prove the robustness of our experiment setup.

Acknowledgment. This research was partially supported by National Science Foundation under Grant 2015254. We thank our colleague Yaying Shi for providing comments about using ML/DL methods for this task. We appreciate Dr. Edward Castillo for sharing his idea with us, and we thank the reviewers for their insights.

References

1. Avants, B.B., Epstein, C.L., Grossman, M., Gee, J.C.: Symmetric diffeomorphic image registration with cross-correlation: evaluating automated labeling of elderly and neurodegenerative brain. Med. Image Anal. **12**(1), 26–41 (2008)
2. Avants, B.B., Tustison, N.J., Song, G., Cook, P.A., Klein, A., Gee, J.C.: A reproducible evaluation of ants similarity metric performance in brain image registration. Neuroimage **54**(3), 2033–2044 (2011)
3. Baheti, B., et al.: The brain tumor sequence registration challenge: establishing correspondence between pre-operative and follow-up MRI scans of diffuse glioma patients. arXiv preprint arXiv:2112.06979 (2021)
4. Balakrishnan, G., Zhao, A., Sabuncu, M.R., Guttag, J., Dalca, A.V.: VoxelMorph: a learning framework for deformable medical image registration. IEEE Trans. Med. Imaging **38**(8), 1788–1800 (2019)
5. Beg, M.F., Miller, M.I., Trouvé, A., Younes, L.: Computing large deformation metric mappings via geodesic flows of diffeomorphisms. Int. J. Comput. Vision **61**(2), 139–157 (2005)
6. Castillo, E.: Quadratic penalty method for intensity-based deformable image registration and 4dct lung motion recovery. Med. Phys. **46**(5), 2194–2203 (2019)
7. Chen, J., Frey, E.C., He, Y., Segars, W.P., Li, Y., Du, Y.: TransMorph: transformer for unsupervised medical image registration. arXiv preprint arXiv:2111.10480 (2021)
8. Chung, J., Gulcehre, C., Cho, K., Bengio, Y.: Empirical evaluation of gated recurrent neural networks on sequence modeling. arXiv preprint arXiv:1412.3555 (2014)
9. Fan, J., Cao, X., Yap, P.T., Shen, D.: BIRNet: brain image registration using dual-supervised fully convolutional networks. Med. Image Anal. **54**, 193–206 (2019)
10. Guéziec, A., Ayache, N.: Smoothing and matching of 3-D space curves. In: Sandini, G. (ed.) ECCV 1992. LNCS, vol. 588, pp. 620–629. Springer, Heidelberg (1992). https://doi.org/10.1007/3-540-55426-2_66
11. Hochreiter, S., Schmidhuber, J.: Long short-term memory. Neural Comput. **9**(8), 1735–1780 (1997)
12. Kim, Y., Denton, C., Hoang, L., Rush, A.M.: Structured attention networks. arXiv preprint arXiv:1702.00887 (2017)
13. Levin, D.: The approximation power of moving least-squares. Math. Comput. **67**(224), 1517–1531 (1998)
14. Lipton, Z.C.: The mythos of model interpretability: in machine learning, the concept of interpretability is both important and slippery. Queue **16**(3), 31–57 (2018)
15. Mahapatra, D.: Gan based medical image registration. arXiv preprint arXiv:1805.02369 (2018)
16. Mahapatra, D., Sedai, S., Garnavi, R.: Elastic registration of medical images with gans. arXiv preprint arXiv:1805.02369 7 (2018)
17. Nocedal, J., Wright, S.J.: Numerical Optimization. Springer, New York (1999). https://doi.org/10.1007/978-0-387-40065-5
18. Oh, S., Kim, S.: Deformable image registration in radiation therapy. Radiat. Oncol. J. **35**(2), 101 (2017)

19. Rister, B., Horowitz, M.A., Rubin, D.L.: Volumetric image registration from invariant keypoints. IEEE Trans. Image Process. **26**(10), 4900–4910 (2017)
20. Shen, Z., Vialard, F.X., Niethammer, M.: Region-specific diffeomorphic metric mapping. Adv. Neural Inf. Process. Syst. **32**, 1–11 (2019)
21. Thirion, J.P.: Image matching as a diffusion process: an analogy with Maxwell's demons. Med. Image Anal. **2**(3), 243–260 (1998)
22. Vaswani, A., et al.: Attention is all you need (2017)
23. Vercauteren, T., Pennec, X., Perchant, A., Ayache, N.: Diffeomorphic demons: efficient non-parametric image registration. Neuroimage **45**(1), S61–S72 (2009)

WSSAMNet: Weakly Supervised Semantic Attentive Medical Image Registration Network

Sahar Almahfouz Nasser[1]([✉]), Nikhil Cherian Kurian[1], Mohit Meena[1], Saqib Shamsi[2], and Amit Sethi[1]

[1] Indian Institute of Technology Bombay, Mumbai, India
sahar.almahfouz.nasser@gmail.com
[2] Whirlpool, Pune, India

Abstract. We present WSSAMNet, a weakly supervised method for medical image registration. Ours is a two step method, with the first step being the computation of segmentation masks of the fixed and moving volumes. These masks are then used to attend to the input volume, which are then provided as inputs to a registration network in the second step. The registration network computes the deformation field to perform the alignment between the fixed and the moving volumes. We study the effectiveness of our technique on the BraTSReg challenge data against ANTs and VoxelMorph, where we demonstrate that our method performs competitively.

Keywords: Deep-learning · MRI · Medical Image Registration · Segmentation · Semantic Attention

1 Introduction

Image registration is the process of finding spatial correspondence between two or more images [21]. It has various applications in medical imaging problems such as in multi-modal image fusion or digital subtraction angiography (DSA), where it is used to map structural changes in tumors before and after treatment or identifying tissue atrophy in degenerative diseases [18]. Brain Tumor Sequence Registration (BraTSReg) challenge [1] is the first challenge to address the problem of registering post-treatment follow-up scans of the magnetic resonance imaging (MRI) to the pre-operative MRI scans of patients treated for glioma. The change in the tissue appearance caused by the pathologies makes this registration very challenging even though we are dealing with a single imaging modality.

In general, registration comprises multiple steps such as feature detection and matching, designing the mapping function, image transformation, and image resampling. For the registration methods, the detected features should be distinctive features such as closed-boundary regions, edges, contours, line intersections, and corners.

S. Bakas et al. (Eds.): BrainLes 2022, LNCS 14092, pp. 15–24, 2023.
https://doi.org/10.1007/978-3-031-44153-0_2

However, unlike natural images medical images are often sparse in features; thus the registration methods for medical images, in general, are region-based methods. For feature matching, the registration methods depend on the similarity measures between the descriptors of the detected features, such as cross-correlation, mutual information, cross-power spectrum. These descriptors should be robust to the noise and the absence of some of the anatomical structures in one of the images to be registered.

2   Related Work

Deep learning-based medical image registration is still in its nascent stages in contrast to other well-studied tasks such as segmentation or classification. Before the advent of deep learning, most registration techniques relied on robust feature matching algorithms such as scale-invariant feature transform (SIFT) [3]. The local interest points generated from these algorithms were inherently scale and rotation invariant. The use of these algorithms enabled robust registration techniques that remain stable against the changes in 3D viewpoint, affine deformations, occlusion, clutter, and noise.

Several successful techniques have been proposed without the use of deep learning [8,11]. In 2016, Lin et al. [12] proposed a registration method based on mimicking the ants foraging for food. Ants algorithm has shown promising results on several medical image registration task in comparison to the other traditional learning techniques. Another well-known method for image registration is the NIFTYReg algorithm which comprises two parts, a global registration followed by a local registration [16]. Machado et al. [14] developed an attribute-matching-based registration method. This method registers intraoperative Ultrasound with preoperative MRI images during image-guided neurosurgery. They utilized Gabor attributes to handle large deformations and absent correspondences.

In the last few years, deep learning has also made its way into image registration [15]. In [10] the authors introduced a weakly supervised CNN for multimodal image registration. The network predicts the displacement field [5] to deform the moving image to match the fixed image, where the labeled images are used during the training and the unlabelled ones are used during the testing. The name weakly supervised derived from the use of anatomical labels to boost the ability of the network to predict the displacement field. The authors proposed this network to tackle the task of registering T2-weighted magnetic resonance images to 3D transrectal ultrasound images from prostate cancer patients. Hu et al. [9] proposed a label-driven weakly supervised learning for multimodal image registration. During the training a cross-entropy loss is computed between the warped moving label and the fixed label. Besides, smoothing over the deformation field is added to the loss function (L2 norm of displacement gradients). To prevent the network from over-fitting due to the direct usage of the binary masks, they proposed a label smoothing technique called one-sided label smoothing. To prevent the network from over-fitting due to the direct usage of the binary masks, they proposed a label smoothing technique called one-sided label smoothing.

In this technique, they provided a spatially smoothed probability map on the background only, keeping the one-hot probabilities of the foreground intact. Lee et al. [12] proposed image-and-spatial transformer networks (ISTNs) for structure-guided image registration.

The proposed ISTNs learn to focus on the structure of interest (SoI). They combined the image transformer network and the spatial transformer network to achieve the registration task. In 2019 Guo proposed a mutual-information-based multi-modal image registration method [7]. A year after, Gunnarsson et al. proposed a Laplacian pyramid for medical image registration [6]. The proposed network starts with a rough estimation of the deformation field and refines it in one or more steps. The fixed and the moving images were downsampled at different levels of the pyramid. A similar method is called deep Laplacian Pyramid Image Registration Network (LapIRN) proposed by Tony et al. [17]. They tried to mimic the traditional multi-resolution-based registration while keeping the non-linearity of the feature maps at different levels of the pyramid. Chen et al. [2] proposed a graph-based registration network. The proposed method consists of two stages. For the first stage a generative adversarial network (GAN) was used for nuclei segmentation. For the second stage a K-nearest neighbors clustring technique was used for constructing the adjacency matrix of the graph.

In this work, we propose a weakly supervised semantic attentive image registration network. WSSAMNet is a segmentation-based registration network. Our proposed method is discussed thoroughly in the following sections.

3   Proposed Work

We propose a weakly supervised method for registering the moving (follow up) scan to the fixed (pre-operative) scan using the landmarks given for every pair of scans. The proposed method consists of two stages, a segmentation stage, followed by a subsequent registration stage as shown in Fig. 1

The segmentation stage consists of two U-Nets with shared parameters [19]. The U-Net architecture is shown in Fig. 2. The U-Nets are alike, each of them contains three levels with residual blocks at every level. Each level of the network has an encoding and a decoding path with a skip connection between them. Data in the encoding path is downsampled using stridden convolutions (2,2,2), and in the decoding path data is upsampled using stridden transpose convolutions. The number of feature maps starts from 8 and gets doubled when moving from one level to the next one. See Fig. 2. Each U-Net segments the regions of interest ROIs, small patches of sizes $(9 \times 9 \times 9)$ around the landmarks of the input volume, for instance, the moving volume or the fixed volume. However, future ablation studies need to be performed to determine the optimal patch size. See Fig. 3.

The segmentation network is followed by an attention block in which the output of the U-Net (a binary segmentation map) is multiplied by the input volume to produce attentive volume. The concatenated outputs (the attentive fixed and moving volumes) of the segmentation network serve as an input to the registration network.

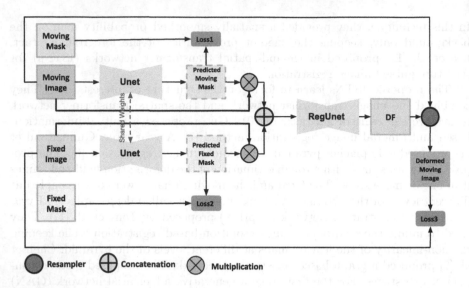

Fig. 1. The architecture of the proposed method. ***Loss1***, ***Loss2*** are the focal loss of the segmentation network of the moving volume and the fixed volume respectively, see equation (1). ***Loss3*** is the registration loss as in equation (5). ***Unet*** refers to the segmentation network, while ***RegUnet*** refers to the registration network.

To tackle the problem of class imbalance between the foreground and the background of the segmentation mask, we used the focal loss between the segmentation masks and the predicted segmentation maps [13], as shown in Eq. 1.

$$FL(p_t) = -(1 - p_t)^{\gamma} log(p_t) \tag{1}$$

Here, γ is a hyperparameter and we set it to 2 in our experiments.

The architecture of the registration network is the same as the U-Net architecture used for segmentation. The difference is that, the network for registration outputs a deformation field instead of a segmentation map. The deformation field is used for deforming the moving volume to match the fixed one.

The loss function of the registration network is a combination of two losses, the similarity loss, and the smoothness loss. The similarity loss is composed of two components with the first one being the mutual information loss calculated between the Laplacian of Gaussian (LoG) of the deformed moving volume and the LoG of the fixed volume, whereas the second component is the local cross-correlation loss calculated between the LoG of deformed moving volume and the LoG of fixed volume. The reason behind using the LoGs of the volumes is due to the changes in the appearance of the tissue caused by the existence of the tumor. Thus, choosing a semantic information-based loss (shape-based loss) works better than an intensity-based loss.

The local cross correlation between the fixed volume f and the moving volume m after deforming it by the deformation field Φ is given by Eq. 2 :

$$cc(f, m \circ \Phi) = \sum_{p \in \Omega} \frac{(\sum_{p_i}(f(p)_i - \hat{f}(p))([m \circ \Phi](p_i) - [\hat{m} \circ \Phi](p)))^2}{(\sum_{p_i}(f(p_i) - \hat{f}(p))^2)(\sum_{p_i}([m \circ \Phi](p_i) - [\hat{m} \circ \Phi](p))^2)} \quad (2)$$

here $\hat{f}(p)$ and $[\hat{m} \circ \Phi](p)$ denote local mean intensity images.

The mutual information between f and $(m \circ \Phi)$ is given by Eq. 3:

$$I(f, m \circ \Phi) = \sum_{a \in f, b \in m \circ \Phi} p(a,b) log(\frac{p(a,b)}{p(a)p(b)}) \quad (3)$$

According to [20] the displacement field is smooth if it does not have severe hops, so it is smooth when there is a gradual change in the direction and the magnitude in a neighborhood. Thus the smoothness loss is the L2 norm of the Laplacian of the deformation field as in Eq. 4.

$$L_{smooth}(\Phi) = \sum_{p \in \Omega} ||\nabla u(p)|| \quad (4)$$

where $\nabla u(p) = (\frac{\partial u(p)}{\partial x}, \frac{\partial u(p)}{\partial y}, \frac{\partial u(p)}{\partial z})$, and $\frac{\partial u(p)}{\partial x} \approx u(p_x + 1, p_y, p_z) - u(p_x, p_y, p_z)$. The total loss function of the registration network is given by 5.

$$Loss = -cc - I + L_{smooth} \quad (5)$$

The provided landmarks were used only for guiding the segmentation network, while the registration network was trained in an unsupervised manner.

4   Data and Experiments

The dataset contains pairs of scans – the pre-operative MRI scans, and the corresponding follow-up MRI scans. Each pair of these scans belongs to the same patient who was cured of glioma. For every patient T1, contrast-enhanced T1-weighted (T1-CE), T2-weighted, and T2 fluid attention inversion recovery (FLAIR) sequences were provided. The training dataset consists of 140 cases and the validation dataset contains 20 cases. Anatomical markers such as blood vessels bifurcations, the shape of the cortex, and the midline of the brain were used to define the landmarks of the scans of every case. The number of the landmarks differs from one case to another, ranging from 6 to 50 landmarks per case. We trained our network end to end using two 24 GB GPUs. All the U-Nets consist of three levels.

Before combining the segmentation and the registration networks in a single pipeline and training it end-to-end, we trained each network independently for around 50 epochs. We trained the segmentation network on segmenting both the baseline volumes as well as the follow-up volumes. Similarly, we trained the registration network to register a volume (before surgery or a follow-up) to its

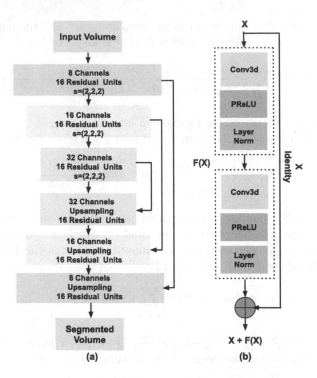

Fig. 2. In this figure (a) represents the U-Net architecture, and (b) represents the residual block. Here S=(2,2,2) refers to the stride of the 3D convolution.

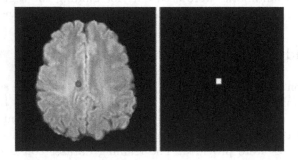

Fig. 3. A 2D MRI slice with a keypoint in red to the left, and the corresponding segmentation mask to the right. (Color figure online)

augmented version; to learn the affine transformation (rotation, scaling, and translation) besides the identity transformation. We used these weights as pre-trained weights of the network trained on registering the follow-up images to the images before the surgery. We used Adam optimizer and step-learning rate scheduler with an initial learning rate of 10^{-4} to train our architecture.

We used only T1-CE volumes for all our experiments as we got the best results for this imaging sequence. Concatenating the four sequences and giving them as channels to the segmentation and registration networks might give better results, but unfortunately, due to the limited computation resources, we could not perform such an experiment.

5 Results

There were two evaluation metrics. The first metric measured the registration error between the follow-up scan (F) and the preoperative scan (B) for a pair of scans (p) using the median absolute error of the landmarks, which is given by:

$$MAE = Median_{l \in L}(|x_l^B - \hat{x}_l^{\,B}|) \tag{6}$$

where x_l^B, x_l^F are the coordinates of corresponding landmarks of $l \in L$ the set of landmarks identified in both B and F.

Table 1. The results of the proposed method versus ANTs and VoxelMorph are reported by the organizers of the challenge on the validation dataset, which consists of 20 pairs. AE refers to absolute error. The average runtime for ANTs when applying an affine transformation is around 1.95 min, and its average runtime is around 4.58 min when applying a combination of an affine transformation and a rigid one. The average runtime of the segmentation model on the CPU is 0.5 min, while the average runtime of the registration model is 0.56 min.

Evaluation Metric	ANTs	VoxelMorph	Proposed Method
Median of Median AE	**3.77**	6.25	**5.00**
Mean of Median AE	**4.59**	9.10	8.37
Median of Mean AE	**4.97**	6.86	6.68
Mean of Mean AE	**5.48**	9.29	9.09
Mean Robustness	**0.64**	0.31	0.32
Average Running time on CPU in minutes	4.58	**0.56**	1.56

The second metric measured the robustness of registration. For a pair of scans (p) the robustness is given by the ratio of the successfully registered landmarks to the total number of landmarks in p, which is given by:

$$R^{B,F}(p) = \frac{|K^{B,F}|}{|L^F|} \tag{7}$$

where $k^{B,F} \subseteq L^F$ are the successfully registered landmarks. The total robustness is given by:

$$R = \frac{1}{P} \sum_{(B,F) \in P} R^{B,F}(p) \tag{8}$$

As shown in Table 1, the absolute errors of ANTs are better than the ones of our proposed method. Besides, the robustness of ANTs is higher than the robustness of our proposed method. However, the runtime of our proposed method is much smaller than the runtime of ANTs. The performance of our proposed method is better than the performance of VoxelMorph for all the evaluation metrics except the average runtime. We reported the average registration time of a pair of volumes on the CPU as we could not find an implementation of ANTs on the GPU. The average runtime of our proposed method on the GPU is around 6.98 s.

6 Ablation Study

To check the effect of the mask size on the performance of WSSAMNet, we trained and tested our method on MRI-to-Ultrasound registration of prostate data. The dataset [4] contains masks of the prostate of the MRI images and the corresponding Ultrasound images of three subjects. We used the data of two subjects for training and validation, while the data of the third subject was kept for testing. The initial overlap between the moving and fixed images over the test dataset is 0.25 ± 0.20.

Our proposed architecture WSSAMNet which is an attention based architecture, surpasses the state-of-the-art technique (LapIRN) in terms of the evaluation score (dice score) for MRI-US fusion problem.

The dice score over the testing dataset, which contains 15 examples are as follows: the dice score of the State-of-the-art (LapIRN) algorithm is 0.35 ± 0.20, while the dice score of our proposed method (WSSAMNet) is 0.48 ± 0.20. So there is a significant improvement around 13% when using WSSAMNet rather than LapIRN. See Fig. 4.

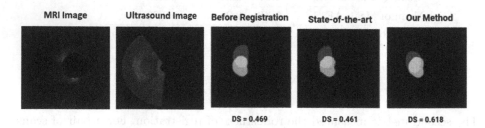

Fig. 4. A visual comparison between the registration results of our proposed method and the state-of-the-art registration algorithm (LapIRN). DS stands for the dice score.

7 Conclusion

We proposed a novel attention-based network for brain MRI registration. Our proposed method surpasses VoxelMorph in terms of median absolute error and robustness. We showed the benefit of training the network to give more attention to the regions around the landmarks in improving the robustness and reducing the registration error.

The size of the segmentation masks affects the performance of our proposed method significantly. As our ablation study revealed, our proposed method beat the state-of-the-art registration algorithms when trained on a dataset with balanced masks of the moving and fixed images.

Acknowledgement. This work would not have been possible without the financial support of the Qualcomm Innovation Fellowship Award, India. We are especially indebted to Mr. Bhargava Chintalapati from Qualcomm for his feedback and support.

References

1. Baheti, B., et al.: The brain tumor sequence registration challenge: establishing correspondence between pre-operative and follow-up MRI scans of diffuse glioma patients. arXiv preprint: arXiv:2112.06979 (2021)
2. Chen, R.J., et al.: Pathomic fusion: an integrated framework for fusing histopathology and genomic features for cancer diagnosis and prognosis. IEEE Trans. Med. Imaging **41**, 757–770 (2020)
3. Crawford, R.: Automated image stitching using sift feature matching (2012)
4. Fedorov, A., Nguyen, P.L., Tuncali, K., Tempany, C.: Annotated MRI and ultrasound volume images of the prostate (2015). https://doi.org/10.5281/zenodo.16396
5. Fischer, B., Modersitzki, J.: Curvature based image registration. J. Math. Imaging Vis. **18**(1), 81–85 (2003)
6. Gunnarsson, N., Sjölund, J., Schön, T.B.: Learning a deformable registration pyramid. In: Shusharina, N., Heinrich, M.P., Huang, R. (eds.) MICCAI 2020. LNCS, vol. 12587, pp. 80–86. Springer, Cham (2021). https://doi.org/10.1007/978-3-030-71827-5_10
7. Guo, C.K.: Multi-modal image registration with unsupervised deep learning. Ph.D. thesis, Massachusetts Institute of Technology (2019)
8. Han, X., et al.: Patient-specific registration of pre-operative and post-recurrence brain tumor MRI scans. In: Crimi, A., Bakas, S., Kuijf, H., Keyvan, F., Reyes, M., van Walsum, T. (eds.) BrainLes 2018. LNCS, vol. 11383, pp. 105–114. Springer, Cham (2019). https://doi.org/10.1007/978-3-030-11723-8_10
9. Hu, Y., et al.: Label-driven weakly-supervised learning for multimodal deformable image registration. In: 2018 IEEE 15th International Symposium on Biomedical Imaging (ISBI 2018), pp. 1070–1074. IEEE (2018)
10. Hu, Y., et al.: Weakly-supervised convolutional neural networks for multimodal image registration. Med. Image Anal. **49**, 1–13 (2018)
11. Klein, S., Staring, M., Murphy, K., Viergever, M.A., Pluim, J.P.: Elastix: a toolbox for intensity-based medical image registration. IEEE Trans. Med. Imaging **29**(1), 196–205 (2009)
12. Lin, T.X., Chang, H.H.: Medical image registration based on an improved ant colony optimization algorithm. Int. J. Pharma. Med. Biol. Sci. **5**(1), 17–22 (2016)
13. Lin, T.Y., Goyal, P., Girshick, R., He, K., Dollár, P.: Focal loss for dense object detection. In: Proceedings of the IEEE International Conference on Computer Vision, pp. 2980–2988 (2017)

14. Machado, I., et al.: Deformable MRI-ultrasound registration via attribute matching and mutual-saliency weighting for image-guided neurosurgery. In: Stoyanov, D., et al. (eds.) POCUS/BIVPCS/CuRIOUS/CPM -2018. LNCS, vol. 11042, pp. 165–171. Springer, Cham (2018). https://doi.org/10.1007/978-3-030-01045-4_20

15. Mahapatra, D., Antony, B., Sedai, S., Garnavi, R.: Deformable medical image registration using generative adversarial networks. In: 2018 IEEE 15th International Symposium on Biomedical Imaging (ISBI 2018), pp. 1449–1453. IEEE (2018)

16. Modat, M., McClelland, J., Ourselin, S.: Lung registration using the NiftyReg package. Med. Image Anal. Clin.-a Grand Challenge **2010**, 33–42 (2010)

17. Mok, T.C.W., Chung, A.C.S.: Large deformation diffeomorphic image registration with Laplacian Pyramid networks. In: Martel, A.L., et al. (eds.) MICCAI 2020. LNCS, vol. 12263, pp. 211–221. Springer, Cham (2020). https://doi.org/10.1007/978-3-030-59716-0_21

18. Noble, J.A.: Reflections on ultrasound image analysis (2016)

19. Ronneberger, O., Fischer, P., Brox, T.: U-net: convolutional networks for biomedical image segmentation (2015). https://doi.org/10.48550/ARXIV.1505.04597

20. Schwarz, L.A.: Non-rigid registration using free-form deformations. Technische Universität München **6**, 4 (2007)

21. Zitova, B., Flusser, J.: Image registration methods: a survey. Image Vis. Comput. **21**(11), 977–1000 (2003)

Self-supervised iRegNet for the Registration of Longitudinal Brain MRI of Diffuse Glioma Patients

Ramy A. Zeineldin[1,2,3(✉)], Mohamed E. Karar[2], Franziska Mathis-Ullrich[3], and Oliver Burgert[1]

[1] Research Group Computer Assisted Medicine (CaMed), Reutlingen University, Reutlingen, Germany
Ramy.Zeineldin@Reutlingen-University.DE
[2] Faculty of Electronic Engineering (FEE), Menoufia University, Menof, Egypt
[3] Department Artificial Intelligence in Biomedical Engineering, Friedrich-Alexander-University Erlangen-Nürnberg, Erlangen, Germany

Abstract. Reliable and accurate registration of patient-specific brain magnetic resonance imaging (MRI) scans containing pathologies is challenging due to tissue appearance changes. This paper describes our contribution to the registration of the longitudinal brain MRI task of the Brain Tumor Sequence Registration Challenge 2022 (BraTS-Reg 2022). We developed an enhanced unsupervised learning-based method that extends our previously developed registration framework iRegNet. In particular, incorporating an unsupervised learning-based paradigm as well as several minor modifications to the network pipeline, allows the enhanced iReg-Net method to achieve respectable results. Experimental findings show that the enhanced self-supervised model improves the initial mean median registration absolute error (MAE) from 8.20 ± 7.62 mm to the lowest value of 3.51 ± 3.50 for the training set while achieving an MAE of 2.93 ± 1.63 mm for the validation set. Additional qualitative validation of this study was conducted through overlaying pre-post MRI pairs before and after the deformable registration. The proposed method scored 5th place during the testing phase of the MICCAI BraTS-Reg 2022 challenge. The docker image to reproduce our BraTS-Reg submission results will be publicly available.

Keywords: Brain · BraTS · CNN · Glioma · MRI · Longitudinal · Registration

1 Introduction

Glioblastoma (GBM), and diffuse glioma, are the most common and aggressive malignant primary tumors with high and heterogeneous infiltration rates [1]. The registration of longitudinal brain Magnetic Resonance Imaging (MRI) scans is crucial in the treatment and follow-up procedures of brain tumors to find map correspondences between pre-operative and post-recurrence. This would support research into the early detection of tumor infiltration and subsequent tumor [2]. Therefore, an automatic, fast, robust fusion

S. Bakas et al. (Eds.): BrainLes 2022, LNCS 14092, pp. 25–34, 2023.
https://doi.org/10.1007/978-3-031-44153-0_3

of follow-up with the pre-operative MRI scans becomes highly important to assist in the early detection of tumor recurrence. However, the registration of MRI brain glioma patients is still a complex and challenging problem due to the inconsistent intensity and missing correspondences between both scans, especially with large deformations caused by large tumors (glioma grade III and IV).

Over the past years, many approaches have been applied to medical image registration that can be classified into classical and learning-based approaches [3, 4]. Classical or non-learning methods are formulated as an iterative pair-wise optimization problem that requires proper feature extraction, choosing a similarity measurement, defining the used transformation model, and finally an optimization mechanism to investigate the search space. Over time, extensive literature has developed using diverse combinations of the aforementioned elements [5–9]. Still, the traditional iterative process is computationally expensive, requiring long processing times ranging from tens of minutes to hours even with an efficient implementation on a regular central processing unit (CPU) or modern graphic processing unit (GPU).

To overcome the limitations of classical methods, learning-based approaches have been proposed in recent years. Learning methods formulate the classical optimization problem into a problem of cost function estimation. Instead of finding the map correspondence for every input MRI scanning separately, learning approaches make a general optimization over all the training datasets [4]. Recently, deep learning has been widely adopted in various medical image analysis tasks outperforming other methods [10]. Supervised deep learning methods were initially proposed [11–13] to learn similar features from the training data using different imaging modalities. Then, unsupervised learning was developed as a demand for faster registration procedures and to eliminate the challenges related to ground truth data generation and optimization techniques [14–17]. In general, once the deep learning networks are trained, they can provide a faster registration than classical optimization methods, without the need for fine-tuning parameters at the test time, in addition to being more robust to outliers.

In this paper, we propose a fully automatic, patient-specific registration approach for pre- and post-operative brain MRI sequences of only a single modality using iRegNet [18]. In particular, we introduce an unsupervised approach of iRegNet (see Fig. 1) in which only moving and fixed MRI pairs are utilized. Then, our proposed method optimizes deformation fields directly from input images using backpropagation. Extensive experiments of our model on the BraTS-Reg challenge data of 160 patients show that the proposed method can provide accurate results with the advantage of having a very fast runtime.

The remainder of the paper is organized as follows: Sect. 2 describes the BraTS-Reg 2022 dataset and our patient-specific registration framework. Qualitative and quantitative evaluations are presented in Sect. 3; Sect. 4 concludes the paper with an outlook on future work.

2 Material and Methods

2.1 Dataset

The BraTS-Reg 2022 dataset [19] comprises 250 patient-specific pairs of pre-operative and follow-up brain multi-institutional MRI scans. For each patient, i) native T1-weighted (T1), ii) contrast-enhanced T1 (T1ce), iii) T2-weighted (T2), and iv) T2 Fluid Attenuated Inversion Recovery (FLAIR) sequences are provided for the pre-operative and follow-up with a time-window in the range of 27 days to 37 months. Reference landmark annotations for the validation set are not made available to the participants. Instead, participants can use the online evaluation platform[1] to evaluate their models and compare their results with other teams on the online leaderboard[2].

Standard pre-processing techniques were applied such as rigid registration to the same anatomical template, resampling to the same isotropic resolution ($1mm^3$), skull removal, and brain extraction. Following these pre-processing steps, we applied the image cropping stage where all brain pixels were cropped. Afterward, z-score normalization was applied by subtracting the mean value and dividing it by the standard deviation individually for each input MRI image.

2.2 Medical Image Registration

Medical image registration is the process of aligning two or more sets of imaging data acquired using mono- or multi-modalities into a common coordinate system. Let I_F and I_M denote the fixed and the moving images, respectively, and let ϕ be the deformation field that relates the two images. Then, our goal is to find the minimum energy function ε as:

$$\varepsilon = S(I_F, I_M.\phi) + R(\phi) \qquad (1)$$

where $(I_M.\phi)$ is the moving image I_M warped by the deformation field ϕ, the dissimilarity metric is denoted by S, and $R(\phi)$ represents the regularization parameter. In this work, follow-up and pre-operative MRI scans are utilized as the moving and fixed images, respectively, since our goal is to reflect the brain shift in the follow-up MRI data.

2.3 iRegNet Workflow

Figure 1 presents an outline of the baseline iRegNet registration method. iRegNet consists of two steps: First, I_F and I_M are fed into our convolutional neural network (CNN) that then predicts ϕ. Second, I_M is transformed into a warped image $(I_M.\phi)$ using a spatial re-sampler. Further details are described as follows.

---

[1] https://ipp.cbica.upenn.edu/.
[2] https://www.cbica.upenn.edu/BraTSReg2022/lboardValidation.html/.

CNN Architecture. The developed cnn architecture utilized in experiments is based on u-net [20, 21]. Using backpropagation, which is a feedback loop that estimates the network weighting parameters, the network can automatically learn the optimal features and the deformation field. The network contains two main paths: a feature extractor (or encoder) as well as a deformation field estimator (or decoder). 3D convolutions are applied in both encoder and decoder parts instead of the 2D convolutions used in the original u-net architecture. The encoder consists of two consecutive 3D convolutional layers, each followed by a rectified linear unit (ReLU) and 3D spatial max pooling. A stride of 2 is employed to reduce the spatial dimension in each layer by half, similar to the traditional pyramid registration scheme. In the decoding path, each step consists of a 3D up-sampling, a concatenation with the corresponding features from the encoder, 3D up-convolutions, and a batch normalization layer, followed by a rectified linear unit (ReLU). Finally, a 1 x 1 x 1 convolution layer is applied to map the resultant feature vector map into ϕ.

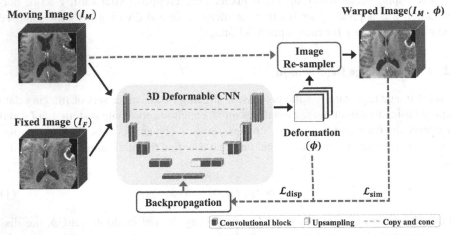

Fig. 1. An overview of the iRegNet workflow for 3D post- to pre-operative MRI image deformable registration. Dashed *red* arrows show the processes applied in the training stage only [18].

Self-Supervised Learning. In contrast to the original iregnet where supervised learning was applied, we incorporated self-supervised learning to compute the optimal deformation field $\hat{\phi}$ corresponding to the smoothness regularization. This model uses only the input mri volume pair, and the registration field is computed accordingly by the cnn network. Formally, this task is defined as:

$$\hat{\phi} = \arg \min_{\phi} \mathcal{L}_{sim}(\mathbf{I_F}, \phi.\mathbf{I_M}) + R(\phi) \tag{2}$$

where $\mathcal{L}_{sim}$ computes the image similarity between the warped image ($\phi.I_M$) and the fixed image I_F,

Loss Function. Owing to the applied two-step approach, the overall loss function $\mathcal{L}_{overall}$ has two components, as shown in eq. (3). $\mathcal{L}_{disp}$ corresponds to the deformation field gradient error.

$$\mathcal{L}_{overall} = \mathcal{L}_{sim} + \mathcal{L}_{disp} \tag{3}$$

where $\mathcal{L}_{sim}$ employs the similarity metric of the local normalized correlation coefficient (*NCC*), which is calculated as follows:

$$\mathcal{L}_{sim} = \mathrm{NCC}(\mathbf{I_F}, \phi.\mathbf{I_M}) = \frac{1}{N} \sum_{p \varepsilon X} \frac{\sum_i \left(\mathbf{I_F}(\mathbf{p}) - \overline{\mathbf{I_F}(\mathbf{p})}\right) \sum_i \left(\phi.\mathbf{I_M}(\mathbf{p}) - \overline{\phi.\mathbf{I_M}(\mathbf{p})}\right)}{\sqrt{\sum_i \left(\mathbf{I_F}(\mathbf{p}) - \overline{\mathbf{I_F}(\mathbf{p})}\right)^2} \sqrt{\sum_i \left(\phi.\mathbf{I_M}(\mathbf{p}) - \overline{\phi.\mathbf{I_M}(\mathbf{p})}\right)^2}} \tag{4}$$

where $(\phi.I_M(p))$ and $I_F(p)$ are the voxel intensities of a corresponding patch p in the warped image and the fixed truth, respectively, whereas $\overline{(\phi.I_M(p))}$ and $\overline{I_F(p)}$ are the mean pixel intensities for both images. $\mathcal{L}_{disp}$ measures spatial gradients differences in the predicted displacement d as follows:

$$\mathcal{L}_{disp} = \sum_{p \varepsilon X} \|\nabla d(p)\| \tag{5}$$

3 Experimental Results

3.1 Experimental Setup

To ensure computational efficiency for the GPU, MRI scans for each patient were center cropped to $160 \times 192 \times 160$ pixels. For training and validation, sets, respectively, the BraTS-Reg dataset was randomly split into 112 (80%) and 28 (20%) volumes. Another 20 MRI volumes were provided by the BraTS-Reg organizers as online validation set with landmarks provided only for the fixed MRI scans. Finally, we performed an affine alignment on moving and fixed MRI volumes using the BRAINSFit toolkit [9] to focus on the non-linear misalignment between volumes. For the experiments, our model was implemented in Python 3.7 using the TensorFlow 2.4 library. The experiments were run on an AMD Ryzen 2920X (32M Cache, 3.50 GHz) CPU with 64 GB RAM and a single NVIDIA GPU (RTX 3060 12 GB or RTX 2080 Ti 11 GB). The ADAM optimizer [22] with an initial learning rate of 1e-4 and a batch size of 2 was used.

To compare with other studies, the mean target registration error (mTRE), which represents the average distance between the corresponding landmarks in each pre-post MRI pair before and after registration, was used. In addition, the proposed method was evaluated by the online submission platform using the following metrics, namely Median Absolute Error (MAE), robustness, and smoothness of the displacement field.

3.2 Ablation Study

To explore the MRI modality which achieves the best performance for the task of longi-tudinal registration, an ablation study has been carried out. The BRAINSFit toolkit was utilized to perform affine alignments on moving and fixed MRI volumes. As listed in Table 1., T1ce has obtained the overall best results on the validation dataset in terms of the mean and median MAE scores while FLAIR achieved the best robustness. There-fore, in our experiments, we only use the T1ce volumes from each patient. Theoretically, using multiple modalities could increase the accuracy of the image registration, and this would be further investigated in future work.

Table 1. The ablation study of MRI modalities on the BraTS-Reg 2022 validation cases. Bold highlights the best scores.

Modality	MAE$_{median}$	MAE$_{mean}$	Robustness
Initial	8.20	8.65	–
T1	4.74	5.65	0.66
T1ce	**4.35**	**5.23**	0.62
T2	4.85	5.60	0.63
FLAIR	4.64	5.40	**0.67**

3.3 Registration Results

Figure 2 shows example results from three patients, where the registration of post- to pre-operative MRI scans is achieved using the self-supervised iRegNet method and the comparing baseline method. From the visual results, it can be seen that warped MRI scans are significantly improved after applying iRegNet. Note that, Fig. 2 (c) shows the FLAIR scans for the follow-up MRI images, only for visualization purposes, to better depict the surgically imposed cavities of these illustrated examples. All the applied registration methods use only the T1ce modality as discussed in Sect. 3.2.

Moreover, Table 2. reports the registration performance of the proposed method as well as the baseline on the BraTS-Reg challenge validation database. The baseline denotes the BRAINSFIT affine transformation between the full-resolution images of pre-operative and follow-up MRI. Compared with the affine method, our proposed self-supervised method effectively improves registration performance. It is notable that the average runtime of the proposed method is 1 s and does not require any manual interaction or supervision. Besides, only one sequence (T1ce) is required in our case.

The statistics of the paired landmark errors before and after the registration are displayed in Fig. 3. For the training database, our model reduced the initial mean MAE (computed by the evaluation platform) from 8.20 ± 7.62 mm to 3.51 ± 3.50 mm. Similarly, an MAE of 2.93 ± 1.63 mm was achieved on the validation database which has an initial 7.80 ± 5.62 mm. This result highlights that our method delivers significantly better results than both initial alignment and affine registration.

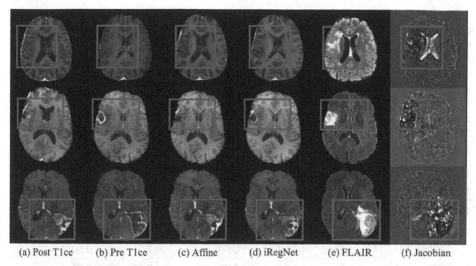

(a) Post T1ce   (b) Pre T1ce   (c) Affine   (d) iRegNet   (e) FLAIR   (f) Jacobian

Fig. 2. Example registration results from three validation cases (patients 141, 148, and 152). From left to right: (a) and (b) the post- and pre-operative MRI T1ce, (c) the follow-up to pre-operative affine registration of BRAINSFit, (d) the follow-up to pre-operative deformable registration of our iRegNet, (e) the pre-operative FLAIR scans, only for visualization purposes, and (f) determinant of the Jacobian of the displacement field are shown, respectively. The red box highlights regions of major differences.

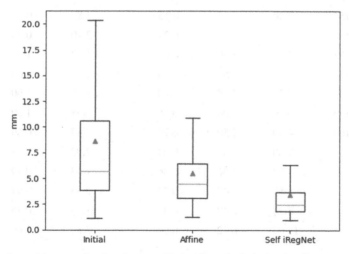

Fig. 3. Boxplots of the mean landmark errors. For each method, the landmark errors are computed against the fixed landmarks of the BraTS-Reg dataset. From left to right, mean absolute registration errors are shown for the initial dataset, affine, and the enhanced iRegNet, respectively. On each box, the red line is the median and the green triangle is the mean. (Color figure online)

Table 2. Quantitative results of the proposed method and the baseline affine method on the BraTS-Reg challenge validation set. MAE denotes the average of median absolute error between the predicted coordinates and the ground truth coordinates, whereas Robustness represents the successful rate of measuring how many landmarks have improved MAE after the registration.

Case	Initial	Affine		Enhanced iRegNet	
	MAE	MAE	Robustness	MAE	Robustness
BraTSReg_141	13.50	3.64	1.00	2.18	1.00
BraTSReg_142	14.00	5.98	0.88	7.18	0.75
BraTSReg_143	16.00	8.85	0.88	4.89	1.00
BraTSReg_144	15.00	9.44	0.88	5.64	1.00
BraTSReg_145	17.00	5.36	1.00	4.71	1.00
BraTSReg_146	17.00	7.13	1.00	2.62	1.00
BraTSReg_147	1.50	2.50	0.00	2.53	0.50
BraTSReg_148	3.50	3.06	0.30	2.61	0.75
BraTSReg_149	9.00	2.18	1.00	1.38	1.00
BraTSReg_150	4.00	4.00	0.11	2.20	0.74
BraTSReg_151	3.00	2.00	0.45	1.47	0.75
BraTSReg_152	5.00	2.00	0.95	1.61	0.95
BraTSReg_153	2.00	2.00	0.33	1.68	0.75
BraTSReg_154	2.00	2.10	0.15	1.83	0.55
BraTSReg_155	2.00	2.63	0.21	2.10	0.53
BraTSReg_156	7.00	3.30	1.00	1.62	1.00
BraTSReg_157	10.00	6.52	0.90	4.58	1.00
BraTSReg_158	4.50	3.75	0.40	1.65	1.00
BraTSReg_159	6.00	8.00	0.36	3.58	1.00
BraTSReg_160	4.00	2.50	0.70	2.47	0.60
Mean	7.80	4.35	0.62	2.93	0.84
StdDev	5.62	2.46	0.36	1.63	0.19
Median	5.50	3.47	0.79	2.33	0.97
25quantile	3.38	2.42	0.33	1.67	0.75
75quantile	13.63	6.12	0.96	3.83	1.00

4   Conclusion

In this paper, we proposed a patient-specific registration framework based on iRegNet, which aligns pre-operative and post-recurrence MRI T1ce sequences. The enhanced iRegNet framework uses deep unsupervised learning for deformable image registration driven by the regularization hyperparameter. The proposed method is evaluated on the

BraTS-Reg challenge dataset brain MR images comprising 140, 20, and 40 divided into training, validation, and testing cohorts. The validation results show that our framework can provide respectable results and is more effective than the classical affine registration with the advantage of being a self-supervised learning approach. In addition, iRegNet provided a faster approach (1 s for 3D brain MRI pair registration) compared to conventional approaches that can last for minutes and hours in some tasks. The results clearly validate the effectiveness of using unsupervised deep-learning techniques in image registration.

Further research work should be conducted to investigate the optimal cropping radius for MRI sequences to minimize the missing data as possible. Automating this procedure will contribute toward rendering iRegNet an end-to-end pipeline. Further analysis of augmenting a supervised loss using weakly-supervised annotations and comparison against other deep learning methods is left for future work.

Acknowledgments. The first author is supported by the German Academic Exchange Service (DAAD) [scholarship number 91705803]. The authors acknowledge the help of the BraTS-Reg challenge organizers for submitting the Singularity container.

References

1. Louis, D.N., et al.: CIMPACT-NOW update 6: new entity and diagnostic principle recommendations of the cIMPACT-Utrecht meeting on future CNS tumor classification and grading. Brain Pathol. **30**, 844–856 (2020)
2. Han, X., et al.: Patient-specific registration of pre-operative and post-recurrence brain tumor mri scans. brainlesion: glioma, multiple sclerosis, stroke and traumatic brain injuries, pp. 105–114 (2019)
3. Liu, J., et al.: Image registration in medical robotics and intelligent systems: fundamentals and applications. Adv. Intell. Syst. **1**(6), 100098 (2019)
4. Haskins, G., Kruger, U., Yan, P.: Deep learning in medical image registration: a survey. Mach. Vision Appl. **31**(1–2), 1–18 (2020). https://doi.org/10.1007/s00138-020-01060-x
5. Modat, M., et al.: Fast free-form deformation using graphics processing units. Comput. Methods Progr. Biomed. **98**, 278–284 (2010)
6. Modat, M., Cash, D.M., Daga, P., Winston, G.P., Duncan, J.S., Ourselin, S.: Global image registration using a symmetric block-matching approach. J. Med. Imag. **1**(2), 024003 (2014)
7. Ou, Y., Sotiras, A., Paragios, N., Davatzikos, C.: DRAMMS: deformable registration via attribute matching and mutual-saliency weighting. Med. Image Anal. **15**, 622–639 (2011)
8. Avants, B.B., Tustison, N., Song, G.: Advanced normalization tools (ANTS). Insight j **2**, 1–35 (2009)
9. Johnson, H., Harris, G., Williams, K.: BRAINSFit: mutual information registrations of whole-brain 3D Images, using the insight toolkit. Insight J. **57**(1), 1–0 (2007)
10. Zeineldin, R.A., Karar, M.E., Coburger, J., Wirtz, C.R., Burgert, O.: DeepSeg: deep neural network framework for automatic brain tumor segmentation using magnetic resonance FLAIR images. Int. J. Comput. Assist. Radiol. Surg. **15**, 909–920 (2020)
11. Cheng, X., Zhang, L., Zheng, Y.: Deep similarity learning for multimodal medical images. Comput. Methods Biomech. Biomed. Eng.: Imag. Visual. **6**, 248–252 (2018)

12. Zeineldin, R.A., Karar, M.E., Mathis-Ullrich, F., Burgert, O.: A hybrid deep registration of MR scans to interventional ultrasound for neurosurgical guidance. In: Lian, C., Cao, X., Rekik, I., Xuanang, Xu., Yan, P. (eds.) Machine Learning in Medical Imaging: 12th International Workshop, MLMI 2021, Held in Conjunction with MICCAI 2021, Strasbourg, France, September 27, 2021, Proceedings, pp. 586–595. Springer International Publishing, Cham (2021). https://doi.org/10.1007/978-3-030-87589-3_60

13. Zeineldin, R.A., Karar, M.E., Coburger, J., Wirtz, C.R., Mathis-Ullrich, F., Burgert, O.: Towards automated correction of brain shift using deep deformable magnetic resonance imaging-intraoperative ultrasound (MRI-iUS) registration. Curr. Direct. Biomed. Eng. 6(1), 20200039 (2020)

14. Balakrishnan, G., Zhao, A., Sabuncu, M.R., Guttag, J., Dalca, A.V.: VoxelMorph: A learning framework for deformable medical image registration. IEEE Trans. Med. Imaging 38(8), 1788–1800 (2019)

15. de Vos, B.D., Berendsen, F.F., Viergever, M.A., Sokooti, H., Staring, M., Isgum, I.: A deep learning framework for unsupervised affine and deformable image registration. Med. Image Anal. 52, 128–143 (2019)

16. Chen, J., Frey, E.C., He, Y., Segars, W.P., Li, Y., Du, Y.: TransMorph: transformer for unsupervised medical image registration. Med. Image Anal. 82, 102615 (2022)

17. Abbasi, S., et al.: Medical image registration using unsupervised deep neural network: a scoping literature review. Biomed. Signal Process. Contr. 73, 103444 (2022)

18. Zeineldin, R.A., et al.: IRegNet: non-rigid registration of MRI to interventional us for brain-shift compensation using convolutional neural networks. IEEE Access 9, 147579–147590 (2021)

19. Baheti, B., et al.: The brain tumor sequence registration challenge: Establishing correspondence between pre-operative and follow-up MRI scans of diffuse glioma patients. arXiv preprint arXiv:2112.06979 (2021)

20. Ronneberger, O., Fischer, P., Brox, T.: U-Net: convolutional networks for biomedical image segmentation. In: Medical Image Computing and Computer-assisted Intervention – MICCAI 2015, pp. 234–241 (2015)

21. Çiçek, Ö., Abdulkadir, A., Lienkamp, S.S., Brox, T., Ronneberger, O.: 3D U-Net: learning dense volumetric segmentation from sparse annotation. In: Medical Image Computing and Computer-assisted Intervention – MICCAI 2016, pp. 424–432 (2016)

22. Kingma, D.P., Ba, J.: Adam: a method for stochastic optimization. arXiv preprint arXiv:1412.6980 (2014)

3D Inception-Based TransMorph: Pre- and Post-operative Multi-contrast MRI Registration in Brain Tumors

Javid Abderezaei, Aymeric Pionteck, Agamdeep Chopra, and Mehmet Kurt$^{(\boxtimes)}$

Department of Mechanical Engineering, University of Washington, Seattle, USA
mkurt@uw.edu

Abstract. Deformable image registration is a key task in medical image analysis. The Brain Tumor Sequence Registration challenge aims at establishing correspondences between pre-operative and follow-up scans of the same patient diagnosed with an adult brain diffuse high-grade glioma and intends to address the challenging task of registering longitudinal data with major tissue appearance changes. In this work, we proposed a two-stage cascaded network based on Inception and TransMorph models. The dataset for each patient was comprised of a native pre-contrast (T1), a contrast-enhanced T1-weighted (T1-CE), a T2-weighted (T2), and a Fluid Attenuated Inversion Recovery (FLAIR). The Inception model was used to fuse the 4 image modalities together and extract the most relevant information. Then, a variant of the TransMorph architecture was adapted to generate the displacement fields. The Loss function was composed of a standard image similarity measure, a diffusion regularizer, and an edge-map similarity measure added to overcome intensity dependence and reinforce correct boundary deformation. We observed that the addition of the Inception module substantially increased the performance of the network. Additionally, performing an initial affine registration before training the model showed improved accuracy in the landmark error measurements between pre and post-operative MRIs.

Keywords: Registration · Glioma · MRI · Longitudinal · Diffuse glioma · Glioblastoma · Deep Learning · Transformers · CNN · Neural Network · U-Net

1 Introduction

In many medical image analysis applications, deformable image registration is a key task. It is often used in a number of clinical applications such as image reconstruction [1, 2], segmentation [3, 4], motion tracking [5, 6], tumor growth monitoring, image guidance [7–9], and co-registration of MR brain images [10]. Using the deformation field, images of the same organ from different patients (inter-patient registration) or images of the same organ from the same person taken at different times or from different medical imaging equipment (intra-patient registration) are aligned for better visualization

---

J. Abderezaei and A. Pionteck—Contributed equally to this paper

S. Bakas et al. (Eds.): BrainLes 2022, LNCS 14092, pp. 35–45, 2023.
https://doi.org/10.1007/978-3-031-44153-0_4

and comparison. The moving (source) image is warped with the deformation field to match the fixed (target) image. Conventional image registration has been framed as an optimization problem to maximize a similarity measure that indicates the closeness of the moving image to the fixed image [10, 11]. Deep Convolutional Neural Networks (CNN) obtained significant success in several image analysis tasks such as object detection and recognition [12, 13], image classification [14, 15], and image segmentation [16, 17]. In image registration, several methods have been proposed to improve the performance in terms of registration accuracy and computation efficiency [18–23]. However, little attention has been given to the specific task of registering longitudinal brain Magnetic Resonance Imaging (MRI) scans containing pathologies. This task is particularly challenging due to major tissue appearance changes, and still an unsolved problem.

Previous Brain Tumor Segmentation challenges (BraTS) were aimed at evaluating state-of-the-art methods for the segmentation of brain tumors. The Brain Tumor Sequence Registration (BraTS-Reg) challenge [24] aims at establishing correspondences between pre-operative and follow-up scans of the same patient diagnosed with an adult brain diffuse high-grade glioma. The BraTS-Reg challenge intends to establish a public benchmark environment for deformable registration algorithms. The associated dataset comprises de-identified multi-institutional multi-parametric MRI (mpMRI) data, curated for each scan's size and resolution, according to a common anatomical template. For each patient, a native precontrast (T1), a contrast-enhanced T1-weighted (T1-CE), a T2-weighted (T2) and a Fluid Attenuated Inversion Recovery (FLAIR) are provided. Clinical experts have generated extensive annotations of landmarks points within the scans descriptive of distinct anatomical locations across the temporal domain. A number of metrics such as Median Absolute Error (MAE), Robustness, and the Jacobian determinant are used to measure the performance of the algorithms proposed by participants.

In this work, inspired by the TransMorph [25] architecture, we propose a novel two-stage cascaded network. In the first stage, we use a variant of the Inception model [26] to merge the 4 image modalities together and extract the most relevant information

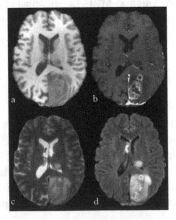

Fig. 1. Example set of provided images, a) T1 weighted b) T1-CE c) T2 weighted d) Flair

from each type of the imaging contrasts. In the second stage, we use a variant of the TransMorph architecture to generate the displacement field used to warp the moving image.

2 Methods

2.1 Model Architecture

An example image set of provided data is presented in Fig. 1, which shows a native precontrast (T1), a contrast-enhanced T1-weighted (T1-CE), a T2-weighted (T2) and a Fluid Attenuated Inversion Recovery (FLAIR) of one of the subjects. A cascaded network was developed by using 2 blocks derived from the Inception architecture [26] to combine the imaging modalities and the output was then fed into the TransMorph model [25] responsible for the image registration (Fig. 2).

The Inception model [26] consists of 2 separate pipelines for both moving and target modalities (Figs. 2, 3). Each Inception pipeline consists of 4 input inception blocks corresponding to T1-CE, T1, Flair, and T2 as shown in Fig. 2. The outputs of the inception blocks are concatenated and passed through a sequential layer of another inception block followed by a single 3d convolution layer with kernel size = stride = 1, which outputs the desired single channel merged image. As described in [26], the main idea of the Inception architecture is finding out how an optimal local sparse structure in a convolutional vision network can be approximated and covered by readily available dense components. The goal is to find the optimal local construction and to repeat it spatially. We used the Inception module with dimension reductions described in Fig. 3 [26]. The advantage of the Inception module was that it allowed us to first process each contrast separately and extract the relevant information before concatenating them. The concatenated data was then passed through more Inception modules that merged the contrasts together and output new moving and target images. This approach had several advantages compared to a simple concatenation of the different contrast images. First, it added more training parameters corresponding to the data merging layers, which in the end should improve the results. It also helped reduce the memory requirements by merging 4 volumetric images into a single one.

The output of the Inception module was then passed to the TransMorph model as described in [25]. The output of the TransMorph model is a displacement field, which was then used as an input to a spatial transformer to register the moving images on the target images. TransMorph [25] is a hybrid TransformerConvNet framework designed for volumetric medical image registration. Transformer, initially designed for natural language processing tasks [27], has shown its potential in computer vision tasks. A Transformer determines which parts of the input sequence are essential based on contextual information by using self-attention mechanisms. Vision Transformer (ViT) [28], which applied the Transformer encoder directly to images, achieved state-of-the-art performance in image recognition. Transformer has also a strong potential for image registration as it can better comprehend the spatial correspondences between the moving and fixed images. Bridging of ViT and V-Net provided good performance in image registration [29]. In this method described in [25], the Swin Transformer [30] is employed as the encoder to capture the spatial correspondence between the input moving and fixed images. Then, a

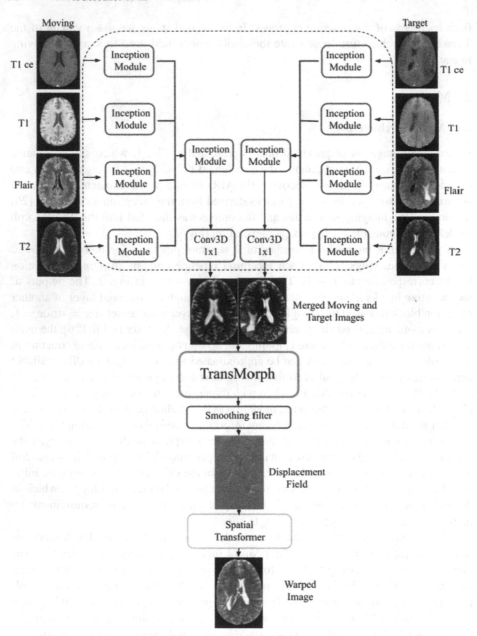

Fig. 2. Architecture of the proposed registration network

ConvNet decoder processed the information provided by the Transformer encoder into a dense displacement field. Long skip connections are used to maintain the flow of localization information between the encoder and decoder stages. Diffeomorphic variations of

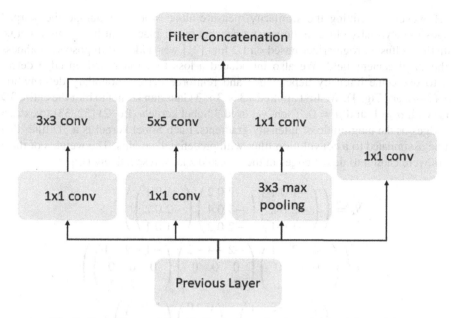

Fig. 3. Inception module with dimension reductions (adapted from [26])

TransMorph were also introduced to ensure a smooth and topology-preserving deformation. The final output of the TransMorph model is a displacement field, which was used to warp the moving image (pre-operative) to match the target image (post-operative).

2.2 Training of the Network

We performed multiple preprocessing steps on the input dataset before training the deep learning network. Because MRI intensity values are not normalized, we applied intensity normalization to each MRI modality of each patient independently by subtracting the mean and dividing by the standard deviation of the brain region. For each specific imaging modality, we also performed a histogram match between pre and post-surgery datasets. Finally, we divided our training into two trials. In the first trial, we trained the networks using the preprocessed dataset, while in the second trial, we first performed an affine registration between the pre and post-surgery images and then trained the networks.

Our network was implemented using PyTorch 1.1.1 [31]. The update of the weights of the network was done using Adam optimizer, with a batch size of 1 and a decaying learning rate with an initial value of $\alpha = 1e^{-4}$.

Training was performed on $2 \times$ NVIDIA A40 GPU 2×48 GB memory. The initial loss function was based on a widely-used image similarity measure which computes the similarity between the deformed moving and the fixed images. We used the mean square error metric (Eq. 1), which was the mean of the squared differences in voxel (i) values between the moving (Y) and the target images ($\hat{Y}$)

$$L_{MSE} = \frac{1}{N} \sum_{i=1}^{N} \left(Y_i - \hat{Y}_i \right)^2 \tag{1}$$

However, optimizing the similarity measure alone would encourage the warped images to be visually close to the target ones, but the displacement fields might not be realistic. Diffusion regularizer based on L2 loss [21] was added to impose smoothness in the displacement field. We also introduced a loss function based on edge detection to overcome intensity dependence and reinforce correct boundary deformation (Eq. (2–4), and Fig. 4). We first applied a $3 \times 3 \times 3$ Gaussian kernel to blur the entire 3D input with $\sigma = 1$, and $\mu = 0$. Then, we used 3 Sobel kernels (Eq. 2) [32, 33] to extract the edges as the magnitude of intensity gradients. Each Sobel kernel is a 3D filter that can be assimilated to a convolution filter with predefined weights. The weights of the 3 filters were chosen to detect edges in the x, y, and z axis, respectively (Eq. 2)

$$S_x = \left(\begin{pmatrix} -1\,0\,1 \\ -2\,0\,2 \\ -1\,0\,1 \end{pmatrix} \begin{pmatrix} -2\,0\,2 \\ -4\,0\,4 \\ -2\,0\,2 \end{pmatrix} \begin{pmatrix} -1\,0\,1 \\ -2\,0\,2 \\ -1\,0\,1 \end{pmatrix} \right)$$

$$S_y = \left(\begin{pmatrix} -1\,-2\,-1 \\ 0\ \ 0\ \ 0 \\ 1\ \ 2\ \ 1 \end{pmatrix} \begin{pmatrix} -2\,-4\,-2 \\ 0\ \ 0\ \ 0 \\ 2\ \ 4\ \ 2 \end{pmatrix} \begin{pmatrix} -1\,-2\,-1 \\ 0\ \ 0\ \ 0 \\ 1\ \ 2\ \ 1 \end{pmatrix} \right)$$

$$S_z = \left(\begin{pmatrix} -1\,-2\,-1 \\ -2\,-4\,-2 \\ -1\,-2\,-1 \end{pmatrix} \begin{pmatrix} 0\,0\,0 \\ 0\,0\,0 \\ 0\,0\,0 \end{pmatrix} \begin{pmatrix} 1\,2\,1 \\ 2\,4\,2 \\ 1\,2\,1 \end{pmatrix} \right) \tag{2}$$

These edges were located where there is a dramatic change in intensity within the filter. The final edge map was obtained by computing and normalizing the magnitude of the extracted intensity gradients (Eq. 3).

$$\mathcal{E}(A) = \sqrt{(S_x * A)^2 + (S_y * A)^2 + (S_z * A)^2} \tag{3}$$

The edge loss was calculated by comparing the edges of the predicted warped image to the target image edges using a standard mean square error loss function (Eq. 4).

$$L_{Edge} = \frac{1}{N} \sum_{i=1}^{N} \left(\mathcal{E}(Y_i) - \mathcal{E}(\hat{Y}_i) \right)^2 \tag{4}$$

The outputs of each function were finally weighted and summed to calculate the final loss value (Eq. 5).

$$L_{Total} = L_{Edge} + L_{MSE} + L_{Diffusion} \tag{5}$$

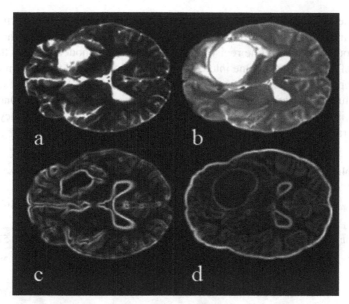

Fig. 4. Example of edge filter application, a) Initial moving image, b) initial target image, c) edges extracted from moving image, and d) edges extracted from target image

3   Results and Discussion

We analyzed 3 different variations of Inception-Transmorph for the task of image registration. We performed two sets of training on our dataset. In the first set of training, the raw dataset after normal preprocessing steps was used to train each model from scratch. In the second set of training, we initially performed an affine registration between pre and post-surgery datasets and then continued training similar to the first step. Finally, we selected the best model according to its performance on the evaluation data. The evaluation of the results was performed on an online evaluation platform (https://ipp.cbica.upenn.edu/). Each model was trained on 140 multi-modal MRI datasets composed of T1, T1-CE, T2, and Flair images. After training the models, we observed that it can successfully warp the moving images into the target ones (Fig. 5). Transmorph + Inception after initial affine registration of the dataset was our best-performing model, which was able to decrease the initial landmark median absolute error of 7.8 mm to 2.91 mm (Table 1). When the dataset was not initially affine registered, we found that the combination of Inception and TransMorph with the addition of edge maps in the training had the best performance compared to the other models (Table 1). Adding the edge maps in the loss function improved the results compared to initial TransMorph and TransMorph + Inception, by 15.6% and 21.8% respectively. The addition of the edge maps also dramatically improved the robustness results (about 25% increased performance; Table 1). This is primarily due to the edge map's ability to enforce the boundary of the deformation and hence more accurately drive the displacement direction.

In the second set of training where we initially performed an affine registration and then trained the models, we observed that the models perform substantially better than without affine registration. Here, TransMorph + Inception had the best performance with a landmark median absolute error of 2.91 mm which is about 28% better than the best model without the initial affine registration (Table 1). This model also had the highest robustness of 0.82 (Table 1). One interesting observation we had was that in this set of training as opposed to the previous one (after affine registration), the use of edge maps in the loss function decreased the performance of the model (Table 1). One possible explanation is that the edge maps contribute more to improving the accuracy of affine registration rather than the general nonlinear warping of the images.

Table 1. Evaluation of the trained models with the BraTS-Reg 2022 datasets

		Median Absolute Error (mm)	Mean Absolute Error (mm)	Robustness
Without Affine Registration	TransMorph	7.29	7.82	0.57
	TransMorph + Inception	7.66	8.09	0.59
	TransMorph + Inception + Edge Maps	6.15	6.48	0.76
With Affine Registration	TransMorph	4.06	5.09	0.72
	TransMorph + Inception	**2.91**	**3.62**	**0.82**
	TransMorph + Inception + Edge Maps	3.51	4.00	0.79

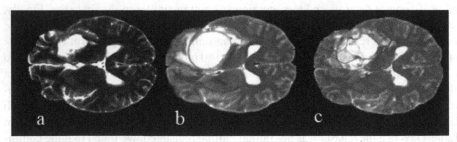

Fig. 5. Example of warped image with output displacement field of the network: a) Moving image, b) target image, c) warped image

4   Conclusion

In this paper, we proposed a two-stage cascaded network. Our approach first merged the 4 image modalities through an Inception model to extract the most relevant features from the different contrasts. Then the output of the first stage went through a model adapted from TransMorph to extract the displacement field. Experiments on the BraTS-Reg 2022 validation set demonstrated that our method could obtain results very close to the target. Adding the edge maps in the loss function improved the results only when we trained the model without using the affine-registered dataset. However, the inclusion of the edge maps resulted in worse performance when we used an affine registration prior to training the model. This is probably due to the effectiveness of edge maps loss function in helping with the affine registration rather than the nonlinear deformation of the images. We believe that with further fine-tuning of hyperparameters as well as a higher number of training epochs, and adopting a multi-scale approach to account for localized deformations, we can achieve improved results with the introduced Inception-Transmorph network.

References

1. Dang, H., Wang, A.S., Sussman, M.S., Siewerdsen, J.H., Stayman, J.W.: DPIRPLE: a joint estimation framework for deformable registration and penalized-likelihood CT image reconstruction using prior images. Phys. Med. Biol. **59**(17), 4799 (2014)
2. McClelland, J.R., et al.: A generalized framework unifying image registration and respiratory motion models and incorporating image reconstruction, for partial image data or full images. Phys. Med. Biol. **62**(11), 4273 (2017)
3. Yang, X., Rossi, P.J., Jani, A.B., Mao, H., Curran, W.J., Liu, T.: "3D transrectal ultrasound (TRUS) prostate segmentation based on optimal feature learning framework," In: Medical Imaging 2016: Image Processing, vol. 9784, pp. 654–660 (2016)
4. Fu, Y., Liu, S., Li, H.H., Yang, D.: Automatic and hierarchical segmentation of the human skeleton in CT images. Phys. Med. Biol. **62**(7), 2812 (2017)
5. Fu, Y.B., Chui, C.K., Teo, C.L., Kobayashi, E.: Motion tracking and strain map computation for quasi-static magnetic resonance elastography. In: Fichtinger, G., Martel, A., Peters, T. (eds.) MICCAI 2011. LNCS, vol. 6891, pp. 428–435. Springer, Heidelberg (2011). https://doi.org/10.1007/978-3-642-23623-5_54
6. Yang, X., Ghafourian, P., Sharma, P., Salman, K., Martin, D., Fei, B.: "Nonrigid registration and classification of the kidneys in 3D dynamic contrast enhanced (DCE) MR images," In: Medical Imaging 2012: Image Processing, 2012, vol. 8314, pp. 105–112 (2012)
7. Taylor, R.H., Menciassi, A., Fichtinger, G., Fiorini, P., Dario, P.: Medical robotics and computer-integrated surgery. In: Siciliano, B., Khatib, O. (eds.) Springer handbook of robotics, pp. 1657–1684. Springer International Publishing, Cham (2016). https://doi.org/10.1007/978-3-319-32552-1_63
8. Sarrut, D.: Deformable registration for image-guided radiation therapy. Z. Für Med. Phys. **16**(4), 285–297 (2006)
9. De Silva, T., et al.: 3D–2D image registration for target localization in spine surgery: investigation of similarity metrics providing robustness to content mismatch. Phys. Med. Biol. **61**(8), 3009 (2016)
10. Gaser, C.: Structural MRI: Morphometry. In:Neuroeconomics, M. Reuter and C. Montag, Eds. Berlin, Heidelberg: Springer (2016). https://doi.org/10.1007/978-3-642-35923-1_21
11. Ashburner, J.: A fast diffeomorphic image registration algorithm. Neuroimage **38**(1), 95–113 (2007). https://doi.org/10.1016/j.neuroimage.2007.07.007
12. Avants, B.B., Epstein, C.L., Grossman, M., Gee, J.C.: Symmetric diffeomorphic image registration with cross-correlation: evaluating automated labeling of elderly and neurodegenerative brain. Med. Image Anal. **12**(1), 26–41 (2008). https://doi.org/10.1016/j.media.2007.06.004

13. Li, J., Liang, X., Shen, S., Xu, T., Feng, J., Yan, S.: Scale-aware fast R-CNN for pedestrian detection. IEEE Trans. Multimed. **20**(4), 985–996 (2018). https://doi.org/10.1109/TMM.2017.2759508
14. Wu, Y., et al.: "Rethinking Classification and Localization for Object Detection," 2020, pp. 10186–10195 (2020). Accessed 15 Jul 2022. https://openaccess.thecvf.com/content_CVPR_2020/html/Wu_Rethinking_Classification_and_Localization_for_Object_Detection_CVPR_2020_paper.html
15. Krizhevsky, A., Sutskever, I., Hinton, G.E.: ImageNet classification with deep convolutional neural networks. In: Advances in Neural Information Processing Systems, vol. 25 (2012). Accessed 15 Jul 2022. https://proceedings.neurips.cc/paper/2012/hash/c399862d3b9d6b76c8436e924a68c45b-Abstract.html
16. Xie, Q., Luong, M.T., Hovy, E., Le, Q.V.: Self-training with noisy student improves imagenet classification. In: 2020 IEEE/CVF Conference on Computer Vision and Pattern Recognition (CVPR), Seattle, WA, USA, Jun. 2020, pp. 10684–10695. https://doi.org/10.1109/CVPR42600.2020.01070
17. Tao, A., Sapra, K., Catanzaro, B.: Hierarchical multi-scale attention for semantic segmentation. ArXiv Prepr. arXiv:200510821 (2020)
18. Chen, L.C., Yang, Y., Wang, J., Xu, W., Yuille, A.L.: Attention to scale: scale-aware semantic image segmentation (2016), pp. 3640–3649. Accessed Jul 15 2022. [Online]. Available: https://openaccess.thecvf.com/content_cvpr_2016/html/Chen_Attention_to_Scale_CVPR_2016_paper.html
19. Yang, X., Kwitt, R., Styner, M., Niethammer, M.: Quicksilver: fast predictive image registration – a deep learning approach. Neuroimage **158**, 378–396 (2017). https://doi.org/10.1016/j.neuroimage.2017.07.008
20. Dalca, A.V., Balakrishnan, G., Guttag, J., Sabuncu, M.R.: Unsupervised Learning for Fast Probabilistic Diffeomorphic Registration. arXiv, 2018, Accessed: Jul 15 2022 https://doi.org/10.1007/978-3-030-00928-1_82 https://dspace.mit.edu/handle/1721.1/137585
21. Balakrishnan, G., Zhao, A., Sabuncu, M.R., Guttag, J., Dalca, A.V.: An unsupervised learning model for deformable medical image registration. ArXiv180202604 Cs (2018) https://doi.org/10.1109/CVPR.2018.00964
22. Balakrishnan, G., Zhao, A., Sabuncu, M.R., Guttag, J., Dalca, A.V.: VoxelMorph: a learning framework for deformable medical image registration. IEEE Trans. Med. Imaging **38**(8), 1788–1800 (Aug.2019). https://doi.org/10.1109/TMI.2019.2897538
23. Estienne, T., et al.: U-ReSNet: Ultimate Coupling of Registration and Segmentation with Deep Nets. In: Shen, D., Liu, T., Peters, T.M., Staib, L.H., Essert, C., Zhou, S., Yap, P.-T., Khan, A. (eds.) MICCAI 2019. LNCS, vol. 11766, pp. 310–319. Springer, Cham (2019). https://doi.org/10.1007/978-3-030-32248-9_35
24. Cao, X., Yang, J., Zhang, J., Nie, D., Kim, M., Wang, Q., Shen, D.: Deformable Image Registration Based on Similarity-Steered CNN Regression. In: Descoteaux, M., Maier-Hein, L., Franz, A., Jannin, P., Collins, D.L., Duchesne, S. (eds.) MICCAI 2017. LNCS, vol. 10433, pp. 300–308. Springer, Cham (2017). https://doi.org/10.1007/978-3-319-66182-7_35
25. Baheti, B., et al.: The brain tumor sequence registration challenge: establishing correspondence between pre-operative and follow-up MRI scans of diffuse glioma patients. arXiv (2021). https://doi.org/10.48550/arXiv.2112.06979
26. Chen, J., Frey, E.C., He, Y., Segars, W.P., Li, Y., Du, Y.: TransMorph: Transformer for unsupervised medical image registration (2022). Accessed 15 Jul 2022. http://arxiv.org/abs/2111.10480
27. Szegedy, C., et al.: Going Deeper with Convolutions (2014). Accessed 15 Jul 2022. http://arxiv.org/abs/1409.4842

28. Vaswani, A., et al.: Attention is all you need. In: Advances in Neural Information Processing Systems, vol. 30 (2017). Accessed 21 Apr 2022. https://papers.nips.cc/paper/2017/hash/3f5 ee243547dee91fbd053c1c4a845aa-Abstract.html
29. Dosovitskiy, A., et al.: An Image is Worth 16x16 Words: Transformers for Image Recognition at Scale. ArXiv201011929 Cs, Jun 2021, Accessed: Apr. 21 2022. http://arxiv.org/abs/2010. 11929
30. Chen, J., He, Y., Frey, E.C., Li, Y., Du, Y.: ViT-V-Net: Vision transformer for unsupervised volumetric medical image registration. ArXiv210406468 Cs Eess, Apr 2021, Accessed 21 Apr 2022. http://arxiv.org/abs/2104.06468
31. Liu, Z., et al.: Swin transformer: hierarchical vision transformer using shifted windows 2021, pp. 10012–10022 (2021). Accessed Jul 22 2022. https://openaccess.thecvf.com/content/ICC V2021/html/Liu_Swin_Transformer_Hierarchical_Vision_Transformer_Using_Shifted_W indows_ICCV_2021_paper.html
32. Paszke, A., et al.: PyTorch: an imperative style, high-performance deep learning library. In: Advances in Neural Information Processing Systems, 2019, vol. 32 (2019). Accessed 22 Jul 2022. https://proceedings.neurips.cc/paper/2019/hash/bdbca288fee7f92f2bfa9f7012727740-Abstract.html
33. Kanopoulos, N., Vasanthavada, N., Baker, R.L.: Design of an image edge detection filter using the Sobel operator. IEEE J. Solid-State Circuits **23**(2), 358–367 (1988). https://doi.org/ 10.1109/4.996
34. Xu, Z., Wu, Z., Feng, J.: CFUN: combining faster R-CNN and U-net network for efficient whole heart segmentation (2018)

CrossMoDa

Unsupervised Cross-Modality Domain Adaptation for Vestibular Schwannoma Segmentation and Koos Grade Prediction Based on Semi-supervised Contrastive Learning

Luyi Han[1,3], Yunzhi Huang[4], Tao Tan[2,3(✉)], and Ritse Mann[1,3]

[1] Department of Radiology and Nuclear Medicine, Radboud University Medical Center, Geert Grooteplein 10, 6525, Nijmegen, GA, The Netherlands
[2] Faculty of Applied Sciences, Macao Polytechnic University, Macao 999078, Macao, Special Administrative Region of China
[3] Department of Radiology, The Netherlands Cancer Institute, Plesmanlaan 121, 1066, Amsterdam, CX, The Netherlands
taotanjs@gmail.com
[4] School of Automation, Nanjing University of Information Science and Technology, Nanjing 210044, China

Abstract. Domain adaptation has been widely adopted to transfer styles across multi-vendors and multi-centers, as well as to complement the missing modalities. In this challenge, we proposed an unsupervised domain adaptation framework for cross-modality vestibular schwannoma (VS) and cochlea segmentation and Koos grade prediction. We learn the shared representation from both ceT1 and hrT2 images and recover another modality from the latent representation, and we also utilize proxy tasks of VS segmentation and brain parcellation to restrict the consistency of image structures in domain adaptation. After generating missing modalities, the nnU-Net model is utilized for VS and cochlea segmentation, while a semi-supervised contrastive learning pre-train approach is employed to improve the model performance for Koos grade prediction. On CrossMoDA validation phase Leaderboard, our method received rank 4 in task1 with a mean Dice score of 0.8394 and rank 2 in task2 with Macro-Average Mean Square Error of 0.3941. Our code is available at https://github.com/fiy2W/cmda2022.superpolymerization.

Keywords: Domain Adaptation · Semi-supervised Contrastive Learning · Segmentation · Vestibular Schwannoma

1 Introduction

Domain adaptation has recently been employed in various clinical settings to improve the applicability of deep learning approaches. The goal of Cross-Modality Domain Adaptation (CrossMoDA) challenge[1] is to segment two key

---

[1] https://crossmoda2022.grand-challenge.org/.

L. Han and Y. Huang—Contributed equally to this work.

brain structures, namely vestibular schwannoma (VS) and cochlea. It also requires predicting the Koos grading scale for VS. The two tasks are required for the measurement of VS growth and evaluation of the treatment plan (surveillance, radiosurgery, open surgery). And an automatic pipeline for VS segmentation and Koos classification on MRIs has been proposed to improve clinical workflow [13]. Although contrast-enhanced T1 (ceT1) MR imaging is commonly used for patients with VS in diagnosis and surveillance, the research on non-contrast imaging, such as high-resolution T2 (hrT2), is growing due to lower risk and more efficient cost. Therefore, to avoid additional annotation, CrossMoDA aims to transfer the learnt knowledge from ceT1 to hrT2 images by building up domain adaptation between unpaired ceT1 and hrT2.

2   Related Work

Weakly supervised and unsupervised domain adaptation for VS and cochlea segmentation has been extensively validated in previous research [7, 8]. Most of them employ an image-to-image translation method, *e.g.* CycleGAN [19], to generate pseudo-target domain images from source domain images. And then generated images and the corresponding manual annotations are used to train the segmentation models. Dong *et al.* [6] utilize NiceGAN [3], which is trained by reusing discriminators for encoding, to improve the performance of domain adaptation and further segmentation. Choi [5] proposes a data augmentation method by halving the intensity in the tumor area for generated hrT2. Shin *et al.* [15] employ an iterable self-training strategy in their method: (1) train the student model with annotated generated hrT2 and pseudo-labeled real hrT2; (2) make the student a new teacher and update the pseudo label for real htT2. Following these works, our proposed method focuses more on extracting joint representations from multi-modality MRIs, which can reduce the distance between different modalities in the latent space.

Classification task for medical images can be very challenging due to insufficient instances. In recent years, contrastive learning has led to state-of-the-art performance in self-supervised representation learning [1,9,12,17]. In contrastive learning, a data sample is first selected as the anchor, and samples with the same class as the anchor are positive samples, while others are negative samples. The key idea is to reduce the distance between an anchor and a positive sample in latent space, and distinguish the anchor from other negative samples. Contrastive learning is often applied to medical image pretraining. Huang *et al.* [10] develop an attentional contrastive learning framework for global and local representation learning between images and radiology reports. You *et al.* [18] introduce lesion and normal contrastive losses to the multi-task approach to learn inter- and intra-variations, which improves the performance of cancer detection. Apart from contrastive learning on pixel-level features, Wang *et al.* [16] propose graph-level contrastive learning to handle population-based fMRI classification. Inspired by these works, contrastive learning is employed at the pretraining phase to mine multi-modality representation strategically for different types of samples.

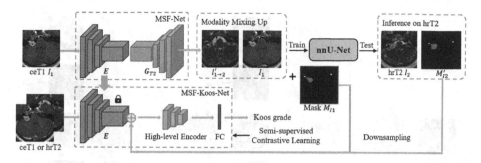

Fig. 1. Overview of the proposed unsupervised domain adaptation segmentation and classification framework.

3 Method

3.1 Framework Overview

Figure 1 illustrates the proposed unsupervised domain adaptation segmentation and classification framework. We first employ a multi-sequence fusion network (MSF-Net) to generate the corresponding hrT2 image from a given ceT1 image. To train a robust segmentation network, we pool real ceT1 images and generated hrT2 images together, instead of pairing them, to ensure the nnU-Net [11] model is able to predict ceT1 and hrT2 images blindly. By leveraging the predicted segmentation mask and pre-trained MSF-Net, we propose MSF-Koos-Net based on semi-supervised contrastive learning to predict Koos grade.

3.2 Cochlea and VS Segmentation Based on Unsupervised Domain Adaptation

Figure 2 illustrates the architecture of the proposed MSF-Net. Although ceT1 and hrT2 MRI images differ in image resolution and appearance, organs' representations from an identical subject are commonly embedded in the latent space. Based on this, we employed a share-weighted encoder $\mathbf{E}$ to extract the domain-free representations from both ceT1 and hrT2 images. Then, two decoders ($\mathbf{G}_{T1}$ and $\mathbf{G}_{T2}$) was constructed to recover the different parametric MRI sequences from the latent representations. The reconstruction loss is as follows,

$$\mathcal{L}_{rec} = \lambda_r \cdot (\|I_1' - I_1\|_1 + \|I_2' - I_2\|_1) + \lambda_p \cdot (\mathcal{L}_p(I_1', I_1) + \mathcal{L}_p(I_2', I_2)) \quad (1)$$

where $I_1' = \mathbf{G}_{T1}(\mathbf{E}(I_1))$, $I_2' = \mathbf{G}_{T2}(\mathbf{E}(I_2))$, $\|\cdot\|_1$ is a L_1 loss, and $\mathcal{L}_p$ refers to the perceptual loss based on pre-trained VGG19. λ_r and λ_p are weight terms and are set to be 10 and 0.01.

Inspired by Cycle-GAN [19], we utilize the adversarial loss to achieve the domain adaptation and employ cycle consistency loss to force the consistency of

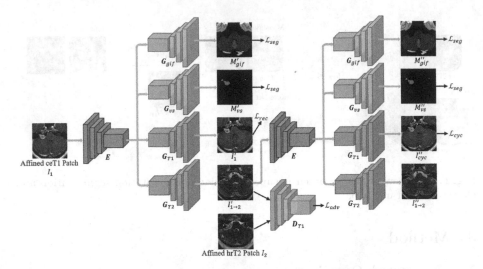

Fig. 2. The architecture of MSF-Net. The reverse transform direction (from real hrT2 to fake ceT1) is omitted for ease of illustration. Note that, both directions share weights for the model, and no proxy paths ($\mathbf{G}_{vs}$ and $\mathbf{G}_{gif}$) are involved in the reverse direction due to lack of annotations.

the anatomical structures.

$$\min_{\mathbf{D}_{T1},\mathbf{D}_{T2}} \max_{\mathbf{G}} \mathcal{L}_{adv} = \|\mathbf{D}_{T1}(I_1) - 1\|_2 + \|\mathbf{D}_{T1}(I'_{2\to1})\|_2 \\ + \|\mathbf{D}_{T2}(I_2) - 1\|_2 + \|\mathbf{D}_{T2}(I'_{1\to2})\|_2 \tag{2}$$

$$\mathcal{L}_{cyc} = \|I''_{1\to2\to1} - I_1\|_1 + \|I''_{2\to1\to2} - I_2\|_1 \tag{3}$$

where $I'_{1\to2} = \mathbf{G}_{T2}(\mathbf{E}(I_1))$, $I''_{1\to2\to1} = \mathbf{G}_{T1}(\mathbf{E}(I'_{1\to2}))$, $I'_{2\to1}$ and $I''_{2\to1\to2}$ are formulated similarly, $\|\cdot\|_2$ is a L_2 loss.

To further restrict the image structure during domain adaptation, especially for tumors, we employ two proxy tasks for real ceT1 images, including VS segmentation ($\mathbf{G}_{vs}$) and brain parcellation ($\mathbf{G}_{gif}$) whose labels are obtained with the Geodesic Information Flows (GIF) algorithm [2].

$$\mathcal{L}_{seg} = \mathcal{L}_{ce}(M'_{vs}, M_{vs}) + \mathcal{L}_{dsc}(M'_{vs}, M_{vs}) \\ + \mathcal{L}_{ce}(M'_{gif}, M_{gif}) + \mathcal{L}_{dsc}(M'_{gif}, M_{gif}) \tag{4}$$

where $\mathcal{L}_{ce}$ refers to the cross entropy loss and $\mathcal{L}_{dsc}$ indicates the dice similarity coefficient loss.

The total loss function of the proposed MSF-Net can be summarized as,

$$\mathcal{L}_{total} = \mathcal{L}_{rec} + \lambda_a \cdot \mathcal{L}_{adv} + \lambda_c \cdot \mathcal{L}_{cyc} + \lambda_s \cdot \mathcal{L}_{seg} \tag{5}$$

where we set $\lambda_a = 1$, $\lambda_c = 10$, and $\lambda_s = 1$ with experimental experience.

3.3   Koos Grade Prediction Based on Semi-supervised Contrastive Learning

Figure 3 illustrates the architecture of MSF-Koos-Net. The frozen pre-trained encoder $\mathbf{E}$ from MSF-Net is employed to extract low-level features from both ceT1 and hrT2 images. To pay more attention to the tumor region, we concatenate the low-level image features with the predicted segmentation mask of the tumor. Then followed with a high-level encoder $\mathbf{E}_{\mathcal{H}}$ to extract high- dimension features and a fully connected layer to output the predicted Koos grade. To achieve better performance of Koos grade prediction with limited data, both supervised and self-supervised contrastive learning [12] are utilized to pre-train the MSF-Koos-Net.

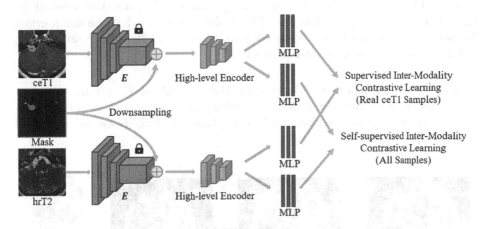

Fig. 3. The architecture of MSF-Koos-Net.

Self-supervised Contrastive Learning. After generating the missing modality, a dataset that includes paired ceT1 and hrT2 is composed. Within a multi-modality batch, let $\mathcal{D}$ be the group of indexes for these samples. For self-supervised contrastive learning, only cross-modality samples with the same indexes as the source sample are positive. The loss function is defined as follows,

$$\mathcal{L}_{self} = -\sum_{i \in \mathcal{D}} \log \frac{\exp\left(z_1^{(i)} \cdot z_2^{(i)}/\tau\right)}{\sum_{j \in \mathcal{D}} \exp\left(z_1^{(i)} \cdot z_2^{(j)}/\tau\right)} \cdot \frac{\exp\left(z_1^{(i)} \cdot z_2^{(i)}/\tau\right)}{\sum_{j \in \mathcal{D}} \exp\left(z_1^{(j)} \cdot z_2^{(i)}/\tau\right)} \tag{6}$$

where $z_1 = \mathcal{F}_{self}(\mathbf{E}_{\mathcal{H}}(\mathbf{E}(I_1)))$ and $z_2 = \mathcal{F}_{self}(\mathbf{E}_{\mathcal{H}}(\mathbf{E}(I_2)))$ refer to features extracted from ceT1 and hrT2 images, $\mathcal{F}_{self}$ indicates the projection network [4] for self-supervised contrastive learning, the $\cdot$ symbol denotes Scalar Product, τ refers to the scalar temperature parameter.

Supervised Contrastive Learning. To leverage Koos grade for pretraining, supervised contrastive learning is employed to enlarge the inter-grade difference and intra-grade similarity. We use samples from real ceT1 and the corresponding fake hrT2 pairs, and let $\mathcal{A}$ be the index group for the annotated samples in a multi-modality batch. The loss takes the following form,

$$
\mathcal{L}_{sup} = -\sum_{i \in \mathcal{A}} \frac{1}{|\mathcal{P}(i)|} \sum_{p \in \mathcal{P}(i)}
$$

$$
\log \frac{\exp\left(q_1^{(i)} \cdot q_2^{(p)}/\tau\right)}{\sum_{j \in \mathcal{A}} \exp\left(q_1^{(i)} \cdot q_2^{(j)}/\tau\right)} \cdot \frac{\exp\left(q_1^{(p)} \cdot q_2^{(i)}/\tau\right)}{\sum_{j \in \mathcal{A}} \exp\left(q_1^{(j)} \cdot q_2^{(i)}/\tau\right)} \tag{7}
$$

where $q_1 = \mathcal{F}_{sup}(\mathbf{E}_{\mathcal{H}}(\mathbf{E}(I_1)))$ and $q_2 = \mathcal{F}_{sup}(\mathbf{E}_{\mathcal{H}}(\mathbf{E}(I_2)))$ refer to features extracted from ceT1 and hrT2 images, $\mathcal{F}_{sup}$ indicates the projection network [4] for supervised contrastive learning, $\mathcal{P}(i) = \{p \in \mathcal{A}|y_p = y_i\}$ is the index group for positive samples whose Koos grades are the same as the source sample $I^{(i)}$, $|\mathcal{P}(i)|$ refers to the number of samples in $\mathcal{P}(i)$.

Koos Grade Prediction. By freezing the pre-trained $\mathbf{E}$ and $\mathbf{E}_{\mathcal{H}}$, we only fine-tune the final fully connected layer with annotated real ceT1 and the corresponding generated hrT2 images. In this phase, the MSF-Koos-Net is trained with a cross-entropy loss.

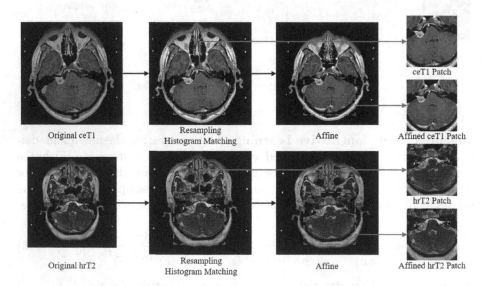

Fig. 4. The pipeline of image preprocessing. Both ceT1 and hrT2 images are resampled and applied with histogram matching respectively. And then the images are registered to the same atlas by affine transformation. Finally, patches with the fixed region of interest are extracted from affined and non-affined images.

4 Experimental Results

4.1 Materials and Implementation Details

Dataset. The dataset for the CrossMoDA challenge is an extension of the publicly available Vestibular-Schwannoma-SEG collection released on The Cancer Imaging Archive (TCIA) [8,14], which is divided into the training dataset (210 subjects with ceT1 images and other unpaired 210 subjects with hrT2 images) and the validation dataset (64 subjects with hrT2 images). All imaging datasets were manually segmented for cochlea and VS, and automated GIF parcellation masks were provided for the training source dataset.

Data Preprocessing. Figure 4 illustrates the pipeline of image preprocessing. All the images are first resampled to the spacing of $1 \times 0.4102 \times 0.4102$ mm. Then we utilize histogram matching to normalize ceT1 and hrT2 images, separately. To improve the performance of domain adaptation, we select an identical hrT2 image as the atlas and employ intra- and inter-modality affine transformation on all the ceT1 and hrT2 images, respectively. Here, we utilize mutual information (MI) loss for ceT1 images and normalized cross-correlation (NCC) loss for hrT2 images. Finally, based on the distribution of tumor areas in the training set, we crop the images to the size of $80 \times 256 \times 256$ by setting a fixed region. Limited by the device, we train the model in 2.5D mode – adjacent three slices are treated as a three-channel 2D input.

Implementation Details. We implemented our method using Pytorch with NVIDIA 3090 RTX. We optimized MSF-Net and MSF-Koos-Net with ADAM. MSF-Net is trained with a learning rate of 2×10^{-4}, a default of 1,000 epochs, and a batch size of 1. nnU-Net is trained with its default settings. MSF-Koos-Net is first pre-trained based on semi-supervised contrastive learning with a learning rate of 1×10^{-2}, a default of 100 epochs, and a batch size of 4. And then we fine-tune MSF-Koos-Net with a learning rate of 1×10^{-4} and a default of 20 epochs.

4.2 Results

Cross-modality domain adaptation results between ceT1 and hrT2 are shown in Fig. 5. Real ceT1 images are correctly transferred to the hrT2 domain keeping the tumor structure unchanged. To evaluate the influence of different generation performances for further segmentation, we compare our proposed method with CycleGAN [19] on ceT1 and hrT2 domain adaptation. And all the comparisons are based on the same segmentation process. Table 1 shows the segmentation results for the nnU-Net models training with fake hrT2 images generated by different methods. The proposed MSF-Net achieve better segmentation results than CycleGAN on the validation set, and the ablation study shows that adding the proxy task of VS and GIF can improve the performance of cross-modality domain

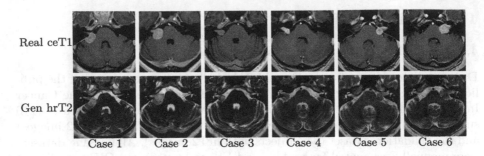

Real ceT1

Gen hrT2

Case 1   Case 2   Case 3   Case 4   Case 5   Case 6

Fig. 5. Examples of real ceT1 images and corresponding generated hrT2 images from the proposed MSF-Net.

adaptation. For Koos grade prediction, the proposed MSF-Koos-Net achieves the best Macro-Average Mean Square Error (MAMSE) of 0.3940. MAMSE increases to 0.6805 when the pre-trained weights are not frozen. And further MAMSE increases to 0.8371 without pretraining with semi-supervised contrastive learning.

Table 1. Segmentation results for nnU-Net utilizing generated hrT2 images with different domain adaptation methods.

Methods	VS Dice ↑	VS ASSD ↓	Cochlea Dice ↑	Cochlea ASSD ↓
CycleGAN	0.7402 ± 0.2504	1.7556 ± 5.3276	0.8202 ± 0.0253	0.2325 ± 0.1545
MSF-Net w/o VS&GIF	0.7764 ± 0.2025	0.6905 ± 0.6437	0.8220 ± 0.0510	0.3097 ± 0.2986
MSF-Net w/o GIF	0.8288 ± 0.0838	0.7901 ± 1.0765	0.8285 ± 0.0354	0.2507 ± 0.1828
MSF-Net	0.8493 ± 0.0683	0.5202 ± 0.2288	0.8294 ± 0.0268	0.2454 ± 0.2102

5   Discussion

In this study, we develop a cross-modality domain adaptation approach for VS and cochlea segmentation and also Koos grade prediction. In practice, our proposed MSF-Net is verified to convert the images from the ceT1 domain to the hrT2 domain and keep the anatomy unchanged. With a weight-shared encoder, MSF-Net is capable of learning joint multi-modality representation, given the ability of modality identification. The constraints on self-supervised modality recovery provide more structure consistency for the model training. Based on this, the proposed MSF-Net achieves better performance on domain adaptation than CycleGAN. This further affects the follow-up segmentation task, making the segmentation results of MSF-Net higher than that of CycleGAN. In addition, proxy tasks also have an important contribution to cross-modality domain adaptation. Segmentation of VS and brain structure can help less structural bias during image-to-image transformation and improve the segmentation accuracy. Our proposed MSF-Koos-Net also achieves high accuracy in the cross-modality classification task. Self-supervised medical image pretraining by contrastive learning has been proven to lead to Koos grade prediction performance improvements. It is shown that freezing the pre-trained weights during finetuning stage of the model is effective for limited training data. It may be because fine-tuning the last layer requires fewer parameters to be optimized. Weight-frozen strategy and contrastive learning are helpful in avoiding overfitting and capturing more representative information from images.

Acknowledgement. Luyi Han was funded by Chinese Scholarship Council (CSC) scholarship. This work was supported by the National Natural Science Foundation of China under Grant No. 62101365 and the startup foundation of Nanjing University of Information Science and Technology.

References

1. Bachman, P., Hjelm, R.D., Buchwalter, W.: Learning representations by maximizing mutual information across views. In: Advances in Neural Information Processing Systems 32 (2019)
2. Cardoso, M.J., et al.: Geodesic information flows: spatially-variant graphs and their application to segmentation and fusion. IEEE Trans. Med. Imaging **34**(9), 1976–1988 (2015)
3. Chen, R., Huang, W., Huang, B., Sun, F., Fang, B.: Reusing discriminators for encoding: towards unsupervised image-to-image translation. In: Proceedings of the IEEE/CVF Conference on Computer Vision And Pattern Recognition, pp. 8168–8177 (2020)
4. Chen, T., Kornblith, S., Norouzi, M., Hinton, G.: A simple framework for contrastive learning of visual representations. In: International Conference on Machine Learning, pp. 1597–1607. PMLR (2020)
5. Choi, J.W.: Using out-of-the-box frameworks for contrastive unpaired image translation for vestibular schwannoma and cochlea segmentation: an approach for the crossmoda challenge. In: Crimi, A., Bakas, S. (eds.) Brainlesion: Glioma, Multiple Sclerosis, Stroke and Traumatic Brain Injuries: 7th International Workshop, BrainLes 2021, Held in Conjunction with MICCAI 2021, Virtual Event, September 27, 2021, Revised Selected Papers, Part II, pp. 509–517. Springer International Publishing, Cham (2022). https://doi.org/10.1007/978-3-031-09002-8_44
6. Dong, H., Yu, F., Zhao, J., Dong, B., Zhang, L.: Unsupervised domain adaptation in semantic segmentation based on pixel alignment and self-training. arXiv preprint arXiv:2109.14219 (2021)
7. Dorent, R., et al.: Scribble-based domain adaptation via co-segmentation. In: Martel, A.L., et al. (eds.) Medical Image Computing and Computer Assisted Intervention – MICCAI 2020: 23rd International Conference, Lima, Peru, October 4–8, 2020, Proceedings, Part I, pp. 479–489. Springer International Publishing, Cham (2020). https://doi.org/10.1007/978-3-030-59710-8_47
8. Dorent, R., et al.: Crossmoda 2021 challenge: benchmark of cross-modality domain adaptation techniques for vestibular schwnannoma and cochlea segmentation. Med. Image Anal. **83**, 102628 (2023)

9. He, K., Fan, H., Wu, Y., Xie, S., Girshick, R.: Momentum contrast for unsupervised visual representation learning. In: Proceedings of the IEEE/CVF Conference on Computer Vision and Pattern Recognition, pp. 9729–9738 (2020)

10. Huang, S.C., Shen, L., Lungren, M.P., Yeung, S.: Gloria: a multimodal global-local representation learning framework for label-efficient medical image recognition. In: Proceedings of the IEEE/CVF International Conference on Computer Vision, pp. 3942–3951 (2021)

11. Isensee, F., Jaeger, P.F., Kohl, S.A., Petersen, J., Maier-Hein, K.H.: nnu-net: a self-configuring method for deep learning-based biomedical image segmentation. Nat. Methods **18**(2), 203–211 (2021)

12. Khosla, P., et al.: Supervised contrastive learning. Adv. Neural. Inf. Process. Syst. **33**, 18661–18673 (2020)

13. Kujawa, A., et al.: Automated koos classification of vestibular schwannoma. Front. Radiol. **2**, 837191 (2022)

14. Shapey, J., et al.: Segmentation of vestibular schwannoma from MRI, an open annotated dataset and baseline algorithm. Sci. Data **8**(1), 1–6 (2021)

15. Shin, H., Kim, H., Kim, S., Jun, Y., Eo, T., Hwang, D.: Cosmos: cross-modality unsupervised domain adaptation for 3d medical image segmentation based on target-aware domain translation and iterative self-training. arXiv preprint arXiv: 2203.16557 (2022)

16. Wang, X., Yao, L., Rekik, I., Zhang, Yu.: Contrastive functional connectivity graph learning for population-based fMRI classification. In: Wang, L., Dou, Q., Fletcher, P.T., Speidel, S., Li, S. (eds.) Medical Image Computing and Computer Assisted Intervention – MICCAI 2022: 25th International Conference, Singapore, September 18–22, 2022, Proceedings, Part I, pp. 221–230. Springer Nature Switzerland, Cham (2022). https://doi.org/10.1007/978-3-031-16431-6_21

17. Wu, Z., Xiong, Y., Yu, S.X., Lin, D.: Unsupervised feature learning via non-parametric instance discrimination. In: Proceedings of the IEEE Conference on Computer Vision and Pattern Recognition, pp. 3733–3742 (2018)

18. You, K., Lee, S., Jo, K., Park, E., Kooi, T., Nam, H.: Intra-class contrastive learning improves computer aided diagnosis of breast cancer in mammography. In: Wang, L., Dou, Q., Fletcher, P.T., Speidel, S., Li, S. (eds.) Medical Image Computing and Computer Assisted Intervention – MICCAI 2022: 25th International Conference, Singapore, September 18–22, 2022, Proceedings, Part III, pp. 55–64. Springer Nature Switzerland, Cham (2022). https://doi.org/10.1007/978-3-031-16437-8_6

19. Zhu, J.Y., Park, T., Isola, P., Efros, A.A.: Unpaired image-to-image translation using cycle-consistent adversarial networks. In: Proceedings of the IEEE International Conference on Computer Vision, pp. 2223–2232 (2017)

Koos Classification of Vestibular Schwannoma via Image Translation-Based Unsupervised Cross-Modality Domain Adaptation

Tao Yang⬤ and Lisheng Wang$^{(\boxtimes)}$ ⬤

Department of Automation, Shanghai Jiao Tong University, Shanghai, China
{yangtao22,lswang}@sjtu.edu.cn

Abstract. The Koos grading scale is a classification system for vestibular schwannoma (VS) used to characterize the tumor and its effects on adjacent brain structures. The Koos classification captures many of the characteristics of treatment decisions and is often used to determine treatment plans. Although both contrast-enhanced T1 (ceT1) scanning and high-resolution T2 (hrT2) scanning can be used for Koos Classification, hrT2 scanning is gaining interest because of its higher safety and cost-effectiveness. However, in the absence of annotations for hrT2 scans, deep learning methods often inevitably suffer from performance degradation due to unsupervised learning. If ceT1 scans and their annotations can be used for unsupervised learning of hrT2 scans, the performance of Koos classification using unlabeled hrT2 scans will be greatly improved. In this regard, we propose an unsupervised cross-modality domain adaptation method based on image translation by transforming annotated ceT1 scans into hrT2 modality and using their annotations to achieve supervised learning of hrT2 modality. Then, the VS and 7 adjacent brain structures related to Koos classification in hrT2 scans were segmented. Finally, handcrafted features are extracted from the segmentation results, and Koos grade is classified using a random forest classifier. The proposed method received rank 1 on the Koos classification task of the Cross-Modality Domain Adaptation (crossMoDA 2022) challenge, with Macro-Averaged Mean Absolute Error (MA-MAE) of 0.2148 for the validation set and 0.26 for the test set.

Keywords: Unsupervised domain adaptation · Image translation · Vestibular schwannoma

1 Introduction

Vestibular schwannoma (VS) is a benign, slow-growing tumor that occurs in the inner auditory canal from the inner ear to the brain [1]. The Koos grading scale is a classification system for vestibular schwannoma used to characterize the tumor and its effects on adjacent brain structures. Specifically, the Koos grading of VS is primarily determined by tumor size, location, and degree of compression of adjacent brain structures. The Koos classification captures many of the characteristics of treatment decisions and is often used to determine treatment plans. Specifically, the Koos grading scale divides vestibular schwannoma into four grades according to criteria, as shown in **Fig. 1**. In recent years, with the advent of deep learning, it has become possible to improve patient outcomes and experience through standardization and personalization of VS treatment, while also significantly reducing physician workload [2]. So far, some deep learning-based VS automatic segmentation frameworks [3, 4] have been developed and demonstrated high segmentation accuracy on large real-world datasets. Meanwhile, a recent work [1] achieves automated classification of Koos rank through accurate segmentation of VS and adjacent brain structures.

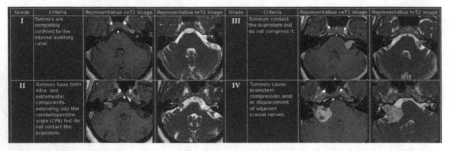

Fig. 1. The Koos grading scale with representative ceT1 and hrT2 images. Image courtesy to Kujawa [1].

However, Koos classification still faces challenges in practical applications, such as unsupervised, since medical data annotation is often time-consuming and expensive, and there is often the problem of domain shift between different imaging modalities. Unsupervised domain adaptation (UDA) has received much attention in the medical field because it does not require any additional annotation. However, the medical field lacks large benchmarks to evaluate the performance of UDA methods. CrossMoDA is the first large multi-class benchmark for unsupervised cross-modality domain adaptation [5, 6]. The goal of the classification task of the crossMoDA 2022 challenge is to automate the Koos classification of VS from magnetic resonance imaging (MRI). The ceT1 scans are commonly used for Koos classification, but recent studies have shown the use of non-contrast imaging sequences, such as hrT2 imaging, can mitigate the risks associated with gadolinium-containing contrast agents. Furthermore, hrT2 imaging is more cost-efficient than ceT1 imaging. Therefore, the classification task of the crossMoDA 2022 challenge aims to automatically determine the Koos grade on unlabeled hrT2 scans using only labeled ceT1 scans based on the unsupervised domain adaptive approach. In this regard, we propose an unsupervised cross-modality domain adaptation method based on image translation by transforming annotated ceT1 scans into hrT2 modality and using their annotations to achieve supervised learning of hrT2 modality. Then, the VS and 7 adjacent brain structures related to Koos classification in hrT2 scans were segmented. Finally, handcrafted features are extracted from the segmentation results, and Koos grade is classified using a random forest classifier. The contributions of this paper are as follows:

- We propose an unsupervised cross-modality domain adaptation method for automatic Koos classification based on image translation.

- Image translation generates target modality images through image contrast transformation, thereby transferring the supervision information from the source domain into the target domain.
- The proposed method is validated on the challenging task of unsupervised cross-modality domain adaptation for Koos classification, outperforming other methods.

2 Related Work

In this section, we will present some work related to our proposed method, including Koos classification and unsupervised cross-modality domain adaptation.

2.1 Koos Classification

Koos classification system has been demonstrated to be a reliable method for vestibular schwannoma classification [7]. However, only recently have the first machine learning frameworks [1] for automatic Koos classification emerged. Before this, Koos grades of vestibular schwannoma could only be hand-labeled by neurosurgeons. Specifically, Kujawa [1] proposed a two-stage approach that implements classification after an initial segmentation stage. In the first stage, the VS and important adjacent brain structures are segmented. The segmentation annotations of these brain structures are obtained by the geodesic information flows (GIF) algorithm [8] rather than by hand. In the second stage, two complementary methods are used to perform Koos classification. The first method directly uses the dense convolutional network (DenseNet) [9] to classify the segmentation results of the first stage. The second method further extracts handcrafted features from the segmentation and then uses a random forest [10] for classification. Experimental results on a large dataset show that the performance of the method is comparable to that of neurosurgeons [1]. However, this method is based on supervised learning and lacks the ability of cross-modality domain adaptation for the unsupervised Koos classification task.

2.2 Unsupervised Cross-modality Domain Adaptation

Unlike natural images, medical images often have multiple complementary but heterogeneous modalities. Using the annotation information of one modality to help another modality build a task model can effectively reduce the annotation cost. Therefore, to bridge the differences between different imaging modalities, many cross-modality adaptation methods have emerged. Yang [11] proposed to find a shared content space through disentangled representations, enabling cross-modality domain adaptation between computed tomography (CT) and MRI images. The method embeds images from each domain into two spaces, a shared domain-invariant content space, and a domain-specific style space, and then performs tasks with representations in the content space. Chen [12] proposed synergistic image and feature alignment (SIFA), an unsupervised domain adaptation framework between MRI and CT images for cardiac substructure segmentation and abdominal multi-organ segmentation. However, these unsupervised cross-modality domain adaptation methods did not aim at our topic of the adaptation between ceT1 and hrT2 modalities.

For the adaptation between ceT1 and hrT2 modalities, Shin [13] proposed a self-training based unsupervised domain adaptation framework (COSMOS) for 3D medical image segmentation and validate it with automatic segmentation of VS and cochlea. The COSMOS realizes the modality transformation of the image through the target-aware contrast conversion network, while preserving the task features in the image during the transformation process. In addition, the method utilizes self-training [14] to iteratively improve segmentation performance. For the same task, Dong [15] proposed an unsupervised cross-modality domain adaptation approach based on pixel alignment and self-training (PAST). During training, pixel alignment is applied to transfer ceT1 scans to hrT2 modality to reduce the domain shift. Besides, Choi [16] proposed a domain adaptation method based on out-of-the-box deep learning frameworks for image translation and segmentation. In this method, an unpaired image-to-image translation model (CUT) based on patch-wise contrastive learning and adversarial learning is used for cross-modality domain adaptation. These unsupervised cross-modality adaptation methods achieve good results on VS and cochlea segmentation tasks. However, these adaptation methods that focus on segmentation tasks cannot be directly applied to the Koos classification task.

3 Methods

Our method consists of two parts: image translation and Koos classification, and the overall framework is shown in **Fig. 2**.

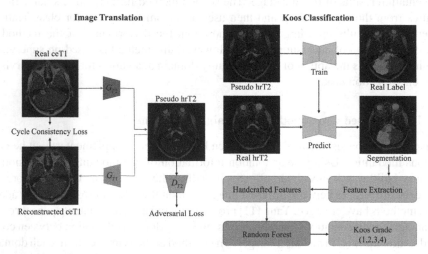

Fig. 2. The framework of Koos classification via image translation-based unsupervised cross-modality domain adaptation.

As shown in **Fig. 2**, image translation converts real ceT1 scans to the modality of hrT2 scans through an adversarial network, thus generating pseudo hrT2 scans. Koos classification consists of three steps. 1) Training a segmentation model in a supervised manner by using pseudo hrT2 scans and real labels. The trained segmentation model is used to predict the real hrT2 scans to generate brain structural segmentation. 2) Extracting handcrafted features from brain structure segmentation. 3) Training a random forest classifier for Koos grade prediction with handcrafted features extracted from the training set.

3.1 Image Translation

Since the source and target domain images in the training set provided by the cross-MoDA 2022 challenge are unpaired, we choose cycle-consistent adversarial networks (CycleGAN) [17] for image translation, i.e., we use CycleGAN to convert annotated ceT1 scans to hrT2 scans. CycleGAN achieved good results in the crossMoDA 2021 challenge [6, 13], which demonstrated the effectiveness of CycleGAN in bridging the gap between ceT1 scans and hrT2 scans. The typical CycleGAN is applied to 2D images, so all 3D images in the training set (including ceT1 scans and hrT2 scans) are sliced along the z-axis to obtain 2D images. Due to the different scanners used, the in-plane matrix sizes of the 3D images in the source and target domains do not match, which also leads to inconsistent sizes of the acquired 2D images. In this regard, we resize the image to a uniform size and do not crop the image so that CycleGAN has a global receptive field for the input image. In addition, considering the large computational effort of CycleGAN for image translation, we resize the original 2D image to the smallest size among all image sizes in the source and target domains. Specifically, the original 2D image is down-sampled to the smallest size among all image sizes in the source and target domains using the bicubic interpolation method. Then, the resized 2D images are fed directly into CycleGAN for training. According to previous work [15], the residual neural network (ResNet) was chosen as the generator of CycleGAN instead of U-net, while for the discriminator the default PatchGAN was chosen. After the training is completed, the annotated ceT1 scans can be translated into hrT2 scans using CycleGAN, thus training the segmentation model with the generated hrT2 scans in a supervised manner.

3.2 Koos Classification

We can train the segmentation model in a supervised manner by using the generated pseudo hrT2 scans and their corresponding annotations to be able to segment brain structures relevant to Koos classification in real hrT2 scans. According to previous work [1], there are 8 brain structures most relevant to Koos classification, including VS, pons, brainstem, cerebellar vermal lobules I-V, VI-VII, and VIII-X, left cerebellum (including the left cerebellum exterior and the left cerebellum white matter) and right cerebellum (including the right cerebellum exterior and the right cerebellum white matter). As in the previous work [16], we use the default 3D full resolution U-Net configuration of the nnU-Net [18] framework for training and inference for the brain structures segmentation task. The segmentation annotations of these brain structures are provided by the crossMoDA 2022 challenge and are initially obtained by the geodesic information flows (GIF) algorithm [8]. nnU-Net automates and condenses the critical decisions required to construct a successful segmentation pipeline for any given dataset [18]. Specifically, it is an out-of-the-box standardized segmentation framework that can self-configure the preprocessing, network architecture, and training pipeline for a given task without the need for manual intervention [13]. Therefore, we keep all automated configurations of nnU-Net without any modification to them. It is worth mentioning that, to reduce the large amount of training time caused by the nnU-Net's default 5-fold cross-validation, we did not use cross-validation, but used all the data to train a single segmentation model.

Eight brain structures and backgrounds are segmented on real hrT2 scans using the trained U-Net segmentation model. According to previous work [1], three handcrafted features are extracted for some structural segmentation masks and background masks, including volume, the shortest distance to the VS (DistVS), and contact surface with the VS (SurfVS). The left and right labels (left cerebellum and right cerebellum) are then transformed into ipsilateral and contralateral labels (ipsilateral cerebellum and contralateral cerebellum) related to the VS position to improve the classification performance. All the handcrafted features extracted are shown in Table 1. Based on these handcrafted features, a random forest classifier was trained on the training set and used to predict the Koos grade of patients.

Table 1. Handcrafted features extracted for Koos classification.

Structures	Handcrafted features		
	Volume	DistVS	SurfVS
Vestibular schwannoma (VS)	✓		
Pons		✓	
Brain stem		✓	
Cerebellar vermal lobules I-V		✓	
Cerebellar vermal lobules VI-VII		✓	
Cerebellar vermal lobules VIII-X		✓	
Ipsilateral cerebellum		✓	
Contralateral cerebellum		✓	
Background			✓

4 Experiments

4.1 Dataset

All experimental data are provided by the crossMoDA 2022 challenge. The experimental data were obtained from two different hospitals, London hospital, and Tilburg hospital. For the London hospital, all images were obtained on a 32-channel Siemens Avanto 1.5T scanner using a Siemens single-channel head coil. For the Tilburg hospital, all images were obtained on a Philips Ingenia 1.5T scanner using a Philips quadrature head coil. A detailed description of the experimental data is shown in Table 2. All 3D images in the training set (including ceT1 scans and hrT2 scans) are sliced along the z-axis to obtain 2D images. Then, the 2D image is down-sampled to 256×256 using the bicubic interpolation method. Other than that, no other processing of the data is performed.

Table 2. The summary of data characteristics of the dataset.

	Training set					Validation set		
	Source		Target			Target		
Hospital	London	Tilburg	London		Tilburg	London		Tilburg
Sequence	ceT1	ceT1	hrT2	hrT2	hrT2	hrT2	hrT2	hrT2
Number of scans	105	105	83	22	105	28	4	32
Annotation	✓	✓	×	×	×	×	×	×
In-plane matrix	512 × 512	256 × 256	448 × 448	384 × 384	512 × 512	448 × 448	384 × 384	512 × 512

4.2 Evaluation Metrics

The macro-averaged mean absolute error (MA-MAE) [19] was used to evaluate the accuracy of the classification results. The MA-MAE is well-designed for ordinal and imbalanced classification problems and is defined as:

$$MA-MAE = \frac{1}{n} \sum_{j=1}^{n} \frac{1}{|T_j|} \sum_{x_i \in T_j} |P(x_i) - y_i|$$

where n represents the number of all images, T_j is the set of images with the true class label y_j, $P(x_i)$ and y_i are the predicted class label and true class label of the image x_i, respectively.

4.3 Experimental Settings

Image Translation. For CycleGAN, the weights of adversarial loss, cycle consistency loss, and identity loss are set to 1:10:5 by default. The training batch size is set to 10. The network was trained with Adam optimizer for 200 epochs, the first 100 epochs maintain an initial learning rate of 0.00015, and the latter 100 epochs decay linearly.

Koos Classification. The settings for the random forest are default, but the number of trees is 100000, the maximum tree depth is 5, and the minimum number of samples per leaf is 2.

4.4 Experimental Results

All models were implemented in PyTorch 1.10 and trained and inference on an RTX 3090 GPU with 24 GB of memory. The proposed method was trained on the training set (182 non-postoperative cases) and used to predict the Koos grade of patients in the validation and test sets. The proposed method received rank 1 on the Koos classification task of the crossMoDA 2022 challenge, with MA-MAE of 0.2148 for the validation set and 0.26 for the test set.

5 Discussion

Although our proposed method achieves the best results, this still falls short of the performance (0.14 ± 0.06) [1] of fully-supervised random forest classification using hrT2 scans. Currently, the best Koos classification performance (0.11 ± 0.05) in fully-supervised scenarios is already comparable to professional doctors (0.11 ± 0.08) [1]. Therefore, the main bottleneck in unsupervised cross-modality Koos classification performance is the modality difference, the brain structures associated with Koos classification in ceT1 scans, including VS, are not fully converted to hrT2 modality. In addition, the degradation of segmentation performance caused by modality difference will also further increase the error of downstream Koos classification task. Therefore, it is more difficult for the unsupervised cross-modality Koos classification task to achieve fully-supervised accuracy than for the unsupervised cross-modality VS segmentation task. Fortunately, the unsupervised cross-modality segmentation performance of VS is already close to fully-supervised approaches [6, 13, 20]. Therefore, if the adaption performance of other brain structures related to Koos classification can be improved, the performance of unsupervised cross-modality Koos classification will likely be comparable to the fully-supervised approaches and professional doctors.

6 Conclusion

This paper proposed an image translation-based unsupervised cross-modality domain adaptation method for Koos classification of vestibular schwannoma. The classification performance on real datasets confirms that the proposed method has good cross-modality domain adaptability. In clinical practice, this domain adaptation method can effectively process unlabeled hrT2 modality images, thereby reducing the annotation cost and improving the diagnostic efficiency to a certain extent.

References

1. Kujawa, A., et al.: Automated koos classification of vestibular schwannoma, Front. Radiol. **2**, 837191 (2022)
2. Shapey, J., et al.: Artificial intelligence opportunities for vestibular schwannoma management using image segmentation and clinical decision tools. World Neurosurg. **149**, 269–270 (2021)
3. Shapey, J., et al.: An artificial intelligence framework for automatic segmentation and volumetry of vestibular schwannomas from contrast-enhanced T1-weighted and high-resolution T2-weighted MRI. J. Neurosurg. **134**(1), 171–179 (2021)

4. Wang, G., et al.: Automatic segmentation of vestibular schwannoma from T2-weighted MRI by deep spatial attention with hardness-weighted loss. In: Shen, D., Liu, T., Peters, T.M., Staib, L.H., Essert, C., Zhou, S., Yap, P.-T., Khan, A. (eds.) MICCAI 2019. LNCS, vol. 11765, pp. 264–272. Springer, Cham (2019). https://doi.org/10.1007/978-3-030-32245-8_30

5. Shapey, J., et al.: Segmentation of vestibular schwannoma from MRI, an open annotated dataset and baseline algorithm. Sci. Data 8(1), 286 (2021)

6. Dorent, R., et al.: Challenge: benchmark of cross-modality domain adaptation techniques for vestibular schwannoma and cochlea segmentation. Med. Image Anal. **2022**, 102628 (2021)

7. Erickson, N.J., et al.: Koos classification of vestibular schwannomas: a reliability study. Neurosurgery 85(3), 409–414 (2019)

8. Cardoso, M.J., et al.: Geodesic information flows: spatially-variant graphs and their application to segmentation and fusion. IEEE Trans. Med. Imaging 34(9), 1976–1988 (2015)

9. Huang, G., Liu, Z., Van Der Maaten, L., Weinberger, K.Q.: Densely connected convolutional networks. In: Proceedings of the IEEE Conference on Computer Vision and Pattern Recognition, 2017, pp. 4700–4708 (2017)

10. Breiman, L.: Random forests. Mach. Learn. **45**(1), 5–32 (2001)

11. Yang, J., Dvornek, N.C., Zhang, F., Chapiro, J., Lin, MingDe, Duncan, J.S.: Unsupervised domain adaptation via disentangled representations: Application to cross-modality liver segmentation. In: Shen, D., Liu, T., Peters, T.M., Staib, L.H., Essert, C., Zhou, S., Yap, P.-T., Khan, A. (eds.) MICCAI 2019. LNCS, vol. 11765, pp. 255–263. Springer, Cham (2019). https://doi.org/10.1007/978-3-030-32245-8_29

12. Chen, C., Dou, Q., Chen, H., Qin, J., Heng, P.A.: Unsupervised bidirectional cross-modality adaptation via deeply synergistic image and feature alignment for medical image segmentation. IEEE Trans. Med. Imaging **39**(7), 2494–2505 (2020)

13. Shin, H., Kim, H., Kim, S., Jun, Y., Eo, T., Hwang, D.: COSMOS: cross-modality unsupervised domain adaptation for 3d medical image segmentation based on target-aware domain translation and iterative self-training, arxiv preprint arXiv:2203.16557 (2022)

14. Xie, Q., Luong, M.T., Hovy, E., Le, Q.V.: Self-training with noisy student improves imagenet classification. In: Proceedings of the IEEE/CVF Conference on Computer Vision And Pattern Recognition, pp. 10687–10698 (2020)

15. Dong, H., Yu, F., Zhao, J., Dong, B., Zhang, L.: Unsupervised domain adaptation in semantic segmentation based on pixel alignment and self-training, arXiv preprint arXiv:2109.14219 (2021)

16. Choi, J.W.: Using out-of-the-box frameworks for unpaired image translation and image segmentation for the crossmoda challenge, arXiv preprint arXiv:2110.01607 (2021)

17. Zhu, J.Y., Park, T., Isola, P., Efros, A.A.: Unpaired image-to-image translation using cycle-consistent adversarial networks, In: Proceedings of the IEEE International Conference on Computer Vision, pp. 2223–2232 (2017)

18. Isensee, F., Jaeger, P.F., Kohl, S.A.A., Petersen, J., Maier-Hein, K.H.: NnU-Net: a self-configuring method for deep learning-based biomedical image segmentation. Nat. Methods **18**(2), 203–211 (2021)

19. Baccianella, S., Esuli, A., Sebastiani, F.: Evaluation measures for ordinal regression. In: 2009 Ninth International Conference on Intelligent Systems Design and Applications, IEEE, 2009, pp. 283-287 (2009)

20. Dorent, R., et al.: Scribble-based domain adaptation via co-segmentation. In: Martel, A.L., Abolmaesumi, P., Stoyanov, D., Mateus, D., Zuluaga, M.A., Kevin Zhou, S., Racoceanu, D., Joskowicz, L. (eds.) MICCAI 2020. LNCS, vol. 12261, pp. 479–489. Springer, Cham (2020). https://doi.org/10.1007/978-3-030-59710-8_47

MS-MT: Multi-scale Mean Teacher with Contrastive Unpaired Translation for Cross-Modality Vestibular Schwannoma and Cochlea Segmentation

Ziyuan Zhao[1,2,3], Kaixin Xu[1], Huai Zhe Yeo[1,4(✉)], Xulei Yang[1,2], and Cuntai Guan[3]

[1] Institute for Infocomm Research (I2R), A*STAR, Singapore, Singapore
`Zhao_Ziyuan@i2r.a-star.edu.sg`
[2] Artificial Intelligence, Analytics And Informatics (AI3),
A*STAR, Singapore, Singapore
[3] Nanyang Technological University, Singapore, Singapore
[4] National University of Singapore, Singapore, Singapore
`huai.zhe.yeo@gmail.com`

Abstract. Domain shift has been a long-standing issue for medical image segmentation. Recently, unsupervised domain adaptation (UDA) methods have achieved promising cross-modality segmentation performance by distilling knowledge from a label-rich source domain to a target domain without labels. In this work, we propose a multi-scale self-ensembling based UDA framework for automatic segmentation of two key brain structures *i.e.*, Vestibular Schwannoma (VS) and Cochlea on high-resolution T2 images. First, a segmentation-enhanced contrastive unpaired image translation module is designed for image-level domain adaptation from source T1 to target T2. Next, multi-scale deep supervision and consistency regularization are introduced to a mean teacher network for self-ensemble learning to further close the domain gap. Furthermore, self-training and intensity augmentation techniques are utilized to mitigate label scarcity and boost cross-modality segmentation performance. Our method demonstrates promising segmentation performance with a mean Dice score of 83.8% and 81.4% and an average asymmetric surface distance (ASSD) of 0.55 mm and 0.26 mm for the VS and Cochlea, respectively in the validation phase of the crossMoDA 2022 challenge.

Keywords: Medical image segmentation · Unsupervised domain adaptation · Vestibular Schwannoma

1 Introduction

Medical image segmentation plays a vital role in the field of medical image analysis, delivering valuable information for diagnostic analysis and treatment plan-

---

This work was done when Huai Zhe was an intern at I2R, A*STAR.

© The Author(s), under exclusive license to Springer Nature Switzerland AG 2023
S. Bakas et al. (Eds.): BrainLes 2022, LNCS 14092, pp. 68–78, 2023.
https://doi.org/10.1007/978-3-031-44153-0_7

ning [10]. Accurate segmentation and measurement of Vestibular Schwannoma (VS) and Cochlea from MRI can assist in VS treatment planning, improving clinical workflow [24]. To this end, researchers have turned to deep learning as a solution to perform autonomous segmentation of VS and Cochlea. Recent findings also suggest that high-resolution T2 (hrT2) MRI could be a safer and more cost-efficient alternative to contrast-enhanced T1 (ceT1) MRI. However, the large domain shift between MRI images with different contrasts coupled with the costly and laborious process of re-annotating medical image scans on another modality, makes it difficult for deep learning to generalize well across both domains. Therefore, we are encouraged to perform unsupervised domain adaptation (UDA) and conduct VS and Cochlea segmentation in the hrT2 domain by leveraging labeled ceT1 scans and unlabeled hrT2 scans. In this work, we propose an effective and intuitive UDA method based on image translation and self-ensembling learning. Firstly, we translate MRI scans from the ceT1 domain to the hrT2 domain using a modified CUT model [21] for image-level adaptation. Then, a nnU-Net [13] is trained on synthetic hrT2 images to generate pseudo annotations for unlabeled hrT2 images. Finally, we build a multi-scale mean-teacher (MS-MT) network [15,28] to transfer multi-level knowledge from the teacher model to the student model for improving the cross-modality segmentation performance. The experimental results show that the proposed UDA network can greatly reduce the domain gap, achieving promising segmentation performance on hrT2 scans.

2   Related Work

To bridge the domain gap across different modalities, many UDA methods have been developed in the medical imaging field to align the distributions between modalities from different perspectives, including image-level alignment [12,31,36], feature-level alignment [7,18,29,30] and their combinations [2,11]. Image alignment is a practical UDA approach that translates source images to appear as if they were sampled from the target domain or vice versa. CycleGAN [36] is mainly used to achieve unpaired image-to-image translation for UDA in medical image segmentation [12,31]. For instance, Huo et al. [12] leveraged CycleGAN to perform MRI to CT synthesis for enabling CT splenomegaly segmentation without using target labels. Zhang et al. [31] proposed a task-driven generative adversarial network by introducing segmentation consistency into the DRR to X-ray translation process to achieve X-ray segmentation with the pre-trained DRR segmentation models. Recently, contrastive learning has demonstrated a powerful capacity for unsupervised visual representation learning in various computer vision tasks [14]. Park et al. [21] first proposed CUT to use contrastive learning for image synthesis, in which, the mutual information between original and generated patches was maximized to keep the content unchanged after translation. Several studies have applied CUT in cross-domain medical image analysis [3,17]. Therefore, in this study, we use CUT for image-level adaptation. Another line of research in UDA is to align the feature distributions across domains from different aspects, including explicit discrepancy minimization [18,29] and implicit adversarial learning [7,9]. For example, Dou *et al.* [7] proposed to fine-tune specific feature layers via adversarial learning for cross-modality cardiac segmentation. To achieve image and feature adaptation, CyCADA [11] was proposed to bridge the appearance gap using CycleGAN and align the feature spaces with adversarial learning separately. Chen *et al.* [2] further introduced additional discriminators in CycleGAN to achieve concurrent feature and image adaptation. These UDA methods have been used in cross-modality VS and Cochlea Segmentation for closing the domain gap [6]. More recently, the usage of weak labels, such as scribbles on the target domain, for weakly-supervised domain adaptation [5] has also shown much promise, receiving attention from the community.

On the other hand, since the labels on the target domain are not accessible, not-so-supervised learning methods [27], such as semi-supervised learning (SSL) [1,28] can be leveraged to relax the dependence on target labels for improving the adaptation performance [33,34,37]. Zou *et al.* [37] built a self-training pseudo-labeling framework for UDA, in which, pseudo-target labels are generated to retrain the model iteratively for improving the UDA performance. Zhao *et al.* [33,34] investigated the source label scarcity problem in UDA, and leveraged self-ensembling models [28] to address annotation scarcity on both domains for label-efficient UDA. These works suggest that SSL techniques can also be leveraged in UDA to improve adaptation performance. In this regard, pseudo-labeling and self-ensembling learning methodologies were explored in our UDA framework.

3   Methods

Given an unpaired dataset of two modalities, *i.e.*, annotated ceT1 MRI images $\mathcal{D}_s = \{(\mathbf{x}_i^s, y_i^s)\}_{i=1}^{N}$ and non-annotated hrT2 MRI scans $\mathcal{D}_t = \{(\mathbf{x}_i^t)\}_{i=1}^{M}$, sharing the same classes (VS and Cochlea), we aim to exploit $\mathcal{D}_s$ and $\mathcal{D}_t$ for unsupervised domain adaptation to enhance the cross-modality segmentation performance of the VS and Cochlea on hrT2 MRI images. The overview of our UDA framework is shown in Fig. 1.

3.1   Segmentation-Enhanced Translation

To close the domain gap across the modalities, we first conduct image-level domain adaptation to generate synthetic target samples. In this regard, the model trained on the synthetic target images will be used for VS and Cochlea segmentation on real hrT2 scans. For unpaired image-to-image translation, we adopt the Contrastive Unpaired Translation (CUT) [21] as our backbone since it is faster and less memory-intensive than CycleGAN [36]. Moreover, we enhance the 2D CUT with an additional segmentation decoder for maintaining the structural information of VS and Cochlea (see Fig. 1). Specifically, a ResNet-based generator is used to translate images from the source domain to the target domain, while a PatchGAN discriminator is employed to distinguish between

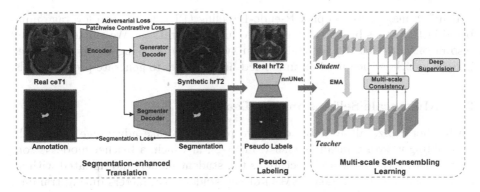

Fig. 1. The overview of our proposed method. First, synthetic hrT2 images are generated with the proposed segmentation-enhanced translation network. Then, we employ a nnU-Net for training on synthetic hrT2 images and generate pseudo labels for unlabeled hrT2 images. Finally, a multi-scale mean teacher network is employed to further close the domain gap.

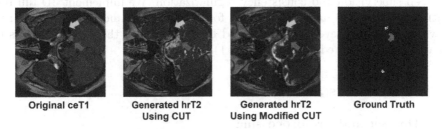

Fig. 2. Visual comparison of the synthetic hrT2 images by different methods.

the real and generated images [21]. We follow the SIFA architecture [2] and connect two layers of the encoder, specifically at the last layer and the layer before the last downsampling, with the segmenter decoder to generate multi-level segmentation predictions. The segmentation loss can help the encoder focus more on areas related to the segmentation task and preserve the structure of VS and Cochlea in the translated images. In Fig. 2, we can observe that the modified CUT can better preserve the shape of the VS and Cochlea in comparison with the original CUT framework.

3.2 Intensity Augmentation and Pseudo-labeling

Considering that tumors exhibit T2 heterogeneous signal intensity [20] and Cochleas show T2 hyperintense signal intensity [16], we perform intensity augmentation (IA) and generate augmented data for diversifying the training distributions, thereby improving the model generalizability. Using the generated hrT2 images and the ground truth annotations, the signal intensities of both the VS and Cochlea were muted and intensified by 50% respectively, doubling the training data. On the other hand, to boost the segmentation performance on real hrT2 images, we adopt a Pseudo-Labeling (PL) strategy to leverage unlabeled hrT2 images by generating pseudo hrT2 annotations. We employ a 3D full resolution nnU-Net [13] for training on synthetic hrT2 images and augmented images, which is then used on unlabeled hrT2 images to generate pseudo-labels.

3.3 Multi-scale Self-ensembling Learning

To further utilize all available data, we propose to take advantage of the self-ensembling network, mean teacher (MT) [28], in which, a teacher model is constructed with the same architecture as the student model, and updated with an exponential moving average (EMA) of the student parameters during training. In our training process, the outputs of the student and teacher models with different perturbations are optimized to be consistent by minimizing the difference using the mean square error (MSE) loss. Inspired by the great success of multi-scale learning in medical image analysis [8,15,32], we follow [15] to construct a multi-scale mean teacher (MS-MT) network to leverage multi-scale predictions for deep supervision and consistency regularization. We implement 3D full resolution nnU-Net [13] as the backbone for both teacher and student networks, in which, auxiliary layers are connected to each block of the last five blocks to obtain multi-scale predictions (see Fig. 1).

4 Experiments and Results

4.1 Dataset and Pre-processing

The training dataset released by the MICCAI challenge crossMoDA 2022 [4,6, 22,23], includes 210 labeled ceT1 images and 210 unlabeled hrT2 images. Due to the varying voxel spacing in the training data, we resampled the images into a common spacing of $0.6 \times 0.6 \times 1.0$ mm and normalized the intensity to $[0, 1]$ using the Min-Max scaling. To remove the noise, the images were cropped into 256×256 pixels in the xy-plane using the 75 percentile binary threshold [3], resulting in $256 \times 256 \times$ N image volumes for 3D nnU-Net training. The processed 3D volumes were sliced along the z-axis to produce N number of 2D image training samples for the 2D CUT. The Dice Score (DSC [%]) [26] and the Average Symmetric Surface Distance(ASSD [voxel]) [19] were used to assess the model performance on VS and Cochlea segmentation.

4.2 Implementation Details

We used single NVIDIA A40 GPU with 48GB of memory for model training. We followed [21] to optimize the proposed segmentation-enhanced CUT network, in which the weights for adversarial loss, contrastive loss, and segmentation loss were set the same. Following [2], the loss weights for additional segmentation in the modified CUT were set to 1 and 0.1 for the last layer and the second last downsampling layers respectively. For pseudo-labeling, we closely followed the

Table 1. Quantitative results on the validation dataset. The metrics are presented in the format of mean ± std.

VS Dice	VS ASSD	Cochlea Dice	Cochlea ASSD	Mean Dice
0.8380 ± 0.097	0.5555 ± 0.3647	0.8139 ± 0.0312	0.2652 ± 0.1553	0.8260 ± 0.0508

nnU-Net optimized settings [13] and trained for 200 epochs with the generated hrT2 images and augmented hrT2 images using cross-validation. The segmentation results from an ensemble of five-fold cross-validations on unlabeled hrT2 images were then used as pseudo labels for the following processes. For the multi-scale mean teacher, the EMA update α was set to 0.9, and the loss weights for consistency regularization were set to $\{0.05, 0.05, 0.05, 0.4, 0.5\}$, assigned to each feature map according to its size in ascending order, and we followed the deep supervision scheme in nnU-Net [13]. The loss weights were ramped up across 160 epochs using the sigmoid function. We used a combination of Dice and cross-entropy losses as our objective function and trained the MS-MT model with an initial learning rate of 0.01 using stochastic gradient descent for 300 epochs. Following [28], the results from the five-fold teacher models were ensembled, and then post-processed by computing the largest connected component (LCC) to remove unconnected labels (The first LCC was preserved for the VS while the first and second LCCs were preserved for the Cochlea) for final submission.

4.3 Experimental Results

The results of our method on the validation dataset are presented in Table 1. With a mean Dice score of 0.826, our method secures a top-10 finish in the Cross-MoDA 2022 competition. Figure 3 highlights some qualitative results produced by our method on the validation set. Finally, our method ranked 5th in the test phase of the crossMoDA 2022 challenge with a mean Dice score of 85.65%, and ranked in 3rd place for the Vestibular Schwannoma segmentation with a mean Dice score of 86.7%.

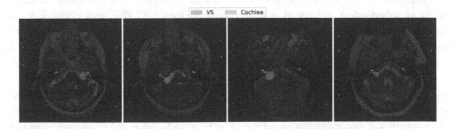

Fig. 3. Qualitative results produced by our method. The VS and Cochlea are indicated in green and yellow color, respectively.

4.4 Ablation Study

Table 2 shows the results of methods of different components, *e.g.*, intensity augmentation(IA), pseudo-labeling (PL), and mean teacher(MT) on the validation dataset. We start by training a 3D nnU-Net on generated images by CUT, *i.e.*, nnU-Net+CUT, which achieves a mean dice of 78.95%. By adding augmented images into the training process, we can observe an improvement in the segmentation performance of both Cochlea and VS. Then, we introduce pseudo-labeling into the training process, which leads to 1.06% increments in mean Dice, and a continued increase was observed with the inclusion of self-ensembling learning. We further build a multi-scale mean teacher, which achieved better performance. Finally, compared to CUT, the model trained on generated images with the proposed segmentation-enhanced CUT (SE-CUT) can achieve better performance.

Table 2. Quantitative results (Dice Score [%]) by different methods on the validation dataset.

Method	Cochlea	VS	Mean
nnU-Net+CUT	79.67 ± 3.72	78.22 ± 21.04	78.95 ± 11.13
nnU-Net+CUT+IA	80.48 ± 4.14	78.31 ± 21.00	79.39 ± 11.28
nnU-Net+CUT+IA+PL	81.06 ± 3.42	79.85 ± 12.88	80.45 ± 6.60
nnU-Net+CUT+IA+PL+MT	81.06 ± 3.28	82.67 ± 11.89	81.86 ± 6.18
nnU-Net+CUT+IA+PL+MS-MT	81.24 ± 3.31	82.98 ± 10.25	82.11 ± 5.39
nnU-Net+SE-CUT+IA+PL+MS-MT	81.39 ± 3.12	83.80 ± 9.72	82.60 ± 5.08

5 Discussion

In this work, we propose to explore image-level domain adaptation and semi-supervised learning to address the unsupervised domain adaptation problem in cross-modality vestibular schwannoma (VS) and cochlea segmentation. Additionally, intensity augmentation is performed to generate additional training data with different VS and cochlea intensities for diversifying the data distributions. Our final submission achieved a mean Dice score of 82.6% and 85.65% in the validation phase and the testing phase, respectively. In particular, our method achieved 5th place for overall segmentation performance and ranked 3rd for Vestibular Schwannoma segmentation. From our experiments, we observe that image adaptation contributes the most to the adaptation performance. We can regard the 3D nnU-Net trained on generated target images with CUT (*i.e.*, nnU-Net+CUT) as a strong baseline, achieving dice scores of approximately 80%, which signifies a competitive result within the leaderboards. However, synthetic images may include noises and artifacts, which would influence the follow-up segmentation performance. Many works [21,25] have been proposed to address the limitations of GANs. In our work, we design a segmentation-enhanced translation network for improved adaptation performance. For data augmentation, we adjust the intensities of VS and cochlea based on clinical characteristics and medical knowledge and achieved better performance. Besides, spatial augmentation methods [35] can be further explored in this UDA task. For SSL, we adopted pseudo-labeling and self-ensembling learning methodologies to improve the adaptation performance. According to our experimental results, both SSL methods are beneficial to improved segmentation performance. However, one limitation of pseudo-labeling is that low-quality pseudo-labels would adversely influence the training process. Since different perturbations are introduced to the self-ensembling models, the influence of noise from synthetic images and pseudo-labels could be weakened to some extent. We further advance multi-level consistency and deep supervision into self-ensembling learning, achieving better UDA performance.

6 Conclusion

In this work, we proposed a three-stage UDA method based on image translation, pseudo-labeling and multi-scale self-ensembling learning to close the gap between two domains and conduct effective image segmentation on the target domain. Specifically, we worked with annotated ceT1 and unannotated hrT2 data to perform segmentation on the target hrT2 domain. In addition, intensity augmentation was implemented to improve the generalizability of the model. With a mean Dice of 0.8216, we achieved a top 10 finish in the CrossMoDA 2022 validation phase and eventually, placed 5th overall in the final competition ranking, demonstrating its effectiveness in bridging the gap between the ceT1 and hrT2 MRI modalities.

References

1. Bai, W., et al.: Semi-supervised learning for network-based cardiac mr image segmentation. In: Descoteaux, M., Maier-Hein, L., Franz, A., Jannin, P., Collins, D.L., Duchesne, S. (eds.) MICCAI 2017. LNCS, vol. 10434, pp. 253–260. Springer, Cham (2017). https://doi.org/10.1007/978-3-319-66185-8_29
2. Chen, C., Dou, Q., Chen, H., Qin, J., Heng, P.A.: Unsupervised bidirectional cross-modality adaptation via deeply synergistic image and feature alignment for medical image segmentation. IEEE Trans. Med. Imaging 39(7), 2494–2505 (2020)
3. Choi, J.W.: Using out-of-the-box frameworks for contrastive unpaired image translation for vestibular schwannoma and cochlea segmentation: an approach for the CrossMoDA challenge. In: Crimi, A., Bakas, S. (eds.) Brainlesion: Glioma, Multiple Sclerosis, Stroke and Traumatic Brain Injuries: 7th International Workshop, BrainLes 2021, Held in Conjunction with MICCAI 2021, Virtual Event, September 27, 2021, Revised Selected Papers, Part II, pp. 509–517. Springer International Publishing, Cham (2022). https://doi.org/10.1007/978-3-031-09002-8_44
4. Clark, K., et al.: The cancer imaging archive (tcia): maintaining and operating a public information repository. J. Digit. Imaging 26(6), 1045–1057 (2013)

5. Dorent, R., et al.: Scribble-based domain adaptation via co-segmentation. In: Martel, A.L., et al. (eds.) Medical Image Computing and Computer Assisted Intervention – MICCAI 2020: 23rd International Conference, Lima, Peru, October 4–8, 2020, Proceedings, Part I, pp. 479–489. Springer International Publishing, Cham (2020). https://doi.org/10.1007/978-3-030-59710-8_47

6. Dorent, R., et al.: Crossmoda 2021 challenge: benchmark of cross-modality domain adaptation techniques for vestibular schwannoma and cochlea segmentation. Medical Image Analysis p. 102628 (2022). https://doi.org/10.1016/j.media.2022.102628

7. Dou, Q., et al.: Pnp-adanet: plug-and-play adversarial domain adaptation network at unpaired cross-modality cardiac segmentation. IEEE Access **7**, 99065–99076 (2019)

8. Dou, Q., et al.: 3D deeply supervised network for automated segmentation of volumetric medical images. Med. Image Anal. **41**, 40–54 (2017)

9. Ganin, Y., et al.: Domain-adversarial training of neural networks. J. Mach. Learn. Res. **17**(1), 2030–2096 (2016)

10. Hesamian, M.H., Jia, W., He, X., Kennedy, P.: Deep learning techniques for medical image segmentation: achievements and challenges. J. Digit. Imaging **32**(4), 582–596 (2019)

11. Hoffman, J., et al.: Cycada: cycle-consistent adversarial domain adaptation. In: International Conference on Machine Learning, pp. 1989–1998. PMLR (2018)

12. Huo, Y., Xu, Z., Bao, S., Assad, A., Abramson, R.G., Landman, B.A.: Adversarial synthesis learning enables segmentation without target modality ground truth. In: 2018 IEEE 15th International Symposium on Biomedical Imaging (ISBI 2018), pp. 1217–1220. IEEE (2018)

13. Isensee, F., Jaeger, P.F., Kohl, S.A., Petersen, J., Maier-Hein, K.H.: nnu-net: a self-configuring method for deep learning-based biomedical image segmentation. Nat. Methods **18**(2), 203–211 (2021)

14. Jaiswal, A., Babu, A.R., Zadeh, M.Z., Banerjee, D., Makedon, F.: A survey on contrastive self-supervised learning. Technologies **9**(1), 2 (2021)

15. Li, S., Zhao, Z., Xu, K., Zeng, Z., Guan, C.: Hierarchical consistency regularized mean teacher for semi-supervised 3d left atrium segmentation. In: 2021 43rd Annual International Conference of the IEEE Engineering in Medicine & Biology Society (EMBC), pp. 3395–3398. IEEE (2021)

16. Lin, E., Crane, B.: The management and imaging of vestibular schwannomas. Am. J. Neuroradiol. **38**(11), 2034–2043 (2017)

17. Liu, H., Fan, Y., Cui, C., Su, D., McNeil, A., Dawant, B.M.: Unsupervised domain adaptation for vestibular schwannoma and cochlea segmentation via semi-supervised learning and label fusion. In: Crimi, A., Bakas, S. (eds.) Brainlesion: Glioma, Multiple Sclerosis, Stroke and Traumatic Brain Injuries: 7th International Workshop, BrainLes 2021, Held in Conjunction with MICCAI 2021, Virtual Event, September 27, 2021, Revised Selected Papers, Part II, pp. 529–539. Springer International Publishing, Cham (2022). https://doi.org/10.1007/978-3-031-09002-8_46

18. Long, M., Cao, Y., Wang, J., Jordan, M.: Learning transferable features with deep adaptation networks. In: International Conference on Machine Learning, pp. 97–105. PMLR (2015)

19. Lu, F., Wu, F., Hu, P., Peng, Z., Kong, D.: Automatic 3D liver location and segmentation via convolutional neural network and graph cut. Int. J. Comput. Assist. Radiol. Surg. **12**(2), 171–182 (2017)

20. Nguyen, D., de Kanztow, L.: Vestibular schwannomas: a review. Appl Radiol **48**(3), 22–27 (2019)

21. Park, T., Efros, A.A., Zhang, R., Zhu, J.-Y.: Contrastive learning for unpaired image-to-image translation. In: Vedaldi, A., Bischof, H., Brox, T., Frahm, J.-M. (eds.) Computer Vision – ECCV 2020: 16th European Conference, Glasgow, UK, August 23–28, 2020, Proceedings, Part IX, pp. 319–345. Springer International Publishing, Cham (2020). https://doi.org/10.1007/978-3-030-58545-7_19

22. Shapey, J., et al.: Segmentation of vestibular schwannoma from magnetic resonance imaging: an open annotated dataset and baseline algorithm. The Cancer Imaging Archive (2021)

23. Shapey, J., et al.: Segmentation of vestibular schwannoma from MRI, an open annotated dataset and baseline algorithm. Sci. Data 8(1), 1–6 (2021)

24. Shapey, J., et al.: An artificial intelligence framework for automatic segmentation and volumetry of vestibular schwannomas from contrast-enhanced t1-weighted and high-resolution t2-weighted mri. J. Neurosurg. 134(1), 171–179 (2019)

25. Shin, H., Kim, H., Kim, S., Jun, Y., Eo, T., Hwang, D.: Cosmos: cross-modality unsupervised domain adaptation for 3D medical image segmentation based on target-aware domain translation and iterative self-training. arXiv preprint arXiv:2203.16557 (2022)

26. Sudre, C.H., Li, W., Vercauteren, T., Ourselin, S., Jorge Cardoso, M.: Generalised dice overlap as a deep learning loss function for highly unbalanced segmentations. In: Cardoso, M.J., et al. (eds.) Deep Learning in Medical Image Analysis and Multimodal Learning for Clinical Decision Support, pp. 240–248. Springer International Publishing, Cham (2017). https://doi.org/10.1007/978-3-319-67558-9_28

27. Tajbakhsh, N., Jeyaseelan, L., Li, Q., Chiang, J.N., Wu, Z., Ding, X.: Embracing imperfect datasets: a review of deep learning solutions for medical image segmentation. Med. Image Anal. 63, 101693 (2020)

28. Tarvainen, A., Valpola, H.: Mean teachers are better role models: weight-averaged consistency targets improve semi-supervised deep learning results. In: Advances in Neural Information Processing Systems 30 (2017)

29. Tzeng, E., Hoffman, J., Zhang, N., Saenko, K., Darrell, T.: Deep domain confusion: Maximizing for domain invariance. arXiv preprint arXiv:1412.3474 (2014)

30. Wang, L., Wang, M., Zhang, D., Fu, H.: Unsupervised domain adaptation via style-aware self-intermediate domain. arXiv preprint arXiv:2209.01870 (2022)

31. Zhang, Y., Miao, S., Mansi, T., Liao, R.: Task driven generative modeling for unsupervised domain adaptation: application to X-ray image segmentation. In: Frangi, A.F., Schnabel, J.A., Davatzikos, C., Alberola-López, C., Fichtinger, G. (eds.) Medical Image Computing and Computer Assisted Intervention – MICCAI 2018: 21st International Conference, Granada, Spain, September 16-20, 2018, Proceedings, Part II, pp. 599–607. Springer International Publishing, Cham (2018). https://doi.org/10.1007/978-3-030-00934-2_67

32. Zhao, Z., et al.: Mmgl: multi-scale multi-view global-local contrastive learning for semi-supervised cardiac image segmentation. In: 2022 IEEE International Conference on Image Processing (ICIP), pp. 401–405 (2022)

33. Zhao, Z., Xu, K., Li, S., Zeng, Z., Guan, C.: MT-UDA: towards unsupervised cross-modality medical image segmentation with limited source labels. In: de Bruijne, et al. (eds.) Medical Image Computing and Computer Assisted Intervention – MICCAI 2021: 24th International Conference, Strasbourg, France, September 27–October 1, 2021, Proceedings, Part I, pp. 293–303. Springer International Publishing, Cham (2021). https://doi.org/10.1007/978-3-030-87193-2_28

34. Zhao, Z., Zhou, F., Xu, K., Zeng, Z., Guan, C., Kevin Zhou, S.: Le-uda: label-efficient unsupervised domain adaptation for medical image segmentation. IEEE Transactions on Medical Imaging (2022)

35. Zhao, Z., Zhou, F., Zeng, Z., Guan, C., Zhou, S.K.: Meta-hallucinator: towards few-shot cross-modality cardiac image segmentation. In: Wang, L., Dou, Q., Fletcher, P.T., Speidel, S., Li, S. (eds.) Medical Image Computing and Computer Assisted Intervention – MICCAI 2022: 25th International Conference, Singapore, September 18–22, 2022, Proceedings, Part V, pp. 128–139. Springer Nature Switzerland, Cham (2022). https://doi.org/10.1007/978-3-031-16443-9_13

36. Zhu, J.Y., Park, T., Isola, P., Efros, A.A.: Unpaired image-to-image translation using cycle-consistent adversarial networks. In: Proceedings of the IEEE International Conference on Computer Vision, pp. 2223–2232 (2017)

37. Zou, Y., Yu, Z., Kumar, B., Wang, J.: Unsupervised domain adaptation for semantic segmentation via class-balanced self-training. In: Proceedings of the European Conference On Computer Vision (ECCV), pp. 289–305 (2018)

An Unpaired Cross-Modality Segmentation Framework Using Data Augmentation and Hybrid Convolutional Networks for Segmenting Vestibular Schwannoma and Cochlea

Yuzhou Zhuang[1], Hong Liu[1(✉)], Enmin Song[1], Coskun Cetinkaya[2], and Chih-Cheng Hung[2]

[1] School of Computer Science and Technology, Huazhong University of Science and Technology, Wuhan, China
hl.cbib@gmail.com
[2] Center for Machine Vision and Security Research, Kennesaw State University, Marietta, MA 30060, USA

Abstract. The crossMoDA challenge aims to automatically segment the vestibular schwannoma (VS) tumor and cochlea regions of unlabeled high-resolution T2 scans by leveraging labeled contrast-enhanced T1 scans. The 2022 edition extends the segmentation task by including multi-institutional scans. In this work, we proposed an unpaired cross-modality segmentation framework using data augmentation and hybrid convolutional networks. Considering heterogeneous distributions and various image sizes for multi-institutional scans, we apply the min-max normalization for scaling the intensities of all scans between -1 and 1, and use the voxel size resampling and center cropping to obtain fixed-size sub-volumes for training. We adopt two data augmentation methods for effectively learning the semantic information and generating realistic target domain scans: generative and online data augmentation. For generative data augmentation, we use CUT and Cycle-GAN to generate two groups of realistic T2 volumes with different details and appearances for supervised segmentation training. For online data augmentation, we design a random tumor signal reducing method for simulating the heterogeneity of VS tumor signals. Furthermore, we utilize an advanced hybrid convolutional network with multi-dimensional convolutions to adaptively learn sparse inter-slice information and dense intra-slice information for accurate volumetric segmentation of VS tumor and cochlea regions in anisotropic scans. On the crossMoDA2022 validation dataset, our method produces promising results and achieves the mean DSC values of 72.47% and 76.48% and ASSD values of 3.42 mm and 0.53 mm for VS tumor and cochlea regions, respectively.

Keywords: Unpaired Cross-modality Segmentation · Data Augmentation · Hybrid Convolutional Networks · Vestibular Schwannoma · Cochlea

S. Bakas et al. (Eds.): BrainLes 2022, LNCS 14092, pp. 79–89, 2023.
https://doi.org/10.1007/978-3-031-44153-0_8

1   Introduction

Unpaired cross-modality medical image segmentation aims to use labeled source scans to segment unpaired target scans without annotations between different modalities [1]. Because of the domain shift caused by different modality imaging techniques, supervised segmentation methods exhibit significant performance degradation in cross-modality segmentation [2]. Recently, unsupervised domain adaptation (UDA) methods based on adversarial learning (e.g., CycleGAN [7] and CUT [27]) are widely employed in unpaired cross-domain image processing [8], which can transfer knowledge between unpaired source and target images in an unsupervised manner. Vestibular schwannoma (VS) is a benign brain tumor originating from the vestibulocochlear nerve, and accurate segmentation of VS tumor and cochlea regions from MRI is desirable for growth detection and treatment planning of the tumor [3, 4]. The crossMoDA challenge [1] aims to automatically segment the VS tumor and cochlea regions of unlabeled high-resolution T2 scans by leveraging labeled contrast-enhanced T1 scans, and the crossMoDA2021 provided the first large cross-modality segmentation benchmark dataset with unpaired and anisotropic MR scans. Recently, the crossMoDA2022 challenge extended the segmentation task by adding multi-institutional scans. In this work, by the combination of two different image synthesis methods and an advanced hybrid convolutional network [6], we proposed an effective unpaired cross-modality segmentation framework with image alignment and multi-dimensional representations for automatically segmenting VS and cochlea regions. Moreover, to improve the robustness of our proposed method, we used various augmentation strategies to simulate the heterogeneity of VS tumor signals and overcome the differences in multi-institutional scans. Experimental results show that our proposed method produces promising results and achieves the mean Dice similarity coefficient (DSC) values of 72.47% and 76.48% and Average symmetric surface distance (ASSD) values of 3.42 and 0.53 mm for VS tumor and cochlea regions on the validation dataset of the crossMoDA2022 challenge, respectively. Our proposed method ranked 9th in the final announced evaluation results of the crossMoDA2022 challenge.

2   Related Works

To automatically perform VS and cochlea segmentation on hrT2 scans, the crossMoDA challenge [1] provides the benchmark datasets [3] and focuses on studying unpaired cross-modality segmentation technologies. Recent works mainly adopt the combinations of domain adaptation methods and segmentation networks for constructing unpaired cross-modality frameworks, which contain the following technologies: image alignment [9, 13]-[11], feature alignment [14, 15], disentangled representation [16] and output space alignment [17, 18]. By generating realistic images for aligning the intensity distribution between source and target domains, SynSeg-Net [13] integrated the cycle-consistent adversarial synthesis and segmentation into an end-to-end framework for cross-modality segmentation. A synergistic image and feature alignment (SIFA) framework [15] adopted the synergistic fusion of alignments from both image and feature perspectives to achieve bidirectional domain adaptation between CT and MR images. However, the standard cycle-consistency constraint assumes that the relationship between the two domains is a strong bijection, which is less effective for unpaired medical images with inconsistent anatomical structure information. To retain the anatomical structure consistency, Liu et al. [19] proposed a bidirectional domain adaptation network with anatomical structure preservation for unpaired cross-modality VS segmentation. Although the above methods have achieved impressive results in unpaired cross-modality segmentation, these methods ignored the abundant spatial information [20] and anisotropic resolutions in volumetric VS tumor brain images. On the other hand, it is hard to simulate the heterogeneity of the VS tumor signal for the methods using only a single image synthesis method [11, 12]. Thus, we integrated two different image synthesis methods with an advanced hybrid convolutional network for constructing a robust and effective cross-modality segmentation framework.

3 Proposed Methods

3.1 Overall Framework

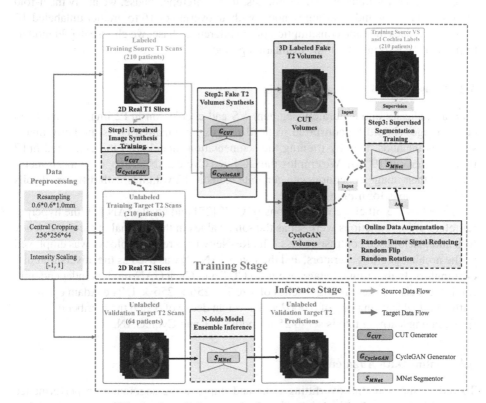

Fig. 1. Overall framework of our proposed method.

We proposed an unpaired cross-modality segmentation framework using various data augmentation and hybrid convolutional networks for segmenting vestibular schwannoma and cochlea, and Fig. 1 displays our proposed framework. Considering heterogeneous distributions and various image sizes for multi-institutional scans, we apply the min-max normalization for scaling the intensities of all scans and use the voxel size resampling and center cropping to obtain fixed-size sub-volumes for training. In the training stage, we first apply the UDA architectures of CUT and CycleGAN for training unpaired image synthesis models between T1 and T2 scans. Then, we use two image generators from CUT and CycleGAN to generate two groups of fake T2 volumes with different details and distributions as training data of the target domain. Finally, considering the anisotropic resolution and various image sizes of the crossMoDA 2022 dataset, we use MNet [6] as the hybrid convolutional segmentation network to segment the VS tumor and cochlea regions, which can represent sparse inter-slice information and dense intra-slice information adaptively and automatically. Besides, to improve the segmentation performance of T2 scans during training, we design a random tumor signal reducing method for simulating the heterogeneity of VS tumor signals, and combine it with random rotation and flipping for online data augmentation. By performing the 10-fold cross-validation on the crossMoDA 2022 training dataset, we can obtain 10 different trained weights for multi-model ensembles. In the inference phase, we apply the n-fold model ensembling and a sliding window with an overlap of 16 to predict unlabeled T2 scans. To reduce the time consumption of the inference phase, we choose 4-fold models to predict the testing data in the evaluation period.

3.2 Cross-Modality Image Synthesis

To automatically and accurately segment VS and cochlea on hrT2 images, annotated ceT1 images should be converted to hrT2 images by unpaired cross-modality image synthesis methods, thereby training the segmentation model with the generated hrT2 images afterward [9, 10]. We employ the CUT and CycleGAN as image synthesis methods, and their image generators can generate realistic T2 volumes with different details and distributions for training.

Based on the official configurations of CUT [27] and CycleGAN [7], the hyperparameters of loss functions were set as the same values in the original cycle-consistency loss and patch-based contrastive loss. The ResNet with 9 residual blocks was employed as the architecture of generators, and the PatchGAN [7] was used as the adversarial discriminators. In the training stage, we train CUT and CycleGAN models independently for 100 epochs by the training batches of size $2 \times 256 \times 256 \times 1$. The Adam optimizer with an initial learning rate of 0.0002 and a weight decay of 0, and the number of epochs for decaying learning rate is set to 25 for both CUT and CycleGAN.

3.3 Online Data Augmentation

To reduce the potential overfitting risks and improve the segmentation performance in multi-institutional and anisotropic scans, we employed the following online data augmentation (ODA) methods:

- **Random Tumor Signal Reducing**. Based on [11], to introduce heterogeneity of tumor signals to mimic such clinical characteristics, we randomly reduce the image intensity of VS tumors between 0% to 50% in synthesized fake T2 scans, which is formulated as:

$$\begin{cases} I_v^{aug} = (1 - 0.5 \cdot \alpha) \cdot I_v^{ori}, v \in S_{VS} \\ I_v^{aug} = I_v^{ori}, v \notin S_{VS} \end{cases} \tag{1}$$

where v is a voxel point in the input scan, S_{VS} represents the voxel set of the VS tumor regions, α is a random factor between 0 and 1, and I_v^{ori} and I_v^{aug} represent the original intensity and the augmented intensity of the voxel point v, respectively.

- **Random Flipping.** Each of three planes is flipped randomly and independently.
- **Random Rotation.** Three different rotation angles of 90°, 180°, 270° on the axial plane are applied.

3.4 The Hybrid Convolutional Network for Volumetric Image Segmentation

Due to the limitations of using vanilla 3D or 2D CNNs for the segmentation of anisotropic volumes, 2.5D segmentation networks [4, 5] perform 2D convolution (3 × 3 × 1) and pooling (2 × 2 × 1) until the spacing of x/y-axis is increased to a similar level of z-axis before performing 3D convolution, thus roughly achieving balanced representation in the 3D field. However, once the spacing ratio of each axis changes, these networks must be adjusted manually and retrained to adapt images. Hence, to overcome the anisotropic resolution and various image sizes of the crossMoDA2022 dataset, as shown in Fig. 2, we use MNet [6] as the segmentation network for accurate volumetric VS and cochlea segmentation. Instead of manually adjusting the network settings according to the spacing ratio before training, MNet adaptively balances the representation inter axes in the

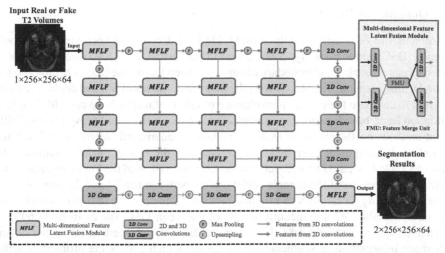

Fig. 2. Network architecture of MNet from the work [6], which simultaneously fuses multi-dimensional and multi-level features by adaptively learning 2D and 3D representations from anisotropic MR brain images. In MNet, 2D and 3D features are passed to the multi-dimensional feature latent fusion module which contains the combination of 2D and 3D convolutions and the feature merging unit (FMU) with element-wise subtraction.

learning process, owing to its free latent extraction and fusion of multi-dimensional representations. By sampling the training batches of size $1 \times 1 \times 256 \times 256 \times 64$, we employ the Adam optimizer with an initial learning rate of 0.0002 and a weight decay of 0.0005 to iteratively train segmentation networks for 250 epochs.

4 Results

4.1 Implement Details

Our proposed methods were implemented using the Pytorch framework, and we performed all experiments on an Ubuntu 18.04 workstation with two 24G NVIDIA GeForce RTX 3090 GPUs and an Intel Xeon Gold 5117 2.00 GHz CPU. The crossMoDA 2022 challenge provides a training dataset with 210 labeled T1 scans and 210 unlabeled T2 scans, a validation dataset with 64 unlabeled T2 scans, and an unseen testing dataset with unlabeled T2 scans for final ranking. Due to different data sources and imaging parameters, this dataset has heterogeneous distributions and various image sizes, and it has the intra-slice spacing of $(0.4–0.8)$ mm $\times$ $(0.4–0.8)$ mm and the inter-slice spacing of $(1.0–1.5)$ mm. In order to obtain the training and testing data with the same voxel size, we resample all cases to a common voxel size of $0.6 \times 0.6 \times 1.0$ mm. Then, we utilize the min-max normalization with a maximum value of 5000 and the minimum value of 0 to scale the intensities of all scans between -1 and 1. To avoid the influence of irrelevant regions such as the eye and the skull, we use a center cropping window of size $256 \times 256 \times 64$ (corresponding to widths, heights, and slices) to sample sub-volumes of T1 and T2 scans for training.

4.2 Quantitative Results

For quantitative comparison on the crossMoDA2022 dataset, the Dice Similarity Coefficiency (DSC) and the Average Symmetric Surface Distances (ASSD) are used to measure the region overlap and boundary distance between the segmentation results and the ground truths, respectively. Meanwhile, the mean DSC values of VS and cochlea regions are used to compare the overall performance of different methods on crossMoDA2022 validation leaderboard. In our experiments, Table 1 shows the quantitative results of different methods on the crossMoDA2022 validation leaderboard, where 'ODA' denotes the online data augmentation, and 'n-folds' denotes the n-fold model ensembles. As shown in Table 1, Method #1 without domain adaptation showed the lowest segmentation performance because of the domain shift problem between the T1 and T2 modalities.

By employing CycleGAN to generate realistic T2 images for unsupervised domain adaptation, Method #2 significantly improves the mean DSC values from 58.69% to 61.76% compared to Method #1. However, the 2D UNet of Method #2 cannot obtain rich space information in segmentation processes, which causes the problem that the segmentation performance of Method #2 is lower than Method #3 and #4 using 3D convolutions. By using MNet to adaptively fuse 2D and 3D representations, Method #5 without model ensembles obtains better overall performance of VS and cochlea regions than Method #3 and #4 with 5-fold model ensembles. By adding generative and online data augmentation, our proposed method (Method #7) gains the best overall DSC value of 74.48% in our experiments, which achieves the DSC values of 72.47% and 76.48% and ASSD values of 3.42 and 0.53 mm for VS tumor and cochlea on the validation dataset, respectively.

Table 1. Quantitative results of different methods on crossMoDA2022 validation leaderboard, where 'ODA' denotes the online data augmentation and 'n-folds' denotes the n-fold model ensembles. Bold values indicate the best results.

#	Methods		DSC (%)↑			ASSD (mm)↓	
	Synthesis	Segment	VS	Cochlea	Mean	VS	Cochlea
1	None	UNet2D (5folds)	36.75 ± 29.30	1.3 ± 2.66	19.05 ± 14.58	9.04 ± 12.19	13.74 ± 10.65
2	CycleGAN	UNet2D (5folds)	65.88 ± 22.27	69.42 ± 6.29	67.65 ± 12.72	4.84 ± 5.24	0.62 ± 1.78
3	CycleGAN	UNet3D (5folds)	64.13 ± 93.53	72.92 ± 4.82	68.52 ± 12.58	6.17 ± 7.78	0.59 ± 1.78
4	CycleGAN	UNet2.5D (5folds)	64.74 ± 27.09	73.33 ± 4.71	69.03 ± 14.25	**2.44 ± 3.21**	0.37 ± 0.16
5	CycleGAN	MNet (1fold)	68.56 ± 21.48	72.23 ± 4.68	70.39 ± 11.29	3.63 ± 6.91	0.59 ± 1.77
6	CycleGAN + CUT	MNet (ODA + 4folds)	68.98 ± 23.56	74.14 ± 4.87	71.56 ± 12.57	2.91 ± 5.88	**0.36 ± 0.17**
7	CycleGAN + CUT	MNet (ODA + 10folds)	**72.47 ± 17.94**	**76.48 ± 4.71**	**74.48 ± 9.99**	3.42 ± 3.53	0.53 ± 1.78

4.3 Qualitative Results

Figure 3 visualizes the segmentation results of different methods in Table 1 for qualitative analysis. As shown in Fig. 3, due to the significant domain gap between training T1 modality and testing T2 modality, Method #1 without domain adaptation hardly segments the cochlea regions, and the segmentation results of the VS region are also incomplete. By generating realistic target domain images for alleviating the intensity distribution gap, Method #2, #3, and #4 obtain more accurate segmentation results than Method #1, especially for the cochlea regions. Unlike the above methods, our proposed Method #6 further aligns the intensity distribution of VS and cochlea regions by various augmentation methods and adaptively obtains multi-dimensional representations, which obtains stable and accurate segmentation results. Finally, our proposed framework (Method #7) with 10-fold model ensembles effectively alleviates the performance degradation of cross-modality VS and cochlea segmentation in Fig. 3.

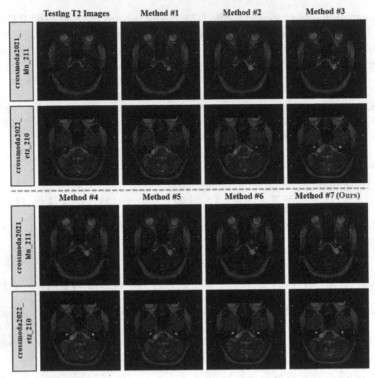

Fig. 3. Qualitative comparison of segmentation results of different methods on the cross-MoDA2022 validation dataset, where the VS and cochlea regions o correspond to red and green colors, respectively.

5 Discussion

In this section, we discuss the advantages and weaknesses of our proposed framework from two main perspectives: 1) Cross-modality Image Synthesis Method, and 2) Segmentation Networks.

5.1 Cross-Modality Image Synthesis Methods

For cross-modality VS and cochlea segmentation in the crossMoDA2022 challenge, current UDA methods (e.g., CycleGAN [7] and CUT [27]) can effectively help segmentation networks to learn the intensity distribution and annotation knowledge of unlabeled target domain by generative adversarial learning between T1 and T2 modalities. However, due to the significant heterogeneity of the VS and cochlea regions in cross-modality multi-institutional scans, it is difficult for a single image synthesis method to overcome the distribution gap among different modalities or scans, resulting in sub-optimal performance. As shown in Fig. 4, we simultaneously employ both CycleGAN and CUT to generate various and realistic target T2 images from labeled T1 images for improving the generalization performance and stability of the segmentation network. On the other hand, in Fig. 4, we observe that the synthesis results of CUT and CycleGAN are different but complementary, which is beneficial for generative data augmentation. The shortcoming of our proposed method is that two individual generative networks need to be trained, which is less efficient compared to other end-to-end methods.

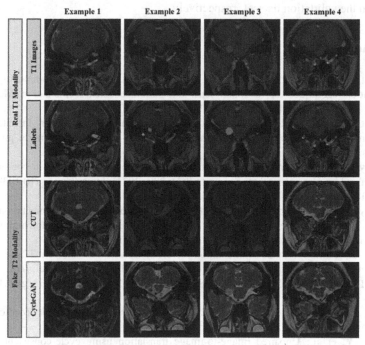

Fig. 4. Comparison of cross-modality image synthesis results for two different image synthesis methods on the crossMoDA2022 training dataset.

5.2 Segmentation Networks

Unlike the existing methods [9]-[12] using nnU-Net, 3D UNet, or 2.D UNet, we used the MNet with the appropriate number of parameters and better multi-dimensional representations as the segmentation network. Compared with other segmentation networks, the method using MNet [6] achieves a better mean DSC value in Table 1. Besides, compared to UNet3D with 22.58M and nnU-Net with 28.50M, MNet with 8.7M parameters shows great superiority in terms of the number of parameters, which means lower model complexity in the crossMoDA2022 challenge.

6 Conclusions

In this work, we proposed an unpaired cross-modality domain adaptation framework for VS and cochlea segmentation. Our proposed framework consists of synthesis and segmentation components. We applied two different image synthesis methods and various data augmentations to deal with the MRIs from different sites and scanners, and we utilized an effective hybrid convolutional network to adaptively integrate sparse inter-slice information with dense intra-slice formation for accurate segmentation. In the validation stage of crossMoDA2022, our method shows promising results and achieves the DSC values of 72.47% and 76.48% and ASSD values of 3.42 and 0.53 mm for VS tumor and cochlea on the validation dataset, respectively.

References

1. Dorent, R., et al.: CrossMoDA 2021 challenge: Benchmark of cross-modality domain adaptation techniques for vestibular schwannoma and cochlea segmentation. Med. Image Anal., 102628 (2022). https://doi.org/10.1016/j.media.2022.102628.
2. Dorent, R., et al.L Scribble-based domain adaptation via co-segmentation. In: International Conference on Medical Image Computing and Computer-Assisted Intervention, pp. 479–489 (2020)
3. Shapey, J., et al.: Segmentation of vestibular schwannoma from MRI, an open annotated dataset and baseline algorithm. Sci. Data **8**(1), 286 (2021). https://doi.org/10.1038/s41597-021-01064-w
4. Shapey, J., et al.: An artificial intelligence framework for automatic segmentation and volumetry of vestibular schwannomas from contrast-enhanced T1-weighted and high-resolution T2-weighted MRI. J. Neurosurg. **134**(1), 171–179 (2019)
5. Wang, G., et al.: Automatic segmentation of vestibular schwannoma from T2-weighted mri by deep spatial attention with hardness-weighted loss. In: Shen, D., et al. (eds.) MICCAI 2019. LNCS, vol. 11765, pp. 264–272. Springer, Cham (2019). https://doi.org/10.1007/978-3-030-32245-8_30
6. Dong, Z., et al.: MNet: rethinking 2D/3D Networks for Anisotropic Medical Image Segmentation (2022). http://arxiv.org/abs/2205.04846
7. Zhu, J.-Y., et al.: Unpaired image-to-image translation using cycle-consistent adversarial networks. In: Proceedings of the IEEE International Conference on Computer Vision, pp. 2223–2232 (2017)
8. Park, T., Efros, A.A., Zhang, R., Zhu, J.-Y.: Contrastive learning for unpaired image-to-image translation. In: Vedaldi, A., Bischof, H., Brox, T., Frahm, J.-M. (eds.) Computer Vision – ECCV 2020: Part IX, pp. 319–345. Springer International Publishing, Cham (2020). https://doi.org/10.1007/978-3-030-58545-7_19
9. Shin, H., Kim, H., Kim, S., Jun, Y., Eo, T., Hwang, D.: COSMOS: cross-modality unsupervised domain adaptation for 3D medical image segmentation based on Target-aware Domain Translation and Iterative Self-Training, arXiv Prepr. http://arxiv.org/abs/2203.16557
10. Dong, H., Yu, F., Zhao, J., Dong, B., Zhang, L.: Unsupervised Domain Adaptation in Semantic Segmentation Based on Pixel Alignment and Self-Training, pp. 4–8 (2021). http://arxiv.org/abs/2109.14219
11. Choi, J.W.: Using Out-of-the-Box Frameworks for Unpaired Image Translation and Image Segmentation for the crossMoDA Challenge, pp. 1–5 (2021). http://arxiv.org/abs/2110.01607
12. Liu, H., Fan, Y., Cui, C., Su, D., McNeil, A., Dawant, B.M.: Unsupervised Domain Adaptation for Vestibular Schwannoma and Cochlea Segmentation via Semi-supervised Learning and Label Fusion, vol. 1, pp. 1–11 (2022). http://arxiv.org/abs/2201.10647
13. Huo, Y., et al.: Synseg-net: Synthetic segmentation without target modality ground truth. IEEE Trans. Med. Imaging **38**(4), 1016–1025 (2018)
14. Dou, Q., et al.: PnP-AdaNet: Plug-and-play adversarial domain adaptation network at unpaired cross-modality cardiac segmentation. IEEE Access **7**, 99065–99076 (2019)

15. Chen, C., et al.: Unsupervised bidirectional cross-modality adaptation via deeply synergistic image and feature alignment for medical image segmentation. IEEE Trans. Med. Imaging **39**(7), 2494–2505 (2020)
16. Pei, C., Wu, F., Huang, L., Zhuang, X.: Disentangle domain features for cross-modality cardiac image segmentation. Med. Image Anal. **71**, 102078 (2021)
17. Tsai, Y.-H., et al.: Learning to adapt structured output space for semantic segmentation. In: Proceedings of the IEEE Conference on Computer Vision and Pattern Recognition, pp. 7472–7481 (2018)
18. Vesal, S., et al.: Adapt Everywhere: Unsupervised Adaptation of Point-Clouds and Entropy Minimization for Multi-Modal Cardiac Image Segmentation. IEEE Trans. Med. Imaging **40**(7), 1838–1851 (2021)
19. Liu, H., et al.: A bidirectional multilayer contrastive adaptation network with anatomical structure preservation for unpaired cross-modality medical image segmentation. Comput. Biol. Med., 105964 (2022)
20. Yao, K., et al.: A novel 3D unsupervised domain adaptation framework for cross-modality medical image segmentation. IEEE J. Biomed. Heal. Inform. 1 (2022)

Weakly Unsupervised Domain Adaptation for Vestibular Schwannoma Segmentation

Shahad Hardan[(✉)], Hussain Alasmawi[(✉)], Xiangjian Hou[(✉)],
and Mohammad Yaqub[(✉)]

Mohamed bin Zayed University of Artificial Intelligence, Abu Dhabi, UAE
{shahad.hardan,hussain.alasmawi,xiangjian.hou,
mohammad.yaqub}@mbzuai.ac.ae
https://mbzuai-biomedia.com/biomedia/

Abstract. Vestibular schwannoma (VS) is a non-cancerous tumor located next to the ear that can cause hearing loss. Most brain MRI images acquired from patients are contrast-enhanced T1 (ceT1), with a growing interest in high-resolution T2 images (hrT2) to replace ceT1, which involves the use of a contrast agent. As hrT2 images are currently scarce, it is less likely to train robust machine learning models to segment VS or other brain structures. In this work, we propose a weakly supervised machine learning approach that learns from only ceT1 scans and adapts to segment two structures from hrT2 scans: the VS and the cochlea from the crossMoDA dataset. Our model 1) generates fake hrT2 scans from ceT1 images and segmentation masks, 2) is trained using the fake hrT2 scans, 3) predicts the augmented real hrT2 scans, and 4) is retrained again using both the fake and real hrT2. The final result of this model has been computed on an unseen testing dataset provided by the 2022 crossMoDA challenge organizers. The mean dice score and average symmetric surface distance (ASSD) are 0.78 and 0.46, respectively. The predicted segmentation masks achieved a dice score of 0.83 and an ASSD of 0.56 on the VS, and a dice score of 0.74 and an ASSD of 0.35 on the cochleas. Among the 2022 crossMoDA challenge participants, our method was ranked the 8th.

Keywords: Domain adaptation · Unsupervised segmentation · Weak supervision · Generative adversarial network · Vestibular schwannoma

1 Introduction

Deep learning (DL) is becoming more popular due to its practicality and its ability to outperform experts in various applications, such as in the medical field. However, unlike humans who can adapt and learn new experiences from different existing ones, DL models are sensitive to the settings they are trained in and do not implicitly adapt to these unseen settings. For instance, changes

---

S. Hardan and H. Alasmawi—These authors contributed equally.

S. Bakas et al. (Eds.): BrainLes 2022, LNCS 14092, pp. 90–99, 2023.
https://doi.org/10.1007/978-3-031-44153-0_9

due to different scanners, image acquisition protocols, and medical centers are among forms of variability [8]. Domain Adaptation (DA) is a field in machine learning (ML) that deals with the distribution changes between different data. The cross-Modality Domain Adaptation (crossMoDA) challenge [4] introduced the first multi-class benchmark for unsupervised cross-modality DA. The challenge consists of two tasks: the segmentation of two structures in the hrT2 scans, and the classification of hrT2 images with vestibular schwannoma (VS) according to the Koos grade. Our work is focused on the first, which involves using contrast-enhanced T1 (ceT1) MRI as a source domain and high-resolution T2 (hrT2) MRI as a target domain to segment two objects: the VS and the cochleas. Vestibular schwannoma is a benign tumor in the brain that, in case of growth, affects the hearing nerves. As an intervention, open surgery or radiosurgery is performed to cure it. These operations require information about the volume and the exact location of the tumor [4]. Therefore, accurate segmentation of the relevant anatomy helps plan the operation properly and consequently increases the chance of patients' recovery.

2   Related Work

Several studies tackled domain adaptation in the medical imaging field. However, they are mostly private, small, and aim for binary image segmentation, unlike the crossMoDA dataset [4]. The challenge started in 2021, providing a total of 242 training images from the two domains (ceT1 and hrT2). In 2021, the winning model achieved a dice score of 0.857 for VS and 0.844 for the cochleas [12]. They applied CycleGAN for domain translation, then used the fakeT2 images to train the nnUNet. After that, they inferred pseudo-labels of the real hrT2, which are used to retrain the model. The second 2021 ranking model used nnUNet while applying the approaches of pixel alignment and self-training [2]. They generated fake hrT2 images using NiceGAN and achieved a mean dice score of 0.839. Finally, the third model used the Contrastive Unpaired Translation (CUT) method to generate fake hrT2, with 3D nnUNET for segmentation to attain a mean dice score of 0.829 [1]. Their approach mainly depends on doubling the number of images by generating augmented images with varying tumor intensities. Aside from the 2021 crossMoDA challenge, several approaches were followed for medical imaging domain adaptation, including weak supervision. In [3], the authors applied a weak supervision methodology based on having partial annotations derived from scribbles on the target domain. They propose a technique that combines structured learning and co-segmentation to segment VS on T2 scans (target domain) from T1 scans (source domain). They achieved a dice score of 0.83 on the target domain.

3   Methods

Our work consists of two public frameworks: Contrastive Unpaired Translation (CUT) [9] for transferring ceT1 to hrT2, and nnUNet [6] for segmentation. All the following work is implemented using PyTorch 1.11 and with the same mathematical formulation proposed in the CUT and nnUNet papers.

3.1 Data

The dataset contains 210 ceT1 MRI scans, 210 hrT2 MRI scans for training, and 64 hrT2 MRI scans for validation [11]. This dataset is an addition to the publicly available Vestibular-Schwannoma-SEG dataset, a part of The Cancer Imaging Archive (TCIA), that was manually segmented [4]. The ceT1 and hrT2 scans are unpaired, and the segmentation masks are only provided for the ceT1 scans. The tumor is on one side of the brain, thus, only one of the cochleas would experience the pressure caused by it. Regardless, the segmentation masks include both the cochleas, as it was found that segmenting the two increases the performance of the models [4]. Image acquisition happened at two institutes in two locations: London and Tilburg. The testing set is made of hrT2 and is not publicly available. Evaluation of the testing set is made by the challenge organizers using the participant's submitted Docker container.

3.2 Pre-processing

The provided 3D scans differ in size and voxel spacing. Thus, we resampled the images into an isotropic resolution of $1 \, mm^3$. During resampling, the interpolation techniques used are a third order b-spline for the images and nearest neighbor for the labels. Based on each image dimension, they were either cropped or padded in the xy-plane to 256×256, with a varying number of slices per image. The scans were normalized on a 3D basis, which led to better results during the domain translation phase. Previous techniques included normalization per slice. Since the slices have different ranges of pixel intensities, 2D normalization resulted in inconsistencies that decreased the quality of the generated hrT2 images during the domain translation phase. We note that domain adaptation processes that rely on generative algorithms are sensitive to the pre-processing techniques, as these results are essentially the input to the segmentation task.

3.3 Domain Translation

Our domain translation work is mainly based on CUT [9] (based on CycleGAN without bijection request) framework to transfer ceT1 images to hrT2 images. In the original CUT paper, ResNet was used as the generator network and a multi-layer perceptron as the discriminator network. In our work, we used StyleGAN2 backbone [7] instead, as it showed more promising results in the literature. Also, the authors trained the CUT for N number of epochs with a fixed learning rate, followed by another N epochs where the learning rate linearly decays to zero. Similarly, we applied this approach during our domain translation phase.

We trained the CUT model in two stages to speed up the training and avoid the discriminator over-shadowing the generator which could make it generate poorly representative hrT2 images. In the first stage, we set a batch size of 32 and a learning rate of 0.001 for the first 50 epochs. Then, for the second 50 epochs, the learning rate was linearly decaying to reach 0 at the final epoch. We used the Fréchet Inception Distance (FID) [10] as a metric to evaluate the proximity of the generated image to the target domain. In the second stage, we re-initialized the discriminator with random weights. This makes it more challenging to the discriminator to distinguish the views, allowing the generator to learn better representation of hrT2 images. If the discriminator was not re-initialized, its effect will dominate, and the generator will produce low-quality hrT2 scans. We trained the CUT for 5 epochs with a learning rate of 0.001, followed by another 5 epochs where the learning rate experienced a linear decay to finally reach 0. The method is summarized in Table 1. In addition, Fig. 1 shows 2D slices of a scan after passing through stage 1 and clarifies how it gets clearer after stage 2. We used these pseudo hrT2 images as the training dataset of the segmentation network.

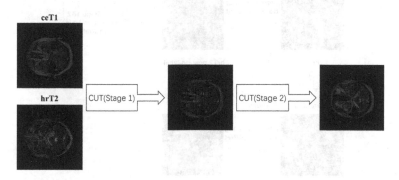

Fig. 1. Overview of our CUT process. Dividing the training of CUT into two parts can speed up the training and avoid the discriminator being too strong. Keeping the batch size as 1 yield the same result.

Table 1. Presented is the methodology followed during the domain translation phase. The table shows the settings of the two training stages of the CUT. BS refers to batch size, while LR refers to the learning rate.

Stage	BS	LR	Generator network baseline	Discriminator network baseline	Epochs	Epochs to decay
1	32	0.001	StyleGAN2 instead of ResNet9	StyleGAN instead of MLP	50	50
2	1	0.0002	StyleGAN2 instead of ResNet9	StyleGAN instead of MLP	5	5

3.4 Segmentation

For the segmentation task, we used the nnUNet framework with the 3D full resolution U-Net configuration. Following the approach of [1], we generated the augmented fake hrT2 images by reducing the tumor signal by 50%, naming them the AT dataset. By that, we had a total of 420 training images. We applied five

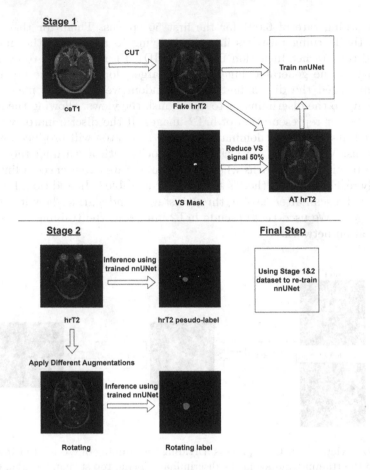

Fig. 2. Overview of the model: Stage 1 includes generating the fake hrT2 images, using them to create the tumor augmented version, and training using fake hrT2 images and the tumor augmented version. Stage 2 involves applying different augmentations to the real hrT2 images and producing their pseudo-labels from the model at stage 1.

fold cross validation using the default nnUNetTrainerV2 which combines two losses: cross entropy and dice, which are

$$\mathcal{L}_{dice} = \frac{-2}{C} \sum_{c \in C} \frac{\sum_i p_i^c g_i^c + \epsilon}{\sum_i p_i^c + \sum_i g_i^c + \epsilon} \tag{1}$$

$$\mathcal{L}_{CE} = \sum_i -g_i \log(p_i) - (1 - g_i)log(1 - p_i) \tag{2}$$

where i refers to the voxel, p is the predicted mask, g is the ground truth, C is the number of classes, and ϵ is the smoothing parameter. In the default setting, ϵ is set to 1. We also used the nnUNet variant that applies the non-smooth dice loss instead of the regular one, having $\epsilon = 0$ in Eq. 1. The non-smooth dice loss proved its effectiveness when the structure of interest is small relative to the scan size, such as the cochlea. We still noticed a gap between the performance on the training and validation datasets. Therefore, to alleviate the generalizability of the model, we used a nnUNet variant which applies multiple augmentation techniques to the training data. Since [12] showed that generating pseudo-labels of real hrT2 images to train on increases the dice score, we followed a similar approach. Thus, our models were then trained on a total of 630 images.

For all the nnUNet variants used in this work, instance normalization was used. Following [5], we applied squeeze-excitation normalization that enhances channel interdependencies. The SE blocks include a global average pooling layer, two fully connected layers (FC), and activation functions. The aim of the pooling layer is to squeeze the channel information into one value, while the FC layers learn the non-linear dependencies between the channels. The model involved a reduction rate ratio of 2 and a ReLU activation function. Other than the normalization approach, all settings were kept the same as in the default nnUNet.

For the final model, we made it depend on augmentations as a weak supervision approach as shown in Fig. 2. We applied eight types of augmentations on the real hrT2 dataset and predicted their pseudo-labels. The augmentation techniques are random rotation of up to $20°$, adding noise, scaling and translating, changing the contrast, and flipping on the three axes. As a result, we had 2100 images with a majority of real hrT2 images. This approach allows our model to better learn the features specific to the hrT2 modality and makes it less prone to the discrepancy arising from the GAN used. All the nnUNet variants apply the deep supervision approach for the loss functions which helps with the gradient vanishing problems for deep networks. Lastly, we ensembled two models involving: the augmentations variant with the combined loss, and the augmentations variant with the non-smooth dice loss. When predicting on an unseen case, we post-process the mask by finding the largest connected component of the VS. This is because the model tends to segment it on both sides of the brain while it is only located on one.

4   Results

As for the CUT model, the first stage achieved an FID of 70.37, while the second stage improved the model, reaching an FID of 51.3. Regarding the nnUNet implementation, Table 2 presents some of the results acquired from the different settings on the validation dataset. The baseline model included the fake hrT2 images with their tumor augmented version. The mean dice score achieved is 0.73, with low performance on segmenting the cochleas. Then, two models were trained after producing the pseudo-labels of the original hrT2 images, giving almost similar results: a mean dice score of 0.76. We then experimented by replacing the instance normalization in the default nnUNet with a squeeze-excitation normalization. However, obtaining a mean dice score of 0.73, we noticed no significant improvement using SE normalization. Thus, we used instance normalization in the rest of the experiments.

After that, we experimented with various augmentation techniques on the training data. Table 2 describes the performance of the augmentations variant models. Relatively, tested on the validation dataset, our analysis concludes that the two models with augmentations during training gave the best results. As a consequence, we produced augmented real T2 images with their pseudo-labels and ran the final ensemble model described in Sect. 3.4. The ensemble model achieved a mean dice score of 0.77 on the validation set, with a considerable improvement on the ASSD of the cochleas, reaching 0.37. As we can see from Table 2, this model has a lower variance compared to the other proposed models, which could be due to its learning to focus on the regions that are shared with the augmented pseudo-label.

Since the testing dataset is not made public, our performance metrics were obtained by the challenge organizers. Our model achieved a mean dice score of 0.78 and an ASSD of 0.46. As to the VS, the dice score is 0.83 and the ASSD is 0.56. The cochleas have a dice score of 0.74 and an ASSD of 0.35.

5 Qualitative Analysis

Our best and worst segmentation results of our final model on the validation set are shown in Fig. 3. The final model is an ensemble of two networks: nnUNet with augmentations and non-smooth dice loss, and nnUNet with augmentations and combined loss. It is still possible to discuss a few points even though we do not have the ground truth mask at hand. As observed in Fig. 3a, the model missed parts of the cochleas during segmentation and over-segmented the background. On the other hand, in the best case scenario for the cochlea in Fig. 3c, the model over-segments the cochlea region. Based on the two VS cases in Figs. 3b and 3c, we can see that the model can segment clear tumors well, while dark tumors are more difficult to segment.

Table 2. Results from different nnUNet variants. The best model is indicated in bold and represents an ensemble of two experiments: nnUNet with augmentations and non-smooth dice loss, and nnUnet with augmentations and combined loss. "Fake hrT2" are generated from the CUT, "AT" represents images where tumor signal is reduced by 50%, "aug var" describes the augmentations variant, and "pseudo-labels" are inferences of the real hrT2 scans.

Model	Dataset	Epoch	Score ↑	VS Dice ↑	VS ASSD ↓	Cochlea Dice ↑	Cochlea ASSD ↓
nnUNetTrainerV2	fake hrT2 + AT	300	0.73 ± 0.08	0.79 ± 0.13	0.73 ± 0.43	0.68 ± 0.07	0.63 ± 1.80
nnUNetTrainerV2	fake hrT2 + AT + pseudo-labels	800	0.76 ± 0.07	0.81 ± 0.11	1.14 ± 1.71	0.71 ± 0.06	0.60 ± 1.80
nnUNetTrainerV2 + non-smooth dice	fake hrT2 + AT+ pseudo-labels	800	0.76 ± 0.07	0.81 ± 0.11	1.28 ± 1.84	0.71 ± 0.06	0.59 ± 1.80
nnUNetTrainerV2 + SE normalization	fake hrT2 + AT	750	0.73 ± 0.09	0.76 ± 0.15	1.74 ± 2.50	0.69 ± 0.07	0.62 ± 1.79
nnUNetTrainerV2 + aug var	fake hrT2 + AT	500	0.75 ± 0.07	0.80 ± 0.11	0.69 ± 0.38	0.70 ± 0.06	0.62 ± 1.80
nnUNetTrainerV2 aug var + non-smooth dice	fake hrT2 + AT	500	0.75 ± 0.08	0.79 ± 0.13	0.71 ± 0.41	0.71 ± 0.06	0.61 ± 1.80
Ensemble of (nnUNetTrainerV2 aug var + non-smooth dice) & (nnUNetTrainerV2 aug var)	fake hrT2 + AT + pseudo-labels	1000	**0.77 ± 0.06**	**0.82 ± 0.09**	**0.61 ± 0.27**	**0.72 ± 0.06**	**0.37 ± 0.18**

6   Discussion

We developed a deep learning algorithm that follows a weak supervision approach to segment two brain structures in the hrT2 modality. The model uses a GAN to generate fake hrT2 images from the ceT1 scans, then these hrT2 images are trained using an nnUNet. After that, the fake hrT2 images are augmented and the nnUNet is used to predict the pseudo-labels of the augmented images. Finally, the model is retrained using the real hrT2 images and the latter augmented hrT2 images as the training dataset, and is validated on the validation dataset provided from the challenge organizers. The applied experiments vary in the loss function, datasets, and augmentations. We observed that the implementation of an accurate GAN model plays a huge role in the success of the unsupervised DA model. Given that the model is predicting an unseen modality, the more generalizable it is, the better. Thus, even if the augmentations increase the size of the training data, it offers the model an optimal chance to diversify the features learned from the target domain. We noticed that the model is more consistent in predicting the cochlea, but less accurate, relative to segmenting the VS. This may be due to the cochlea's size being small in relation to the entire image, but has a fixed location across the patients' scans. However, the VS prediction is not consistent because the tumor intensity, location, and size vary by patient. Moreover, the ASSD metric improved significantly in the final model compared to the improvement noticed in the dice score, especially for the cochleas. We associate it with the different augmentations applied during training, which led

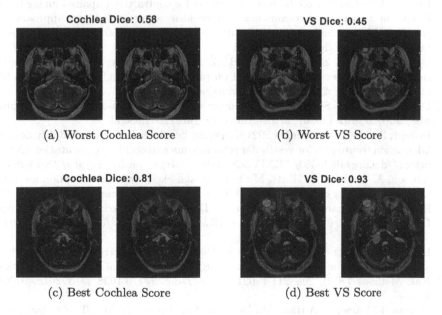

(a) Worst Cochlea Score   (b) Worst VS Score

(c) Best Cochlea Score   (d) Best VS Score

Fig. 3. The best and the worst segmentation according to the dice score for Cochlea (in green) and VS (in red). (Color figure online)

to a better study of the overall shape of the structures in different orientations. The ASSD considers the distance between the boundaries of the ground truth and the predicted mask which is more sensitive to outliers in prediction. Thus, we can conclude that the improvement in ASSD indicates that the final model is more robust than the previous models.

7   Conclusion

The application of domain adaptation enables ML models to aid in cases similar to the VS disease, where there is a growing interest in using hrT2 images, but not enough data. Both the settings of the GAN used and the segmentation network impacts the efficiency, especially for small-size structures, such as the cochleas. In some cases, weak supervision approaches may be computationally expensive. Regardless, they enable the model to learn different properties and views of the target domain scans. Thus, they maximize the learning of features and increase generalizability. Since the augmented hrT2 scans are predicted from the initial nnUNet network, improving it would significantly improve the quality of the prediction. Therefore, further work includes higher performing segmentation models, especially on the cochleas, in order to be combined with our weak supervision approach.

References

1. Choi, J.W.: Using out-of-the-box frameworks for contrastive unpaired image translation for vestibular schwannoma and cochlea segmentation: an approach for the CrossMoDa challenge (2021). https://doi.org/10.48550/ARXIV.2110.01607. https://arxiv.org/abs/2110.01607
2. Dong, H., Yu, F., Zhao, J., Dong, B., Zhang, L.: Unsupervised domain adaptation in semantic segmentation based on pixel alignment and self-training. CoRR abs/2109.14219 (2021). https://arxiv.org/abs/2109.14219
3. Dorent, R., et al.: Scribble-based domain adaptation via co-segmentation. CoRR **abs/2007.03632** (2020). https://arxiv.org/abs/2007.03632
4. Dorent, R., et al.: CrossMoDa 2021 challenge: benchmark of cross-modality domain adaptation techniques for vestibular schwannoma and cochlea segmentation (2022). https://doi.org/10.48550/ARXIV.2201.02831. https://arxiv.org/abs/2201.02831
5. Iantsen, A., Visvikis, D., Hatt, M.: Squeeze-and-excitation normalization for automated delineation of head and neck primary tumors in combined PET and CT images. In: Andrearczyk, V., Oreiller, V., Depeursinge, A. (eds.) HECKTOR 2020. LNCS, vol. 12603, pp. 37–43. Springer, Cham (2021). https://doi.org/10.1007/978-3-030-67194-5_4
6. Isensee, F., Jaeger, P.F., Kohl, S.A.A., Petersen, J., Maier-Hein, K.H.: nnU-Net: a self-configuring method for deep learning-based biomedical image segmentation. Nat. Methods **18**(2), 203–211 (2021). https://doi.org/10.1038/s41592-020-01008-z
7. Karras, T., Laine, S., Aittala, M., Hellsten, J., Lehtinen, J., Aila, T.: Analyzing and improving the image quality of StyleGAN. CoRR abs/1912.04958 (2019). http://arxiv.org/abs/1912.04958

8. van Opbroek, A., Ikram, M.A., Vernooij, M.W., de Bruijne, M.: Transfer learning improves supervised image segmentation across imaging protocols. IEEE Trans. Med. Imaging **34**(5), 1018–1030 (2015). https://doi.org/10.1109/TMI.2014.2366792
9. Park, T., Efros, A.A., Zhang, R., Zhu, J.-Y.: Contrastive learning for unpaired image-to-image translation. In: Vedaldi, A., Bischof, H., Brox, T., Frahm, J.-M. (eds.) ECCV 2020. LNCS, vol. 12354, pp. 319–345. Springer, Cham (2020). https://doi.org/10.1007/978-3-030-58545-7_19
10. Seitzer, M.: PyTorch-FID: FID score for PyTorch, August 2020. https://github.com/mseitzer/pytorch-fid. Version 0.2.1
11. Shapey, J., et al.: Segmentation of vestibular schwannoma from MRI - an open annotated dataset and baseline algorithm (2021). https://doi.org/10.1101/2021.08.04.21261588
12. Shin, H., Kim, H., Kim, S., Jun, Y., Eo, T., Hwang, D.: Self-training based unsupervised cross-modality domain adaptation for vestibular schwannoma and cochlea segmentation (2021). https://doi.org/10.48550/ARXIV.2109.10674. https://arxiv.org/abs/2109.10674

Multi-view Cross-Modality MR Image Translation for Vestibular Schwannoma and Cochlea Segmentation

Bogyeong Kang, Hyeonyeong Nam, Ji-Wung Han, Keun-Soo Heo, and Tae-Eui Kam$^{(\boxtimes)}$

Department of Artificial Intelligence, Korea University, Seoul, Republic of Korea
{kangbk,kamte}@korea.ac.kr

Abstract. In this work, we propose a multi-view image translation framework, which can translate contrast-enhanced T_1 (ceT_1) MR imaging to high-resolution T_2 (hrT_2) MR imaging for unsupervised vestibular schwannoma and cochlea segmentation. We adopt two image translation models in parallel that use a pixel-level consistent constraint and a patch-level contrastive constraint, respectively. Thereby, we can augment pseudo-hrT_2 images reflecting different perspectives, which eventually lead to a high-performing segmentation model. Our experimental results on the CrossMoDA challenge show that the proposed method achieved enhanced performance on the vestibular schwannoma and cochlea segmentation.

Keywords: Multi-view image translation · Cross-modality · MRI segmentation · Unsupervised domain adaptation

1 Introduction

Vestibular schwannoma (VS) is a benign tumor that occurs in the nerve membrane cells of the vestibular nerve [6,11]. For diagnosis and treatment of VS, it is necessary to segment the VS and its surrounding organs, especially the cochleas [6,11]. In general, VS is diagnosed through contrast-enhanced T_1 (ceT_1) MR imaging but there are concerns about side effects such as allergy to gadolinium-containing contrast agents [6,11]. As an alternative, high-resolution T_2 (hrT_2) MR imaging, a non-contrast imaging technique, has shed light on VS segmentation [6,11]. However, it is very time-consuming and expensive to manually annotate newly released data. For this reason, the lack of annotated data can be a big problem for applying deep learning techniques in the medical domain. This issue can be solved by applying unsupervised domain adaptation, which allows a model trained in one domain to be adapted in another unseen domain without supervision [1,5,8]. Recently, some studies [3,4,12] have been conducted based on cross-modality domain adaptation for VS and cochlea segmentation in unseen hrT_2 scans. Previous studies [3,4,12] achieved outstanding

S. Bakas et al. (Eds.): BrainLes 2022, LNCS 14092, pp. 100–108, 2023.
https://doi.org/10.1007/978-3-031-44153-0_10

performance on VS and cochlea segmentation utilizing image translation models such as CycleGAN [14] or CUT [10]. Of note, CycleGAN employs pixel-level consistent constraints, while CUT adopts patch-level contrastive constraints. The former constraint can better reflect the intensity and the texture of VS through cycle-consistency loss, but the structure of VS and cochleas could be distorted. Besides, the latter constraint uses contrastive loss, having an advantage in preserving the structure of VS and cochleas, but could ignore the detailed characteristics such as intensity and texture. Based on these considerations, we believe that we can obtain diverse pseudo-hrT2 images, which can help to improve the segmentation model performance by using the two aforementioned constraint models together.

Therefore, we design a multi-view image translation framework to obtain the pseudo-hrT$_2$ images with different perspectives by adopting two image translation models in parallel, CycleGAN [14] and QS-Attn [7]. CycleGAN employs a pixel-level consistent constraint, and QS-Attn is an advanced patch-level contrastive constraint method that focuses on domain-relevant features [7]. To our best knowledge, QS-Attn [7] is first adopted for image translation from ceT$_1$ to hrT$_2$ images in this work. Based on our multi-view image translation framework, the following segmentation model can learn both structure and texture of VS and cochleas.

2 Related Work

Cross-modality unsupervised domain adaptation has drawn a lot of attention in the CrossMoDA challenge [6]. The goal of this challenge is to construct a VS and cochlea segmentation model on hrT$_2$ images with unpaired annotated ceT$_1$ and non-annotated hrT$_2$ scans. Recent studies [3,4,12] first translated the source ceT$_1$ images to the target hrT$_2$ images, and then trained their segmentation models with the translated hrT$_2$ (i.e., pseudo-hrT$_2$) images. More specifically, Shin et al. [12] translated the ceT$_1$ images to the hrT$_2$ images by adding an additional decoder to CycleGAN to preserve the structures of VS and cochleas. Dong et al. [4] conducted image translation using NiceGAN [2], which is based on CycleGAN [14], and Choi et al. [3] obtained pseudo-hrT$_2$ images using CUT [10]. Of note, they all obtained pseudo-hrT$_2$ images by taking only one constraint model. Besides, Choi et al. [3] performed post-processing to obtain the images with low intensity, similar to the VS in real hrT$_2$ scans.

3 Proposed Method

3.1 Overview

Figure 1 shows an overview of our proposed framework, which consists of three parts; (1) multi-view image translation, (2) segmentation model training, and (3) self-training. Specifically, we first generate the pseudo-hrT$_2$ images with various characteristics through multi-view image translation. After that, we train the

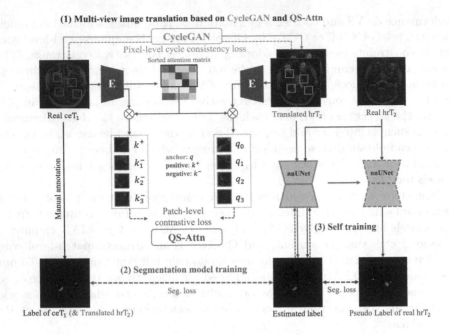

Fig. 1. The overview of our proposed framework.

segmentation model using the multi-view pseudo-hrT$_2$ images and the labels of the ceT$_1$ images. In the self-training, the trained segmentation model first performs pseudo-labeling of real hrT$_2$ images, and then is further trained by including the pseudo-labeled real hrT$_2$ images in the next training phase.

3.2   Multi-view Image Translation

We first translate ceT$_1$ images into multi-view pseudo-hrT$_2$ images by adopting CycleGAN [14] and QS-Attn [7] in parallel.

CycleGAN. CycleGAN uses cycle-consistency loss to translate the source domain ceT$_1$ images into the target domain hrT$_2$ images. Cycle-consistency loss described in Eq. 1 encourages $F(G(x_s))$ to be equal to x_s and $G(F(x_t))$ to be equal to x_t in pixel-level when given the $G : X_s \rightarrow X_t$ and $F : X_t \rightarrow X_s$ generators [14].

$$L_{cycle} = \|F(G(x_s)) - x_s\| + \|G(F(x_t)) - x_t\| \tag{1}$$

QS-Attn. QS-Attn is an unpaired image translation model that is improved from CUT [10]. CUT preserves the structural information by constraining the patches from the same location on the source and the translated images to be close, compared to the different locations. CUT maximizes the mutual information between the source and translated images through the Eq. 2 [10],

$$L_{con} = -\log\left[\frac{\exp(q \cdot k^+/\tau)}{\exp(q \cdot k^+/\tau) + \sum_{i=1}^{N-1}\exp(q \cdot k^-/\tau)}\right] \tag{2}$$

where q is the anchor feature from the translated image and k^+ is a single positive at the same location in the source image and k^- are $(N-1)$ negatives at the other locations, and τ is a temperature [7].

However, CUT [10] calculates the contrastive loss between the randomly selected patches, which could have less domain-relevant information. QS-Attn addresses this limitation by adopting the QS-Attn module, which can select domain-relevant patches. The QS-Attn module constructs the attention matrix A_g using the features in the source images and then obtains the entropy H_g by following Eq. 3 [7].

$$H_g(i) = -\sum_{j=1}^{HW} A_g(i,j)\log A_g(i,j) \tag{3}$$

Of note, the smaller entropy H_g means the more important feature. Thus, A_g is sorted in ascending order according to entropy H_g to select domain-relevant patches [7]. By calculating the contrastive loss using the selected domain-relevant patches, the structures of the source domain better preserve, and more realistic images are generated compared to CUT [10].

We empirically found that CycleGAN with pixel-level cycle-consistency loss allows the model to better reflect the intensity and the texture of the VS and cochleas in the target images, while QS-Attn takes advantage of preserving the structure of them more clearly via patch-level contrastive loss (refer to Sect. 5 for more details). By using them together, our multi-view image translation can augment pseudo-hrT$_2$ images from different perspectives, and it can help improve the performance of the following segmentation model.

3.3   Segmentation and Self-training

Motivated by the previous works [3,4,12], we also utilize nnUNet [9] and self-training procedure [13] to construct the segmentation model. nnUNet is a powerful segmentation framework that automatically performs pre-processing, training, and post-processing with heuristic rules [9]. Self-training is carried out to reduce the distribution gap between real hrT$_2$ and translated hrT$_2$ images and to improve the robustness of the segmentation model for unseen real hrT$_2$ scans. The segmentation and self-training procedure consists of four steps; (1) training the segmentation model using the translated hrT$_2$ scans with labels of the ceT$_1$ scans. (2) Generating pseudo labels of unlabeled real hrT$_2$ scans by using the trained segmentation model. (3) Retraining the segmentation model using both the translated hrT$_2$ scans with labels of the ceT$_1$ scans and the real hrT$_2$ scans with pseudo labels. 4) Repeating Steps 2-3 to achieve further performance improvement.

4   Experiments and Results

4.1   Dataset and Preprocessing

We used the CrossMoDA dataset[1] [6] for training, validation. The CrossMoDA dataset consists of data from two different institutions: London and Tilburg. The London data consists of 105 ceT_1 scans and 105 hrT_2 scans. The ceT_1 scans were acquired with the in-plane resolution of 0.4×0.4 mm, in-plane matrix of 512×512, and slice thickness of 1.0 to 1.5 mm with an MPRAGE sequence (TR=1900 ms, TE=2.97 ms, TI=1100 ms). Meanwhile, hrT_2 scans were acquired with the in-plane resolution of 0.5×0.5 mm, in-plane matrix of 384×384 or 448×448, and slice thickness of 1.0 to 1.5 mm with a 3D CISS or FIESTA sequence (TR = 9.4 ms, TE = 4.23 ms). For the Tilburg data set, ceT_1 scans and hrT_2 scans consist of 105 subjects each. The ceT_1 scans were acquired with the in-plane resolution of 0.8×0.8 mm, in-plane matrix of 256×256, and slice thickness of 1.5 mm with a 3D-FFE sequence (TR=25 ms, TE=1.82 ms). The hrT_2 scans were acquired with the in-plane resolution of 0.4×0.4mm, in-plane matrix of 512×512, and slice thickness of 1.0 mm with a 3D-TSE sequence (TR=2700 ms, TE=160 ms, ETL=50) [6]. The training dataset of the CrossMoDA2022 Challenge[1] contains a total of 210 ceT_1 scans with annotation labels and 210 hrT_2 scans without annotation labels. In addition, they provide 64 scans of hrT_2 images for validation.

Since the voxel spaces vary across scans, all the images were resampled to [0.41, 0.41, 1.5] voxel sizes. For image translation, the 3D MRI images were sliced into a series of 2D images along the axial plane and the images were center-cropped and resized to 256×256. After performing image translation, the translated hrT_2 images were merged into 3D MR imaging and fed into the segmentation model.

4.2   Implementation Details

We implement CycleGAN [14], QS-Attn [7], and nnUNet [9], following their default parameter settings. We also apply a global attention in QS-Attn [7], and ensemble selection in nnUNet [9] for the final prediction. All the implementations are powered by RTX 3090 24GB GPUs. The training of CycleGAN, QS-Attn, and nnUNet is performed with PyTorch 1.8.0, 1.7.1, and 1.10.2, respectively.

4.3   Results

Table 1 and Fig. 2 show the VS and cochlea segmentation results with different image translation methods. The proposed multi-view image translation framework with CycleGAN [14] and QS-Attn [7] shows better performance compared to other methods using each model alone. Moreover, we greatly improved the performance of the segmentation model with self-training. As a result, our proposed method obtained a great achievement with a mean dice score of 0.85040.0466 in the validation period.

---

[1] https://crossmoda-challenge.ml/.

Table 1. Segmentation results with dice and ASSD scores (ST: self-training).

Translation model	Dice score			ASSD	
	VS	Cochlea	Mean	VS	Cochlea
CycleGAN (*w/o.* ST)	0.7798 (±0.1901)	0.8066 (±0.0323)	0.7932 (±0.0972)	0.8750 (±0.9222)	0.2422 (±0.1608)
QS-Attn (*w/o.* ST)	0.7779 (±0.1825)	0.8158 (±0.0287)	0.7968 (±0.0929)	0.6667 (±0.3891)	0.2365 (±0.1573)
Proposed (*w/o.* ST)	0.8043 (±0.1656)	0.8158 (±0.0289)	0.8101 (±0.0863)	0.5742 (±0.2461)	0.2387 (±0.1581)
Proposed (*w.* ST)	**0.8520 (±0.0889)**	**0.8488 (±0.0235)**	**0.8504 (±0.0466)**	**0.4748 (±0.2072)**	**0.1992 (±0.1524)**

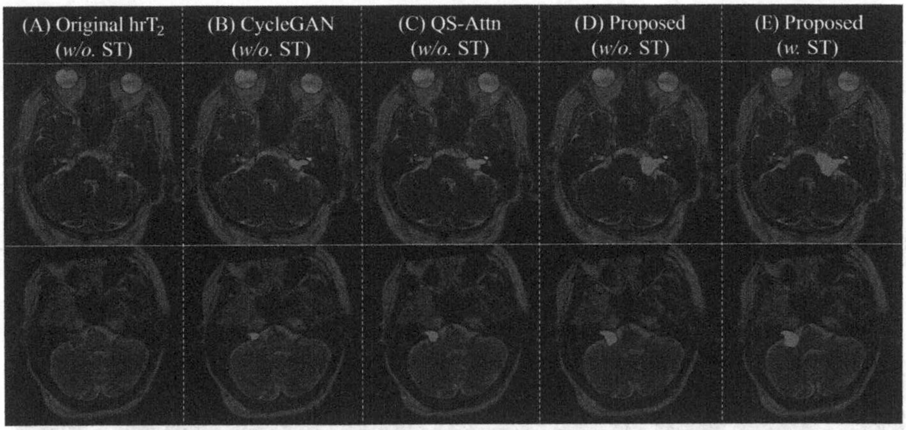

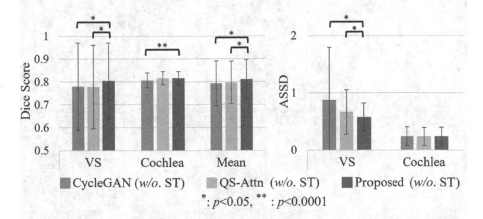

Fig. 2. Qualitative comparison of segmentation results for validation set. We visualize the segmentation results of VS (red) and cochlea (green) (ST: Self-training). (Color figure online)

Fig. 3. Performance comparison of VS and cochlea segmentation models (ST: Self-training).

We conducted paired t-test among CycleGAN [14], QS-Attn [7], and our proposed method (*w/o.* self-training, ST) to compare the segmentation performance, and the results are plotted in Fig. 3. CycleGAN, QS-Attn, and our proposed method (*w/o.* ST) show statistical significance with $p < 0.05$ for the dice score of VS and mean values. In addition, our proposed method (w/o. ST) is statistically better with $p < 0.0001$ than CycleGAN on the dice score of cochleas. Through this statistical comparison, we proved that our proposed framework achieved better performance compared to other methods that use either of the two models alone.

5   Discussion

Figure 4 shows the results of the two separate image translation models utilized in the multi-view image translation framework. For comparison, we randomly picked two ceT_1 images (A&E), their corresponding translated hrT_2 images (B-C&F-G), and two unpaired real hrT_2 images (D&H). We can see that QS-Attn (C) well captured the structure of cochleas with less distortion or blurring compared to CycleGAN (B). Meanwhile, some images translated through QS-Attn (G) have too high intensities for VS, whereas those by CycleGAN (F) have similar intensity and textures to VS in the real hrT_2 image (H). As shown in Fig. 4,

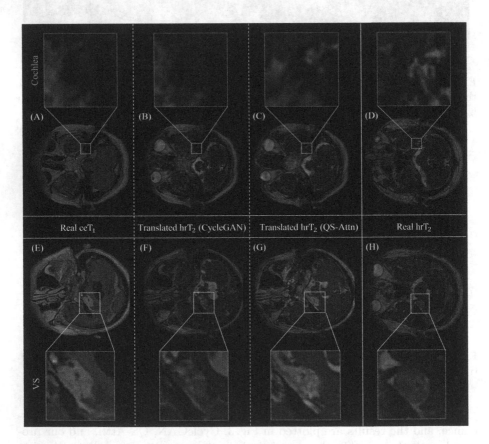

Fig. 4. Comparison results of image translation by CycleGAN and QS-Attn.

the two constraint models have different strengths. Therefore, in the proposed method, the segmentation model can learn both structures and textures of VS and cochleas through our multi-view image translation framework. It allows the segmentation model to consider various perspectives of VS and cochleas and helps improve the performance of the segmentation model.

6 Conclusion

In this work, we design a multi-view image translation framework for VS and cochlea segmentation. Specifically, we adopt CycleGAN and QS-Attn in parallel to translate the given ceT1 images to pseudo-hrT2 images reflecting various perspectives. Based on the pseudo-hrT2 images, the segmentation model can learn both structures and textures of VS and cochleas. Our proposed method obtained great achievement in the CrossMoDA challenge2022.

Acknowledgment. This work was supported by Institute of Information & communications Technology Planning & Evaluation (IITP) grant funded by the Korea government (MSIT) (No. 2019-0-00079, Artificial Intelligence Graduate School Program (Korea University)), and the National Research Foundation of Korea (NRF) grant funded by the Korea government (MSIT) (No. 2020R1C1C1013830, No. 2020R1A4A1018309).

References

1. Chen, C., Dou, Q., Chen, H., Qin, J., Heng, P.A.: Synergistic image and feature adaptation: Towards cross-modality domain adaptation for medical image segmentation. In: Proceedings of the AAAI conference on artificial intelligence, vol. 33, pp. 865–872 (2019)
2. Chen, R., Huang, W., Huang, B., Sun, F., Fang, B.: Reusing discriminators for encoding: Towards unsupervised image-to-image translation. In: Proceedings of the IEEE/CVF Conference on Computer Vision and Pattern Recognition, pp. 8168–8177 (2020)
3. Choi, J.W.: Using out-of-the-box frameworks for unpaired image translation and image segmentation for the crossmoda challenge. arXiv e-prints, pp. arXiv-2110 (2021)
4. Dong, H., Yu, F., Zhao, J., Dong, B., Zhang, L.: Unsupervised domain adaptation in semantic segmentation based on pixel alignment and self-training. arXiv preprint arXiv:2109.14219 (2021)
5. Dorent, R., et al.: Scribble-based domain adaptation via co-segmentation. In: Martel, A.L., et al. (eds.) MICCAI 2020. LNCS, vol. 12261, pp. 479–489. Springer, Cham (2020). https://doi.org/10.1007/978-3-030-59710-8_47
6. Dorent, R., et al.: Crossmoda 2021 challenge: Benchmark of cross-modality domain adaptation techniques for vestibular schwnannoma and cochlea segmentation. arXiv preprint arXiv:2201.02831 (2022)
7. Hu, X., Zhou, X., Huang, Q., Shi, Z., Sun, L., Li, Q.: QS-Attn: query-selected attention for contrastive learning in i2i translation. In: Proceedings of the IEEE/CVF Conference on Computer Vision and Pattern Recognition, pp. 18291–18300 (2022)

8. Huo, Y., et al.: Synseg-net: synthetic segmentation without target modality ground truth. IEEE Trans. Med. Imaging **38**(4), 1016–1025 (2018)

9. Isensee, F., Jaeger, P.F., Kohl, S.A., Petersen, J., Maier-Hein, K.H.: nnU-net: a self-configuring method for deep learning-based biomedical image segmentation. Nat. Methods **18**(2), 203–211 (2021)

10. Park, Taesung, Efros, Alexei A.., Zhang, Richard, Zhu, Jun-Yan.: Contrastive learning for unpaired image-to-image translation. In: Vedaldi, Andrea, Bischof, Horst, Brox, Thomas, Frahm, Jan-Michael. (eds.) ECCV 2020. LNCS, vol. 12354, pp. 319–345. Springer, Cham (2020). https://doi.org/10.1007/978-3-030-58545-7_19

11. Shapey, J., et al.: Segmentation of vestibular schwannoma from MRI, an open annotated dataset and baseline algorithm. Sci. Data **8**(1), 1–6 (2021)

12. Shin, H., Kim, H., Kim, S., Jun, Y., Eo, T., Hwang, D.: COSMOS: cross-modality unsupervised domain adaptation for 3d medical image segmentation based on target-aware domain translation and iterative self-training. arXiv preprint arXiv:2203.16557 (2022)

13. Xie, Q., Luong, M.T., Hovy, E., Le, Q.V.: Self-training with noisy student improves imagenet classification. In: Proceedings of the IEEE/CVF conference on computer vision and pattern recognition, pp. 10687–10698 (2020)

14. Zhu, J.Y., Park, T., Isola, P., Efros, A.A.: Unpaired image-to-image translation using cycle-consistent adversarial networks. In: Proceedings of the IEEE International Conference on Computer Vision, pp. 2223–2232 (2017)

Enhancing Data Diversity for Self-training Based Unsupervised Cross-Modality Vestibular Schwannoma and Cochlea Segmentation

Han Liu[1(✉)], Yubo Fan[1], Ipek Oguz[1,2], and Benoit M. Dawant[2]

[1] Department of Computer Science, Vanderbilt University, Nashville, USA
han.liu@vanderbilt.edu
[2] Department of Electrical and Computer Engineering, Vanderbilt University, Nashville, USA

Abstract. Automatic segmentation of vestibular schwannoma (VS) and cochlea from magnetic resonance imaging can facilitate VS treatment planning. Unsupervised segmentation methods have shown promising results without requiring the time-consuming and laborious manual labeling process. In this paper, we present an approach for VS and cochlea segmentation in an unsupervised domain adaptation setting. Specifically, we first develop a cross-site cross-modality unpaired image translation strategy to enrich the diversity of the synthesized data. Then, we devise a rule-based offline augmentation technique to further minimize the domain gap. Lastly, we adopt a self-configuring segmentation framework empowered by self-training to obtain the final results. On the CrossMoDA 2022 validation leaderboard, our method has achieved competitive VS and cochlea segmentation performance with mean Dice scores of 0.8178 ± 0.0803 and 0.8433 ± 0.0293, respectively.

Keywords: Vestibular schwannoma · Cochlea · Unsupervised domain adaptation · Self-training

1 Introduction

Vestibular schwannoma (VS) is a benign tumor that stems from an overproduction of Schwann cells. It develops from the vestibular nerve which connects the brain and the inner ear and its common symptoms include hearing loss, dizziness, and tinnitus [19]. Magnetic resonance imaging (MRI) is crucial for diagnosis and surveillance of VS and contrast enhanced T1 weighted (ceT1) MRI is currently the most commonly used protocol. However, this involves gadolinium, which may produce side effects ranging from mild to severe. As a possible noncontrast and

---

H. Liu and Y. Fan—Equal contribution.

© The Author(s), under exclusive license to Springer Nature Switzerland AG 2023
S. Bakas et al. (Eds.): BrainLes 2022, LNCS 14092, pp. 109–118, 2023.
https://doi.org/10.1007/978-3-031-44153-0_11

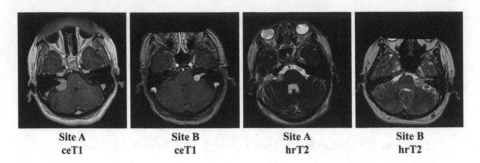

Fig. 1. Two types of domain gaps exist in CrossMoDA 2022 due to the difference in (1) acquisition sites and (2) MRI modalities.

lower-cost alternative, high-resolution T2-weighted (hrT2) imaging has shown promises for follow-up surveillance scans [2,15,17].

To facilitate the clinical workflow, automatic methods to segment the VS in ceT1 and hrT2 have recently emerged [17,20,24]. However, training supervised VS segmentation models requires manual annotation, which is expensive and time-consuming. Weakly-supervised [4] and unsupervised VS segmentation methods [5] have thus drawn increasing interest in the community. In the Cross-MoDA 2021 challenge [5], participants were given the task of unsupervised cross-modality VS and cochlea segmentation, i.e., segmenting these two structures in hrT2, but annotations were only provided in unpaired ceT1 images in the training set. In the CrossMoDA 2022 challenge, an additional set of ceT1 and hrT2 images are acquired at another MRI site. Therefore, two types of domain gaps exist in this challenge due to the difference in (1) acquisition sites, i.e., site A vs. site B, and (2) MRI modalities, i.e., ceT1 vs. hrT2, as shown in Fig. 1. Both domain gaps need to be addressed to achieve robust segmentation performance in CrossMoDA 2022.

In this paper, we present our solution to the segmentation task of CrossMoDA 2022. We approach this task as an unsupervised domain adaptation (UDA) problem where we first train cross-site unpaired image translation models to generate pseudo target domain (hrT2) images, then apply a rule-based augmentation to the pseudo hrT2 images, and finally train nnU-Net [9] segmentation models using a self-training scheme. The results on the challenge leaderboard showed that our method has achieved promising segmentation performances on both VS and cochlea.

2 Related Work

2.1 Unsupervised Domain Adaptation (UDA)

The performance of machine learning models can be affected by data distribution shift between the training/source dataset and test/target dataset [7]. UDA refers to the task of improving model performance on target domain data when their label is not available. Feature alignment-based methods aim to learn domain-invariant features across different domains. Domain Adversarial Neural Network (DANN) [6] is a representative architecture that utilizes adversarial learning between a feature extractor and a domain discriminator. The domain discriminator learns to differentiate whether the extracted features are from the source or target domain, and the feature extractor learns domain-invariant features such that it can fool the discriminator. Another way to align features is by optimizing some divergence metrics [14,21] between the source and target domains. With the emergence of unpaired image-to-image translation approaches such as CycleGAN [23] and UNIT [13], image-level alignment is also used to tackle the UDA problem [8]. By utilizing a cycle-consistency loss between the input and the reconstructed images, the models are trained without paired data. Then, image-level alignment can be achieved by generating pseudo target domain images from the source domain images. In this work, we adopt image-level alignment paradigm to bridge the domain gap between ceT1 and hrT2.

2.2 Self-training in UDA

Self-training strategies have shown promising results in the field of UDA by fully utilizing the unlabeled target domain data. It has been shown to improve the performance of the segmentation models by fine-tuning them on the target images with pseudo labels. Zou et al. [25] propose a confidence regularized self-training framework which encourages the smoothness of the network output and reduces the confidence in false positives during training. Yu et al. [22] use a portion of the pseudo labels with high probability to iteratively fine-tune the model and achieve superior performance on a UDA dataset. This strategy is also used by the top teams in CrossMoDA 2021 [5], further demonstrating its effectiveness in the UDA problem.

3   Methods

3.1   Overview

In this study, we propose to tackle the UDA segmentation problem by following the popular "synthesis-then-segmentation" training strategy [1,3,12,18]. Specifically, we perform unpaired image translation to synthesize the pseudo target domain images in a cross-site and cross-modality fashion. Then we devise a rule-based offline augmentation method to further increase the data variability. Lastly, we adopt the nnU-Net framework and perform self-training to train a target-domain segmentation model with both the synthetic and real target domain data.

3.2   Cross-Site Cross-Modality Unpaired Image Translation

Since our task is to segment the VS and cochlea in hrT2 images while their labels are only available in the unpaired ceT1 images, we adopt an unpaired

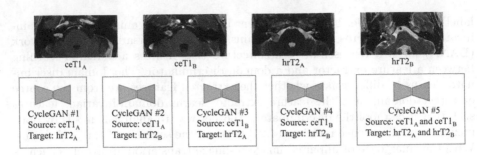

Fig. 2. The diagram of cross-site cross-modality unpaired image translation.

image translation method, i.e., CycleGAN [23], to bridge the gap between the two modalities and synthesize pseudo hrT2 from ceT1. Then the pseudo hrT2 images with the annotations from the corresponding ceT1 can be utilized to train segmentation models. However, MRIs (both ceT1 and hrT2) in the provided dataset were acquired from two different sites, and we observe slight appearance differences within each modality (especially hrT2) across sites. To enrich the diversity of the pseudo hrT2 images, we synthesize them using ceT1 within and across sites. Specifically, as shown in Fig. 2, five CycleGAN models are trained with different source/target domain data configurations to generate pseudo hrT2 images. We use subscripts to denote images from site A or site B, e.g., $hrT2_A$ means hrT2 from site A. Compared to only generating within-site pseudo images, i.e., pseudo $hrT2_A$ from $ceT1_A$ (CycleGAN #1) and pseudo $hrT2_B$ from $ceT1_B$ (CycleGAN #4), our cross-site training scheme can generate twice more pseudo hrT2 data for the downstream task of nnU-Net segmentation. Note that Cycle-GAN #5 has the same network architecture as the other four, and the only difference is that its training set contains images from both site A and site B.

3.3   Rule-Based Offline Augmentation for VS and Cochlea

Thanks to the unpaired image translation, the domain gap between ceT1 and hrT2 can be substantially reduced at the image-level by generating pseudo hrT2 images. However, there is still a domain gap between the pseudo and real hrT2, as we observe that the cochlea and VS in the pseudo hrT2 images do not have the same intensity characteristics as in the real hrT2 images. To overcome this issue, we propose to adjust the intensities of the VS and cochlea regions in pseudo hrT2 images to further minimize the domain gap, as shown in Fig. 3. As suggested by [1], for VS, we reduce the signal intensity of the voxels that are labeled as VS by 50% to further increase the heterogeneity of VS signals [1]. This VS augmentation is randomly applied to 50% of our pseudo hrT2 images. Cochleae typically have high signal intensities in hrT2 images, with values that were empirically found to be within the [85th, 95th] intensity percentile. However, we observe that the generated cochlea in pseudo hrT2 images can have low intensities or can even be absent. To improve the appearance of pseudo hrT2 images with a mean cochlea

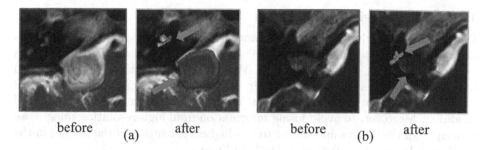

before   (a)   after   before   (b)   after

Fig. 3. An illustration of the rule-based offline augmentation technique on two cases. Orange and blue arrows represent the augmented cochlea and VS, respectively. (Color figure online)

intensity lower than the 85th intensity percentile, we replace the original intensity of the cochlea voxels by a value randomly sampled from a uniform distribution, which is bounded by the 85th and 95th intensity percentile of that image. Lastly, the augmented cochlea region is smoothed by a 3D Gaussian kernel to further refine the cochlea appearance. The cochlea augmentation is applied to all the pseudo hrT2 images.

3.4   Segmentation with NnU-Net and Self-training

With the augmented pseudo hrT2 images, we can train a segmentation model supervised by the paired ceT1 labels. Here, we utilize a popular self-configuring segmentation framework, i.e., nnU-Net, for supervised learning. However, with this approach the real hrT2 images are not involved in training the segmentation model due to the lack of labels. To tackle this problem, we adopt a self-training strategy to make use of the unlabeled real hrT2 images. Specifically, we firstly use the model trained on pseudo hrT2 images to obtain the pseudo labels of the unlabeled real hrT2 images. Next, we re-train the nnU-Net with the combined data, i.e., pseudo hrT2 images with real ceT1 labels and real hrT2 images with pseudo labels. Note that we perform self-training several (in our case, 3) times, since we observe improvements on the validation leaderboard each time the network is re-trained with the updated pseudo labels produced by self-training.

4   Experiments and Results

4.1   Dataset

The dataset was released by the MICCAI challenge CrossMoDA 2022 [16]. 105 ceT1 and 105 hrT2 unpaired images were obtained on a 32-channel Siemens Avanto 1.5T scanner, which are called "London data" or site A data. Another 105 ceT1 and 105 hrT2 unpaired images were obtained on a Philips Ingenia 1.5T scanner, which are called "Tilburg data" or site B data. Image resolutions are different for images from different sequences and sites. The manually segmented mask of the VS and cochlea for the 210 ceT1 images are provided.

4.2   Pre-processing and Network Training

We observe that the fields of view and resolutions vary substantially across different sites and modalities. Inspired by [12], to discard the irrelevant brain regions in our task, we first crop each MRI scan into a region of interest (ROI) by rigid registration with an atlas. Specifically, we use 4 atlases (2 sites × 2 modalities) and we register each scan with the atlas from the same site and modality. Moreover, to avoid losing information from high-resolution images, we resample all the images and masks to the highest resolution of the images in the challenge dataset, i.e., [0.4102, 0.4102, 1.0] mm.

For CycleGANs, we train the 5 models (as in Fig. 2) in both 2D and 3D settings. The patch size for 2D CycleGANs is 256 × 256 and for 3D is 112 × 112 × 24. Random cropping or zero padding is used when the dimension of the resampled ROI does not match the patch size during training. We use Adam optimizer [10] with a fixed learning rate of 2e-4. The training is stopped after 100 epochs for the 2D CycleGANs and after 1000 epochs for the 3D CycleGANs. Sliding window inference with an overlapping ratio of 0.8 is used to generate the final synthesis results. Synthesized 2D slices are then merged into the 3D volumes based on their original positions.

For nnU-Net training, we use the network architecture and patch size provided by the 3D fullres mode. Five-fold cross-validation is used. The Dice loss + cross-entropy loss is used as the loss function. The SGD optimizer with an initial learning rate of 1e-2 is used and the learning rate is decayed by a polynomial function. We do not apply connected component analysis to post-process the segmentation results, as we find that the impact of this post-processing operation on the segmentation results varies across folds.

Overall, we use 4 training stages. In stage 1, we train the nnU-Net with the pseudo hrT2 images generated from 2D and 3D CycleGANs. In stage 2, we replace the images from 2D CycleGANs with real hrT2 images for self-training. In stage 3, we apply offline VS augmentation and oversample the pseudo hrT2 images with small tumors, as we observe on the validation leaderboard that the small-tumor segmentation performance of our network is low. We oversample the pseudo hrT2 images with small tumors based on the VS labels from ceT1 till the training data size reaches 1000 (maximum number that nnU-Net allows). In stage 4, we perform another round of self-training and use the ensemble model from stages 2, 3, and 4 as our final model by averaging softmax probabilities.

4.3   Experimental Results

Synthesis Results. In Fig. 4, we qualitatively show the effectiveness of the cross-site cross-modality unpaired image translation. We select a representative ceT1 image from site A and generate the pseudo hrT2 images using CycleGAN #1, #2, and #5, which generate pseudo hrT2 from site A, site B, and a combination of site A and site B, respectively. Two representative real hrT2 images from site A and from site B are provided in Fig. 4 for comparison. We observe the consistency of the overall image contrast characteristics between the pseudo and real images from the same site.

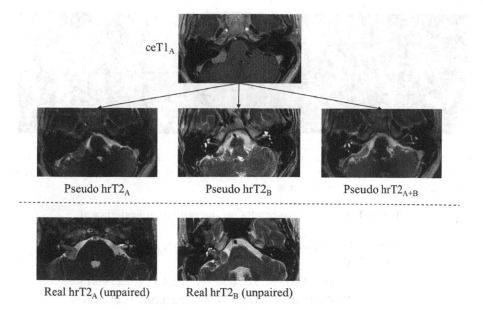

Fig. 4. Synthesis results of the cross-site cross-modality unpaired image translation. First row: source domain (ceT1) image. Second row: pseudo target domain (hrT2) images. Third row: real target domain (hrT2) images as reference.

Segmentation Results. For quantitative evaluation, we submit our segmentation results to the validation leaderboard, where the Dice score and average symmetric surface distance (ASSD) between segmentation results and the ground truth are computed. In Table 1, we show the segmentation results for both VS and cochlea obtained at each training stage (the configurations are described in detail in Sect. 3.2). We notice that the largest improvement is observed from stage 1 to stage 2, when the model is trained on real target domain images for the first time. Moreover, the effectiveness of our proposed offline VS augmentation and small-tumor oversampling is demonstrated by the improvement observed from stage 2 to stage 3. Lastly, the mean Dice scores and ASSDs achieved by our final ensemble model are 0.8178 ± 0.0803 and 0.8433 ± 0.0293, and 0.6673 ± 0.2713 mm and 0.2053 ± 0.1489 mm for VS and cochlea, respectively. For qualitative evaluation, we visualize the segmentation results in Fig. 5 for four representative cases (a and b are from site A; c and d are from site B). We posit that the poor VS segmentation, i.e., f and h, is due to the uncommon appearances of VS in the validation set, which can be difficult to synthesize if such appearances rarely exist in our target domain training dataset.

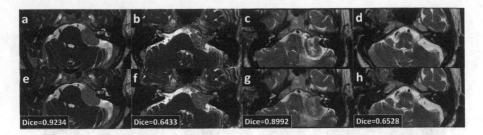

Fig. 5. Qualitative results on the validation set. The first row and the second row correspond to the hrT2 images and their segmentation results, respectively. Note that a, b and c, d are from different sites.

Table 1. Quantitative results on the validation leaderboard

Stage	Dice↑ (%)		ASSD↓ (mm)	
	VS	Cochlea	VS	Cochlea
1	73.54±24.26	81.91±4.33	1.89±8.41	0.25±0.15
2	77.97±18.29	82.42±4.01	0.72±0.29	0.23±0.15
3	80.37±9.64	**84.46±2.97**	1.14±1.73	0.22±0.18
ensemble	**81.78±8.03**	84.33±2.93	**0.67±0.27**	**0.21±0.15**

5   Discussion and Conclusion

In the CrossMoDA 2021 challenge, we have observed that there were three important components used by the top teams including (1) segmentation via nnU-Net [1,3,18], (2) self-training with real target domain data [3,18], and (3) data augmentation for VS and cochlea [1,11]. Based on this observation, our proposed method for CrossMoDA 2022 also incorporates these components to achieve competitive performance on the leaderboard. To address the additional domain gap (multi-site MRI) in CrossMoDA 2022, we synthesize site-specific pseudo target domain images with multiple CycleGAN models. Nevertheless, we conjecture that the segmentation performance might be further improved if we also train site-specific target domain segmentation models; this will be investigated.

In conclusion, we proposed a solution to tackle the UDA problem for VS and cochlea segmentation in CrossMoDA 2022. We developed a cross-site cross-modality unpaired image translation strategy to enrich the diversity of the synthesized data and a rule-based offline augmentation method to further minimize the domain gap. Lastly, we empowered the nnU-Net by self-training to make use of the unlabeled data. According to the validation leaderboard, our method has achieved a promising segmentation performance on both VS and cochlea.

Acknowledgements. This work was supported in part by the NIH grants NIDCD-DC014462, NIDCD-DC008408, NIBIB-T32EB021937, and by the Advanced Computing Center for Research and Education (ACCRE) of Vanderbilt University. This publication contents are solely the responsibility of the authors and do not necessarily represent the official views of the founding institutes.

References

1. Choi, J.W.: Using out-of-the-box frameworks for unpaired image translation and image segmentation for the crossmoda challenge. arXiv e-prints, pp. arXiv-2110 (2021)
2. Coelho, D.H., Tang, Y., Suddarth, B., Mamdani, M.: MRI surveillance of vestibular schwannomas without contrast enhancement: clinical and economic evaluation. Laryngoscope **128**(1), 202–209 (2018)
3. Dong, H., Yu, F., Zhao, J., Dong, B., Zhang, L.: Unsupervised domain adaptation in semantic segmentation based on pixel alignment and self-training. arXiv preprint arXiv:2109.14219 (2021)
4. Dorent, R., et al.: Scribble-based domain adaptation via co-segmentation. In: Martel, A.L., et al. (eds.) MICCAI 2020. LNCS, vol. 12261, pp. 479–489. Springer, Cham (2020). https://doi.org/10.1007/978-3-030-59710-8_47
5. Dorent, R., et al.: Crossmoda 2021 challenge: Benchmark of cross-modality domain adaptation techniques for vestibular schwannoma and cochlea segmentation (2022)
6. Ganin, Y., et al.: Domain-adversarial training of neural networks. In: Csurka, G. (ed.) Domain Adaptation in Computer Vision Applications. ACVPR, pp. 189–209. Springer, Cham (2017). https://doi.org/10.1007/978-3-319-58347-1_10
7. Guan, H., Liu, M.: Domain adaptation for medical image analysis: a survey. IEEE Trans. Biomed. Eng. **69**(3), 1173–1185 (2022). https://doi.org/10.1109/TBME.2021.3117407
8. Hoffman, J., et al.: Cycada: cycle-consistent adversarial domain adaptation. In: Proceedings of the 35th International Conference on Machine Learning, pp. 1989–1998. PMLR, July 2018. https://proceedings.mlr.press/v80/hoffman18a.html
9. Isensee, F., Jaeger, P.F., Kohl, S.A., Petersen, J., Maier-Hein, K.H.: nnU-net: a self-configuring method for deep learning-based biomedical image segmentation. Nat. Methods **18**(2), 203–211 (2021)
10. Kingma, D.P., Ba, J.: Adam: a method for stochastic optimization. arXiv arXiv:1412.6980, January 2017
11. Li, H., Hu, D., Zhu, Q., Larson, K.E., Zhang, H., Oguz, I.: Unsupervised cross-modality domain adaptation for segmenting vestibular schwannoma and cochlea with data augmentation and model ensemble. In: Crimi, A., Bakas, S. (eds.) Brainlesion: Glioma, Multiple Sclerosis, Stroke and Traumatic Brain Injuries. BrainLes 2021. LNCS, vol. 12963, pp. pp. 518–528. Springer, Cham (2022). https://doi.org/10.1007/978-3-031-09002-8_45
12. Liu, H., Fan, Y., Cui, C., Su, D., McNeil, A., Dawant, B.M.: Unsupervised domain adaptation for vestibular schwannoma and cochlea segmentation via semi-supervised learning and label fusion. In: Crimi, A., Bakas, S. (eds.) Brainlesion: Glioma, Multiple Sclerosis, Stroke and Traumatic Brain Injuries, pp. 529–539. Springer International Publishing, Cham (2022)

13. Liu, M.Y., Breuel, T., Kautz, J.: Unsupervised image-to-image translation networks. In: Advances in Neural Information Processing Systems, vol. 30. Curran Associates, Inc. (2017). https://proceedings.neurips.cc/paper/2017/hash/dc6a6489640ca02b0d42dabeb8e46bb7-Abstract.html

14. Long, M., Cao, Y., Wang, J., Jordan, M.I.: Learning transferable features with deep adaptation networks. arXiv arXiv:1502.02791, May 2015. arXiv.org:1502.02791

15. Pizzini, F.B., et al.: Usefulness of high resolution t2-weighted images in the evaluation and surveillance of vestibular schwannomas? Is gadolinium needed? Otol. Neurotol. **41**(1), e103–e110 (2020)

16. Shapey, J.: Segmentation of vestibular schwannoma from MRI, an open annotated dataset and baseline algorithm. Sci. Data **8**(1), 1–6 (2021)

17. Shapey, J., et al.: An artificial intelligence framework for automatic segmentation and volumetry of vestibular schwannomas from contrast-enhanced t1-weighted and high-resolution t2-weighted MRI. J. Neurosurg. **134**(1), 171–179 (2019)

18. Shin, H., Kim, H., Kim, S., Jun, Y., Eo, T., Hwang, D.: COSMOS: cross-modality unsupervised domain adaptation for 3d medical image segmentation based on target-aware domain translation and iterative self-training. arXiv preprint arXiv:2203.16557 (2022)

19. Vestibular schwannoma (acoustic neuroma) and neurofibromatosis. https://www.nidcd.nih.gov/health/vestibular-schwannoma-acoustic-neuroma-and-neurofibromatosis

20. Wang, G., et al.: Automatic segmentation of vestibular Schwannoma from T2-weighted MRI by deep spatial attention with hardness-weighted loss. In: Shen, D., et al. (eds.) MICCAI 2019. LNCS, vol. 11765, pp. 264–272. Springer, Cham (2019). https://doi.org/10.1007/978-3-030-32245-8_30

21. Yan, H., Ding, Y., Li, P., Wang, Q., Xu, Y., Zuo, W.: Mind the class weight bias: weighted maximum mean discrepancy for unsupervised domain adaptation. In: 2017 IEEE Conference on Computer Vision and Pattern Recognition (CVPR). p. 945–954. IEEE, Honolulu, HI, July 2017. https://doi.org/10.1109/CVPR.2017.107, http://ieeexplore.ieee.org/document/8099590/

22. Yu, F., Zhang, M., Dong, H., Hu, S., Dong, B., Zhang, L.: DAST: unsupervised domain adaptation in semantic segmentation based on discriminator attention and self-training. Proc. AAAI Conf. Artif. Intell. **35**(1212), 10754–10762 (2021). https://doi.org/10.1609/aaai.v35i12.17285

23. Zhu, J.Y., Park, T., Isola, P., Efros, A.A.: Unpaired image-to-image translation using cycle-consistent adversarial networks. In: Proceedings of the IEEE International Conference on Computer Vision, pp. 2223–2232 (2017)

24. Zhu, Q., Li, H., Cass, N.D., Lindquist, N.R., Tawfik, K.O., Oguz, I.: Acoustic neuroma segmentation using ensembled convolutional neural networks. In: Medical Imaging 2022: Biomedical Applications in Molecular, Structural, and Functional Imaging, vol. 12036, pp. 228–234. SPIE (2022)

25. Zou, Y., Yu, Z., Vijaya Kumar, B.V.K., Wang, J.: Unsupervised domain adaptation for semantic segmentation via class-balanced self-training. In: Ferrari, V., Hebert, M., Sminchisescu, C., Weiss, Y. (eds.) ECCV 2018. LNCS, vol. 11207, pp. 297–313. Springer, Cham (2018). https://doi.org/10.1007/978-3-030-01219-9_18

FeTS

Regularized Weight Aggregation in Networked Federated Learning for Glioblastoma Segmentation

Muhammad Irfan Khan[1(✉)], Mohammad Ayyaz Azeem[2], Esa Alhoniemi[1],
Elina Kontio[1], Suleiman A. Khan[1], and Mojtaba Jafaritadi[1]

[1] Turku University of Applied Sciences, 20520 Turku, Finland
{irfan.khan,esa.alhoniemi,elina.kontio,
suleiman.alikhan,mojtaba.jafaritadi}@turkuamk.fi
[2] Riphah International University, Islamabad 45210, Pakistan
32175@student.riphah.edu.pk

Abstract. In federated learning (FL), the global model at the server requires an efficient mechanism for weight aggregation and a systematic strategy for collaboration selection to manage and optimize communication payload. We introduce a practical and cost-efficient method for regularized weight aggregation and propose a laborsaving technique to select collaborators per round. We illustrate the performance of our method, regularized similarity weight aggregation (RegSimAgg), on the Federated Tumor Segmentation (FeTS) 2022 challenge's federated training (weight aggregation) problem. Our scalable approach is principled, frugal, and suitable for heterogeneous non-IID collaborators. Using FeTS2021 evaluation criterion, our proposed algorithm RegSimAgg stands at 3rd position in the final rankings of FeTS2022 challenge in the weight aggregation task. Our solution is open sourced at: https://github.com/dskhanirfan/FeTS2022.

Keywords: Brain Tumors · Cancer · Collaborative Learning · Federated Learning · FeTS Challenge · Lesion Segmentation · Weight Aggregation

1 Introduction

Federated learning (FL) is on the horizon to replace the current paradigm of data sharing, allowing for privacy-preserving cross-institutional research including a wide range of biomedical disciplines. In simple terms, FL is a machine learning paradigm in a distributed or decentralized setting. It is particularly favorable because pooling all the curated data from different data silos to a central location is arduous, for training machine learning models. Moreover, sharing sensitive data is becoming increasingly difficult due to data privacy and security concerns, bureaucratic challenges and stringent GDPR (EU) and HIPAA (US) laws [1, 20].

S. Bakas et al. (Eds.): BrainLes 2022, LNCS 14092, pp. 121–132, 2023.
https://doi.org/10.1007/978-3-031-44153-0_12

The implementation of FL in practice requires several distinct clients called *collaborators* to contribute to the creation of a global expert model via a defined server called an *aggregator*. Each collaborator provides some of the information that the aggregator would combine [14]. The aggregator does not have access to the collaborator's private data, which does not egress from the collaborator. The actual training tasks are executed at the collaborators, because each collaborator has a chunk of the whole data. During federation rounds, participating collaborators cartel the parameters combined at the server for a unified consensus model to foster knowledge exchange. This global model is assembled by learned information, in terms of parameters, from a conglomerate of individual participating collaborators that execute the learning task independently. Hence, model training is essentially performed in a distributed fashion on the data hoarded at distinct edge devices. After model training, the generalizable global model or model parameters are dispatched to the collaborators [7]. Consequently, in a federation process, all the participating collaborators get potential benefit from the global model at the aggregator, because they receive the learned model parameters collected from trained models on other collaborators as well. Moreover, the performance and inference of global model, trained on several collaborators, on unseen data is better as compared to the model trained on any individual collaborator data. Figure 1 shows a high-level schema of the federated learning framework.

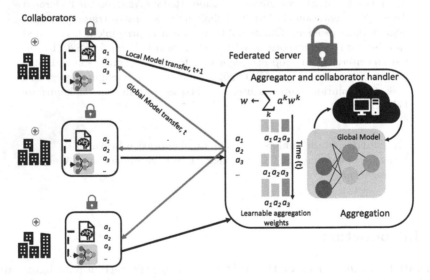

Fig. 1. General workflow of an FL-trained model and the key components in a federated learning setting [23]. Private collaborators communicate the local weight updates with a federated secure server at regularly occurring intervals to learn a global model; the server aggregates the updates and sends back the parameters of the updated global model to the clients. The aggregation weights are learned on the clients and dynamically adjusted throughout the training process when communicating with the federated server.

The utility spectrum of federated learning is quite broad with wide-range applications in telecommunication services, fintech, and healthcare sector. In healthcare, data analytics in radiology and genomics can particularly welfare from harnessing the power of FL ecosystem. A direct clinical impact of FL therefore could be made in the most-effective translation medicine, e.g. privacy-preserving medical image segmentation [11,19]. However, training a shared generalizable global model for medical image segmentation in a federated fashion presents a number of challenges and limitations. These include training local models using different imaging modalities on many scanners from different manufacturers, acquisition times, and various image resolutions and protocols. The improper use of such training data, referred to as not independent and identically distributed (non-IID), thus can result in performance degradation among different clients. FL has been combined with domain adaptation [25], contrastive learning [9], and knowledge distillation [13] in order to learn a more generalizable federated model. Other limitations include cross domain and imbalance of annotated data (limited labeling budgets) [6]. The challenge of data heterogeneity and domain shifting was recently tackled in novel ways by, for example, federated disentanglement learning via disentangling the parameter space into shape and appearance [6] and automated federated averaging based on Dirichlet distribution [22]. Dynamic Re-Weighting mechanisms [12], federated cross ensemble learning [24], and label-agnostic (mixed labels) unified FL formed by a mixture of the client distributions [21] have been recently proposed to relax an unrealistic assumption that each client's training set will be annotated similarly and therefore follows the same image supervision level during the training of an image segmentation model. Although extensive research has been carried out on FL, there is still a need for methods to enable the development of more generalized FL models for clinical use which can effectively deal with statistical heterogeneity in weight aggregation, communication efficiency, and privacy with security.

In this paper, we aim to establish an adaptive regularized weight aggregation by upgrading our previously developed similarity weight aggregation (SimAgg) algorithm [8]. We propose a robust and efficient federated lesion segmentation algorithm applicable in generalized and realistic detection of the "rare" disease of glioblastoma, a form of brain cancerous tumor, and particularly on the delineation of its sub-regions by leveraging multi-modal magnetic resonance imaging (MRI) brain scans [17]. We present an extensive evaluation of the proposed regularized similarity weight aggregation (RegSimAgg) strategy in a networked federated learning fashion. In the light of our previous research in FeTS2021, we propose an efficient yet simple method for addressing FeTS2022 and existing challenges of FL.

The rest of this paper is organized as follows: in Sect. 2, we describe the upgraded methodologies to the previous SimAgg algorithm including collaborator selection and weight aggregation regularization through our experiment setting. In Sect. 3, we describe FL experiments and evaluate the performance of the proposed method quantitatively and in Sect. 4, we discuss about the presented work, potentials and limitations, and describe our future direction in FL. Finally, Sect. 5 concludes this work.

2   Methods

2.1   FeTS 2022 Challenge

Federated Tumor Segmentation (FeTS) 2022 is a continuation to the previous FeTS2021 [17] challenge with the focus on federated training methodologies including weight aggregation, client selection, training per-round, compression, communication efficiency, and algorithmic generalizability on out-of-sample data. It is intended to build and evaluate a consensus model that effectively identifies intrinsically heterogeneous brain tumors.

The FeTS 2022 challenge provides updated multi-institutional multiparametric Magnetic Resonance Imaging (mpMRI) scans of glioblastoma (GBM), the most common primary brain tumor, prior to any kind of resection surgery. The datasets used in the FeTS 2022 challenge are the subset of GBM cases from the Brain Tumor Segmentation (BraTS) Continuous Challenge which aims at identifying state-of-the-art segmentation algorithms for brain diffuse glioma patients and their sub-regions [2–5,15].

All FeTS brain MRI scans, provided as NIfTI files (`.nii.gz`), had four structural MRI sequences including native (T1), post-contrast T1-weighted (T1Gd), T2-weighted (T2), and T2 FLuid Attenuated Inversion Recovery (FLAIR) volumes. Image samples were acquired with different clinical protocols and various scanners from multiple data contributing institutions. One to four raters annotated each of the images manually, following a standardized protocol, and their annotations were approved by neuroradiologists. Annotations comprise the pathologically confirmed segmentation labels with similar volume size of $240 \times 240 \times 155$ including the GD-enhancing tumor (ET—label 4), the peritumoral edematous/invaded tissue (ED—label 2), and the necrotic tumor core (NCR—label 1). All these provided MRI scans including the ground truth data were preprocessed such as rigid registration, brain extraction, alignment, $1 \times 1 \times 1$ mm resolution resampling, and skull stripping were applied as described in [15].

The training and validation datasets include 1251 and 219 subjects, respectively. The training set consists of two partitions each providing information for how to split the training data into non-IID institutional subsets. That is, each patient dataset is linked to a de-identified partitioning label according to the acquiring institutions.

We deployed Intel Federated Learning (OpenFL) [18] framework for training brain tumor segmentation model—an encoder-decoder 3D U-shape type of convolutional neural network provided by FeTS2022 challenge—using the data-private collaborative learning paradigm of FL [16]. OpenFL considers two main components: 1) the collaborator which uses a local dataset to train the global model and 2) the aggregator which receives model updates from each collaborator and fuses them to form the global model.

2.2   Regularized Similarity Weighted Aggregation (RegSimAgg)

In FeTS 2021 challenge, we suggested a novel aggregation method named Similarity Weighted Aggregation (SimAgg) for efficient aggregation of model parameters at the server that is suitable for both IID as well as non-IID data [8]. Here, we propose an extension of SimAgg method which contains a regularization mechanism to speed up convergence, which is a critical issue in the computationally demanding federated learning framework.

Collaborator Selection. We allow collaborators to contribute in a nondeterministic fashion by picking up a subset of the available collaborators (for example, 20%) at each round. To ensure that the model sees all collaborators the same number of times at regular intervals, we use a sliding window over the randomized collaborator index as shown in Fig. 2; once all collaborators have participated in the updates, the order is randomly shuffled. In this manner, we ensure roughly equal participation of all collaborators. However, a particular combination of the collaborators selected in one FL round will not be repeated in the successive rounds.

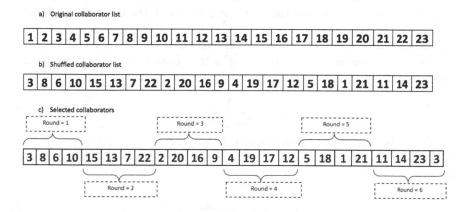

Fig. 2. Strategy for choosing collaborators. In a) Original collaborator list is given to the model, in b) collaborator order is randomized, and in c) collaborators are selected for each round using a sliding window. The collaborator list is reshuffled once it has been fully utilized, and the process repeats step b). The collaborators chosen in a certain combination during one FL round, however, will not be chosen again during subsequent rounds.

Weight Aggregation. The fact that model parameters from the collaborators can differ is a major concern with non-IID data. We employ weighted aggregation of the collaborators at the server to overcome such a scenario. The collaborators' weights are determined by measuring similarity of the collaborators to their non-weighted average. We have also learned that, from the convergence point of view, it is beneficial to add regularization to the weighting process after the initial FL rounds. Our aggregation algorithm is compactly described in Algorithm 1, and the steps are explained in detail below.

At round r, the parameters p_{C^r} of the participating collaborators C^r are sent to the server. At the server, the average of these parameters is calculated as:

$$\hat{p} = \frac{1}{|C^r|} \Sigma_{i \in C^r} p_i. \tag{1}$$

We then calculate the inverse distance (similarity) of each collaborator $c \in C^r$ from the average:

$$sim_c = \frac{\Sigma_{i \in C^r} |p_i - \hat{p}|}{|p_c - \hat{p}| + \epsilon}, \tag{2}$$

where $\epsilon = 1e - 5$ (small positive constant). We normalize the distances to obtain *similarity weights* as follows:

$$u_c = \frac{sim_c}{\Sigma_{i \in C^r} sim_i}. \tag{3}$$

The collaborators close to the average receive a high similarity weight and vice versa. In the extreme case this approach can expel the diverging collaborator.

In order to adjust for the effect of varying number of samples at each collaborator $c \in C^r$, we use *sample size weights* that favor collaborators with large sample sizes:

$$v_c = \frac{N_c}{\Sigma_{i \in C^r} N_i}, \tag{4}$$

where N_c is the number of examples at collaborator c.

Using the weights obtained using Eqs. 3 and 4, the *aggregation weights* are computed as:

$$w_c = \frac{u_c + v_c}{\Sigma_{i \in C^r} (u_i + v_i)}, \tag{5}$$

If we have run enough iterations (e.g., $r > 10$), we also regularize the aggregation weights:

$$w_c = \frac{w_c}{\frac{1}{|C^r|} \Sigma_{i \in C^r} (p_i^{\text{prev}} - p_i)}. \tag{6}$$

Compared to the SimAgg method proposed earlier by us in [8], this is the only but remarkable change in our algorithm. The basic idea is to let the FL system learn fast during the initial FL rounds after which the regularization makes learning somewhat slower but stable by suppressing significant weight adjustments. The FL round iteration limit (here 10) for starting the regularization is a hyperparameter of the FL aggregator, and based on our experience it is sensible to set it to a relatively small value.

The parameters are finally aggregated as a weighted average using the aggregation weights:

$$p^m = \frac{1}{|C^r|} \cdot \Sigma_{i \in C^r} (w_i \cdot p_i). \tag{7}$$

The normalized aggregated parameters p^m are dispatched to the next set of collaborators in the successive federation rounds.

Algorithm 1. RegSimAgg aggregation algorithm

1: **procedure** REGULARIZED SIMILARITY WEIGHTED AGGREGATION(C^r, p_{C^r}, $p_{C^r}^{\text{prev}}$)
2:     $\epsilon \leftarrow 1e - 5$ ▷ C^r = set of collaborators (at round r)
3:     $\hat{p}$ = average(p_{C^r}) using **Eq. 1** ▷ p_{C^r} = parameters of the collaborators in C^r
4:     **for** c in C^r **do**
5:         Compute similarity weights u_c using **Eqs. 2** and **3**
6:         Compute sample weights v_c using **Eq. 4**
7:     **for** c in C^r **do**
8:         Compute aggregation weights w_c using **Eq. 5**
9:     **if** $r > 10$ **then**
10:         Regularize the aggregation weights w_c using **Eq. 6**
11:     Compute master model parameters p^m using **Eq. 7**
12:     **return** p^m

---

3   Experiments

3.1   Setup

Task 1 focuses on efficient aggregation, client selection, training-per-round, and communication efficiency in order to optimize the federation process. We have devised a mechanism for aggregating model updates trained on individual collaborators that is both efficient and effective. A training data set with total of 1251 multi-institutional patients and 219 validation data set was available. Supplementary data shows how patients are divided into distinct partitions. Partition 1 has 23 contributors, whereas partition 2 has 33 collaborators. For the semantic segmentation of the whole tumor, tumor core, and enhancing tumor, the experimental setup leverages Intel's OpenFL platform for federated learning and a preconfigured 3D U-shape neural network. Binary DICE similarity (whole tumor, enhancing tumor, tumor core) and Hausdorff (95 percent) distance are the metrics computed in the aggregation rounds (whole tumor, enhancing tumor, tumor core) as described in [17].

The hyperparameters used are shown in Table 1. Collaborator selection for RegSimAgg is shown in Fig. 2.

Table 1. Hyperparameters used in aggregation algorithms.

Hyperparameter	RegSimAgg
Learning rate	5e−5
Epochs per round	1.0

3.2   Results

In this section, regularized similarity weighted aggregation (RegSimAgg) findings are summarized for partition 2. The results demonstrate that our approach quickly converges and maintains stability as learning advances across all assessed criteria.

Model Training and Performance Using Internal Validation Data. Figure 3 shows the performance of model training on internal validation data for partition 2.

Model Performance Using External Validation Data. Prior to the formal testing phase, challenge organizers provided 219 cases of external validation data that we used to evaluate the performance of our approach RegSimAgg, see Tables 2. Overall, RegSimAgg performs better on whole tumor segmentation as compared to enhancing tumor segmentation and tumor core segmentation.

Model Performance Using Fully Blinded Test Set. Team HT-TUAS submitted RegSimAgg algorithm for the leaderboard ranking. Model training is performed for 500 rounds by challenge organizers. The performance stats on the fully blinded test set for 570 patients are shown in Tables 3. When a weightage of 6 is given to the communication cost, our team achieved third place in the leaderboard.

4   Discussion

Several federated aggregation methods like exponential smoothing aggregation and conditional threshold aggregation methods require user defined threshold parameter settings. Therefore, these algorithms are not easily applicable to new and unexplored data sets. To overcome this issue, we developed regularized similarity weighted aggregation, which adaptively learns the participating collaborator weights.

Our method does not require any participation in the modeling process at the client side but it learns a global model at the server side. It is able to minimize the contribution of diverging collaborators and allows clients with varying settings to join the federation. This is in contrast to Fedprox [10], which performs client side regularization of diverging collaborators. Moreover, studies have shown that training federated learning algorithms using a randomly selected subset of collaborators expedites the process [26]. We expanded on these ideas and developed a sliding window technique that corroborates that all collaborators participate in the training process.

FeTS 2022 data is released in two partitions which split the training data into non-IID data sets based on institution and tumor size. As a result, amount

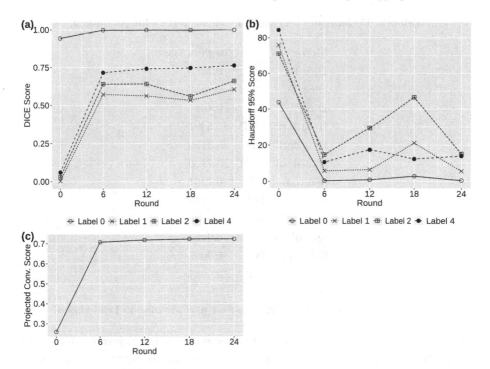

Fig. 3. Performance metrics for model training of RegSimAgg for partition 2 for internal validation. The horizontal axis refers to the number of rounds and the vertical axis to the performance metrics. (a) DICE Score for labels 0, 1, 2, 4; (b) Hausdorff 95% Score for labels 0, 1, 2, 4; (c) Projected Convergence Score. Total simulation time was approximately 154 h.

and characteristics of data may vary for different collaborators. Weighted aggregation strategy helps to learn a model that represents well the majority of the contributors at each round with low impact by outliers. Therefore, our method works well on both partitions. Even though the model works well when data has non-IID splits in general, it could be also be useful to study the performance on outliers further.

A limitation of the current setting is that the number of patients for each collaborator is fixed. In a real-world setting the patient data at a collaborator may change between federation rounds. Additional patient data potentially alters collaborator's data distribution – which might, in turn, affect the learned parameters at the master model: during the FL learning process, a previously diverging collaborator may become similar to the participating collaborators, compelling some other participating collaborators to become outliers. However, our approach takes diverging collaborator weights into account at each round. Hence, this method can be used as a baseline for refined generation of a better model that can be used at scale to newly generated data sets. Moreover, incorporation of our FL approach with a cutting-edge privacy protection AI framework

Table 2. Performance on external validation data for partition 2.

Metrics	RegSimAgg
Dice ET	0.7350
Dice TC	0.7337
Dice WT	0.8091
Hausdorff95 ET	30.3497
Hausdorff95 TC	25.3156
Hausdorff95 WT	23.7706
Sensitivity ET	0.7231
Sensitivity TC	0.7146
Sensitivity WT	0.8144
Specificity ET	0.9998
Specificity TC	0.9998
Specificity WT	0.9988

Table 3. RegSimAgg (HT-TUAS) test set performance on Leaderboard

	Mean	Standard Deviation	Median	25quantile	75quantile
DICE ET	0.6745	0.2920	0.8004	0.5704	0.8866
DICE WT	0.7247	0.2026	0.7820	0.6235	0.8811
DICE TC	0.7169	0.3002	0.8655	0.6154	0.9259
Sensitivity ET	0.7501	0.3087	0.8815	0.6882	0.9612
Sensitivity WT	0.7834	0.2044	0.8546	0.7079	0.9307
Sensitivity TC	0.7592	0.3091	0.9035	0.6990	0.9715
Specificity ET	0.9991	0.0017	0.9997	0.9992	0.9999
Specificity WT	0.9974	0.0033	0.9985	0.9968	0.9994
Specificity TC	0.9992	0.0017	0.9997	0.9994	0.9999
Hausdorff (95%) ET	35.2283	86.9517	3.7417	1.7321	19.1724
Hausdorff (95%) WT	35.9036	30.8538	31.6172	8.4853	58.6204
Hausdorff (95%) TC	33.7853	80.5775	6.4807	3.0000	20.1239
Communication Cost	0.6905	0.6905	0.6905	0.6905	0.6905

is one of our future research directions. We also intend to investigate a potential solution to the communication payload bottleneck between the collaborators and the server. Further, we will also study how a decrease in the payload throughput affects model convergence time-efficiency and task performance optimization.

5 Conclusion

In this paper, we propose regularized similarity weighted aggregation as an improved weight aggregation strategy for federated learning and apply it to imaging in order to achieve robust brain tumor segmentation. In our experiments, the proposed method – deployed in the OpenFL platform – performed well in terms of convergence score and communication costs. Currently, the proposed algorithm is a comprehensive proof-of-concept (POC) solution in the healthcare domain, demonstrated to potentially assist radiologists in diagnostic digital pathology. However, this edge computing infrastructure can easily be scaled to versatile real-world multi-client production level applications for foundational collaborative computation and federated learning workflows in other disciplines like internet-of-things (IoT) and telecommunication. Moreover, this methodology can issue stronger privacy guarantee via integrating differential privacy or secure multi-party computation, or a combination of the two, which is an intriguing future research topic.

Acknowledgements. This work was supported by the Business Finland under Grant 33961/31/2020. We also acknowledge the support and computational resources facilitated by the CSC-Puhti super-computer, a non-profit state enterprise owned by the Finnish state and higher education institutions in Finland.

References

1. Annas, G.J.: HIPAA regulations-a new era of medical—record privacy? (2003)
2. Baid, U., et al.: The RSNA-ASNR-MICCAI BraTS 2021 benchmark on brain tumor segmentation and radiogenomic classification. arXiv preprint arXiv:2107.02314 (2021)
3. Bakas, S., et al.: Segmentation labels and radiomic features for the pre-operative scans of the TCGA-GBM collection. The cancer imaging archive. Nat. Sci. Data **4**, 170117 (2017)
4. Bakas, S., et al.: Segmentation labels and radiomic features for the pre-operative scans of the TCGA-LGG collection. The cancer imaging archive **286** (2017)
5. Bakas, S., et al.: Advancing the cancer genome atlas glioma MRI collections with expert segmentation labels and radiomic features. Sci. Data **4**(1), 1–13 (2017)
6. Bernecker, T., et al.: FedNorm: modality-based normalization in federated learning for multi-modal liver segmentation. arXiv preprint arXiv:2205.11096 (2022)
7. Kairouz, P., et al.: Advances and open problems in federated learning (2019). https://arxiv.org/abs/1912.04977
8. Khan, M.I., Jafaritadi, M., Alhoniemi, E., Kontio, E., Khan, S.A.: Adaptive weight aggregation in federated learning for brain tumor segmentation. In: Crimi, A., Bakas, S. (eds.) Brainlesion: Glioma, Multiple Sclerosis, Stroke and Traumatic Brain Injuries, pp. 455–469. Springer, Cham (2022). https://doi.org/10.1007/978-3-031-09002-8_40
9. Li, Q., He, B., Song, D.: Model-contrastive federated learning. In: Proceedings of the IEEE/CVF Conference on Computer Vision and Pattern Recognition, pp. 10713–10722 (2021)

10. Li, T., Sahu, A.K., Zaheer, M., Sanjabi, M., Talwalkar, A., Smith, V.: Federated optimization in heterogeneous networks. arXiv preprint arXiv:1812.06127 (2018)
11. Li, W., et al.: Privacy-preserving federated brain tumour segmentation. In: Suk, H.-I., Liu, M., Yan, P., Lian, C. (eds.) MLMI 2019. LNCS, vol. 11861, pp. 133–141. Springer, Cham (2019). https://doi.org/10.1007/978-3-030-32692-0_16
12. Liu, D., et al.: MS lesion segmentation: revisiting weighting mechanisms for federated learning. arXiv preprint arXiv:2205.01509 (2022)
13. Liu, Q., Chen, C., Qin, J., Dou, Q., Heng, P.A.: FedDG: federated domain generalization on medical image segmentation via episodic learning in continuous frequency space. In: Proceedings of the IEEE/CVF Conference on Computer Vision and Pattern Recognition, pp. 1013–1023 (2021)
14. McMahan, B., Moore, E., Ramage, D., Hampson, S., Arcas, B.A.: Communication-efficient learning of deep networks from decentralized data. In: Artificial Intelligence and Statistics, pp. 1273–1282. PMLR (2017)
15. Menze, B.H., et al.: The multimodal brain tumor image segmentation benchmark (BRATS). IEEE Trans. Med. Imaging **34**(10), 1993–2024 (2014)
16. Pati, S., et al.: Federated learning enables big data for rare cancer boundary detection. arXiv preprint arXiv:2204.10836 (2022)
17. Pati, S., et al.: The federated tumor segmentation (FeTS) challenge. arXiv preprint arXiv:2105.05874 (2021)
18. Reina, G.A., et al.: OpenFL: an open-source framework for federated learning. arXiv preprint arXiv:2105.06413 (2021)
19. Sarma, K.V., et al.: Federated learning improves site performance in multicenter deep learning without data sharing. J. Am. Med. Inform. Assoc. **28**(6), 1259–1264 (2021)
20. Voigt, P., Von dem Bussche, A.: The EU general data protection regulation (GDPR). A Practical Guide, 1st Edn. Springer, Cham (2017). https://doi.org/10.1007/978-3-319-57959-7
21. Wicaksana, J., et al.: FedMix: mixed supervised federated learning for medical image segmentation. arXiv preprint arXiv:2205.01840 (2022)
22. Xia, Y., et al.: Auto-FedAvg: learnable federated averaging for multi-institutional medical image segmentation. arXiv preprint arXiv:2104.10195 (2021)
23. Xu, J., Glicksberg, B.S., Su, C., Walker, P., Bian, J., Wang, F.: Federated learning for healthcare informatics. J. Healthcare Inf. Res. **5**(1), 1–19 (2021)
24. Xu, X., et al.: Federated cross learning for medical image segmentation. arXiv preprint arXiv:2204.02450 (2022)
25. Yan, Z., Wicaksana, J., Wang, Z., Yang, X., Cheng, K.T.: Variation-aware federated learning with multi-source decentralized medical image data. IEEE J. Biomed. Health Inform. **25**(7), 2615–2628 (2020)
26. Zhao, Y., Li, M., Lai, L., Suda, N., Civin, D., Chandra, V.: Federated learning with non-IID data. arXiv preprint arXiv:1806.00582 (2018)

A Local Score Strategy for Weight Aggregation in Federated Learning

Gaurav Singh[✉]

Varanasi, India
gauravsingh141116@gmail.com

Abstract. Federated Learning is a new paradigm for training a machine learning model without sharing the data. Federated Learning aims to deal with this and achieve a competitive result like in centralised settings. FeTS Challenge is an initiative focusing on federated learning and robustness to distribution shifts between medical institutions for brain tumor segmentation. In this paper, we describe a method based on the local score rate for the weight aggregation of clients. We have reported results based on the Training, Validation and Testing of the FeTS 2022 dataset.

Keywords: Federated Learning · Convolutional Neural Network · MICCAI · Brain Tumor Segmentation · Federated Algorithms

1 Introduction

Traditional machine learning involves a data pipeline that uses a central server (on-premise or cloud) that hosts the trained model in order to make predictions. The downside of this architecture is that all the data collected by local devices and sensors are sent back to the central server for processing, and subsequently returned back to the devices. This round-trip limits a model's ability to learn in real time. Federated learning (FL) in contrast, is an approach that downloads the current model and computes an updated model at the device itself (aka edge computing) using local data. These locally trained models are then sent from the devices back to the central server where they are aggregated, i.e. averaging weights, and then a single consolidated and improved global model is sent back to the devices. There are several key challenges that must be addressed for effective federated training, such as expensive communication, systems and statistical heterogeneity, privacy concerns, effective aggregation and hyper-parameters selection [1,2].

FedAvg (Federated Averaging) [3] is a communication-efficient algorithm for distributed training, using relatively few rounds of communication. It works well empirically, mainly when it is non-convex problem, but it having a problem of convergence i.e. not guaranteed and can be diverged when data are heterogeneous. Another framework for FL, FedProx [4] to tackle heterogeneity in federated networks and it can be viewed as a generalization and re-parametrization

---

G. Singh—Independent Research.

© The Author(s), under exclusive license to Springer Nature Switzerland AG 2023
S. Bakas et al. (Eds.): BrainLes 2022, LNCS 14092, pp. 133–141, 2023.
https://doi.org/10.1007/978-3-031-44153-0_13

of the FedAvg algorithm. It also has more robust convergence than FedAvg. FedNova [5], a normalized averaging method that eliminates objective inconsistency while preserving fast error convergence. In another paper [6], authors proposed federated versions of adaptive optimizers, including adagrad, adam, and yogi, and analyzed their convergence in the presence of heterogeneous data for general non-convex settings. Their results highlighted the interplay between client heterogeneity and communication efficiency. In this paper, we describe a method based on the local score rate for the weight aggregation of clients. In addition, we mainly investigated the effective aggregation and statistical heterogeneity challenges. As part of FeTS Challenge 2022, we have conducted several experiments and reported results on FeTS validation and test dataset.

2   Dataset

We have used FeTS 2022 dataset [2,7–10] in this work. All FeTS mpMRI scans are available as NIfTI files (.nii.gz) and describe a) native (T1) and b) post-contrast T1-weighted (T1Gd), c) T2-weighted (T2), and d) T2 Fluid Attenuated Inversion Recovery (T2-FLAIR) volumes, and were acquired with different clinical protocols and various scanners from multiple data contributing institutions. We intend to release the associated de-identifed DICOM (.dcm) files after the conclusion of the challenge.

All the imaging datasets have been annotated manually, by one to four raters, following the same annotation protocol, and their annotations were approved by experienced neuro-radiologists. Annotations comprise the GD-enhancing tumor (ET—label 4), the peritumoral edematous/invaded tissue (ED—label 2), and the necrotic tumor core (NCR—label 1), as described both in the BraTS 2012–2013 TMI paper and in the latest BraTS summarizing paper. The ground truth data were created after their pre-processing, i.e., co-registered to the same anatomical template, interpolated to the same resolution ($1\,\mathrm{mm}^3$) and skull-stripped. We have 1251 training set and 219 validation set for our experiment.

3   Methods

3.1   Federated Methodology

Our methodology uses a federated learning setting over a multi-institutional dataset by aggregating weighted model updates on a central aggregator server. Each client locally trains and validates its models, and sends its updates to the central server to get aggregated. Afterwards, updated aggregated models will be sent to its participating client in the next federated round. However, in our case, we used our client's selection approach for selecting clients and our weight aggregation strategy for aggregating the weight from each client to each federated round. A simple architecture of federated learning environment can be seen in Fig. 1.

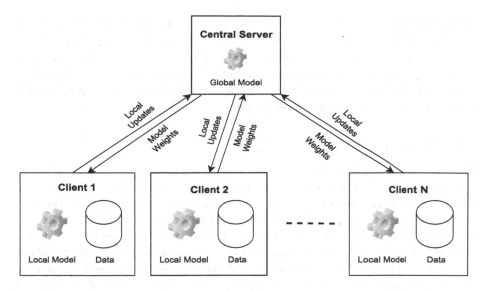

Fig. 1. Simple Architecture of federated learning environment

Clients Selection. Clients' selection is a significant component of training an effective aggregated model in a federated environment. In our experiments, to choose clients in a particular round, we sampled based on a randomly shuffled list of all clients [11]. We first chose the minimum number of clients to participate in a specific round and then made groups from the list of all clients into multiple groups based on the minimum number of clients. By partitioning file 1, we have 23 clients, we chose the minimum number of clients to participate to 6 and divided all clients into groups of 6, 6, 6, 5 and four groups were created from all clients after that we iterated over these different groups in different rounds, 4 FL rounds will take for all clients present in different groups. After iteration is completed, it has accounted for all clients for training. We re-shuffled the list of all clients, and again grouping of clients will be done, and iteration over new groups will be started.

Weight Aggregation Strategy. An effective weight aggregation can lead to a high-performing model in federated settings. We proposed a simple weight aggregation strategy inspired from [12]. In our approach, we added an extra term to the FedAvg algorithm based on the local dice rate corresponding to each client. We took the ratio of local validation dice scores after training clients and local validation dice scores before training the clients (validation dice score on aggregated model coming from FL Server) as an extra term. This helps us to reduce the storage of the history of algorithms and reduces RAM consumption.

$$W^{i+1} = \sum_{j=1}^{N} (\alpha * d_j + \beta * l_j) * W_j^i$$

where N = number of clients participating in specific round, α and β is weighting hyper-parameters (here both are fixed to 0.5), $\alpha + \beta = 1$, $d_j = n_j / \sum_{j=1}^{N} n_j$, $n_j = S_j / \sum_{j=1}^{N} S_j$, S_j = number of samples, $l_j = s_j / \sum_{j=1}^{N} s_j$, $s_j = D_1(W_j^i)/D_2(W_j^i)$, $D_1(.)$ = validation dice scores calculated after training the clients and $D_2(.)$ = validation dice scores calculated before training the clients (means it calculated on the weighted model from the aggregator).

3.2   Model Architecture

We have used the pre-trained ResUNet model Architecture (can be seen in Fig. 2) [13] provided from the challenge [2]. ResUNet is a fully convolutional neural network that is designed to get high performance with fewer parameters. It is an improvement over the existing UNet architecture [14]. ResUNet takes the advantage of both the UNet architecture and Deep Residual Learning. The use of residual blocks helps in building a deeper network without worrying about the problem of vanishing gradients or exploding gradients. It also helps in easy training of the network. The rich skip connections in the ResUNet help in a better flow of information between different layers, which helps in a better flow of gradients while training (backpropagation).

3.3   Implementation Details

We have trained the network for 20 federated rounds, used SGD optimizer with the learning rate = $5e^{-5}$ and it takes one epoch per round to train each client in a given round. We have used our client's selection approach for selecting the clients and our weight aggregation strategy for aggregating the weight from each client on every FL round. The entire network is trained from scratch and does not use other training data other than FeTS 2022 dataset. We have used the dice loss function provided by the organizer of the challenge. The experiments are conducted using 256 RAM Memory and 48 GB Memory NVIDIA A40 GPU.

4   Results

We have reported results on the different metrics provided by Challenge's Platform on FeTS validation and test data.

Figure 3 shows scores of different parameters/metrics (convergence score, round dice, dice label 1, dice label 2 and dice label 4) for different rounds while training on FeTS training data. Figure 4 shows comparison of Ground Truth Segmentation (Top) and Predicted Segmentation from our model (Bottom) on specific slice of patient MRI Image. The mean value of Dice coefficient score for whole tumor, tumor core and enhance tumor regions are 0.78, 0.72 and 0.71 on FeTS 2022 validation data respectively (can be seen Table 1). Dice Scores, Hausdorff Distance (95th percentile), Sensitivity and Specificity of each tumor region shows respectively on FeTS 2022 validation data in Table 1. Figure 5 shows box plot of dice coefficient score on FeTS 2022 validation data. The mean value of

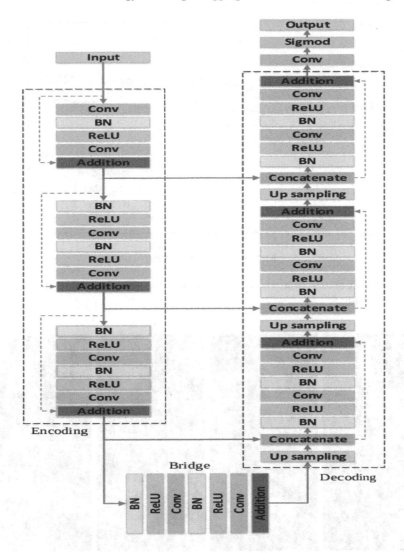

Fig. 2. ResUNet Model Architecture

Dice coefficient score for whole tumor, tumor core and enhance tumor regions are 0.72, 0.68 and 0.66 on FeTS 2022 test data respectively (can be seen Table 2).

5 Discussion

In this paper, we have described a method based on the local score rate for weight aggregation of clients for brain tumor segmentation using federated learning. In our experiments, we achieved a mean value of the dice coefficient for the whole tumor, tumor core and enhance tumor region are 0.78, 0.72 and 0.71 respectively on the validation set and 0.72, 0.68 and 0.66 respectively on the test set.

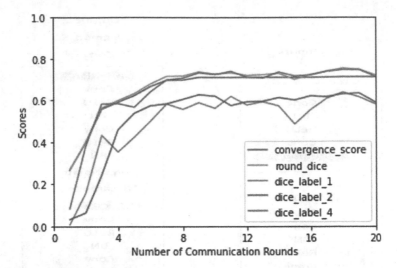

Fig. 3. Different scores from the experiment with respect to different FL rounds in federated training.

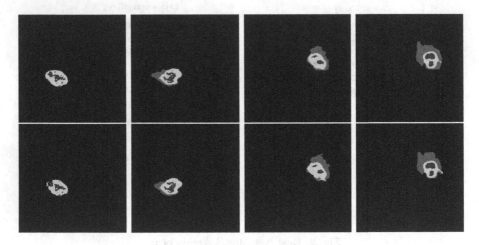

Fig. 4. Ground Truth segmentation (Top) and Predicted segmentation (Bottom) Left-to-Right (Patient ID with slice number): FeTS2022_00000 on slice 60, FeTS2022_00000 on slice 80, FeTS2022_00030 on slice 80 and FeTS2022_00030 on slice 100.

Table 1. Performance of Dice Coefficient, Hausdorff Distance, Sensitivity and Specificity on the FeTS 2022 validation data.

Label	Mean	StdDev	Median	25quantile	75quantile
Dice_ET	0.71	0.28	0.82	0.66	0.89
Dice_TC	0.72	0.31	0.88	0.64	0.92
Dice_WT	0.78	0.16	0.83	0.73	0.89
H95_ET	36.31	93.82	3.16	1.73	8.83
H95_TC	20.68	47.70	5.38	2.44	18.90
H95_WT	25.96	26.93	10.81	6.16	44.22
Sens_ET	0.72	0.30	0.85	0.64	0.94
Sens_TC	0.70	0.33	0.86	0.57	0.95
Sens_WT	0.77	0.17	0.82	0.69	0.90
Spec_ET	0.99	0.00	0.99	0.99	0.99
Spec_TC	0.99	0.00	0.99	0.99	0.99
Spec_WT	0.99	0.00	0.99	0.99	0.99

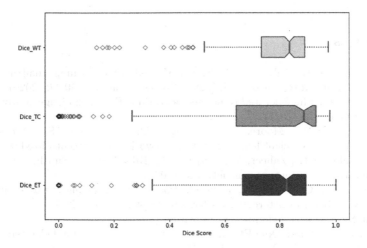

Fig. 5. Box Plot of the Dice Coefficient on the FeTS 2022 validation data.

Table 2. Final Performance of Dice Coefficient, Hausdorff Distance, Sensitivity, Specificity and Communication Cost on the unseen FeTS 2022 testing data.

Label	Mean	StdDev	Median	25quantile	75quantile
Dice_ET	0.66	0.29	0.78	0.55	0.88
Dice_TC	0.68	0.30	0.81	0.54	0.91
Dice_WT	0.72	0.21	0.79	0.63	0.88
H95_ET	32.43	87.65	3.74	2.00	13.66
H95_TC	32.66	81.04	8.00	3.60	18.07
H95_WT	25.23	28.34	13.17	6.16	39.53
Sens_ET	0.66	0.32	0.78	0.47	0.93
Sens_TC	0.70	0.31	0.84	0.53	0.95
Sens_WT	0.69	0.24	0.78	0.56	0.89
Spec_ET	0.99	0.00	0.99	0.99	0.99
Spec_TC	0.99	0.00	0.99	0.99	0.99
Spec_WT	0.99	0.00	0.99	0.99	0.99
Comm_Cost	0.71	0.71	0.71	0.71	0.71

References

1. Li, T., Sahu, A.K., Talwalkar, A., Smith, V.: Federated learning: challenges, methods, and future directions. IEEE Signal Process. Mag. **37**, 50–60 (2020)
2. Pati, S., et al.: The federated tumor segmentation (FeTS) challenge. arXiv preprint arXiv:2105.05874 (2021)
3. McMahan, H.B., Moore, E., Ramage, D., Hampson, S., Arcas, B.A.: Communication-efficient learning of deep networks from decentralized data (2017)
4. Li, T., Sahu, A.K., Zaheer, M., Sanjabi, M., Talwalkar, A., Smith, V.: Federated optimization in heterogeneous networks (2020)
5. Wang, J., Liu, Q., Liang, H., Joshi, G., Poor, H.V.: Tackling the objective inconsistency problem in heterogeneous federated optimization (2020)
6. Reddi, S.: Adaptive federated optimization (2020)
7. Reina, G.A., et al.: OpenFL: an open-source framework for federated learning. arXiv preprint arXiv:2105.06413 (2021)
8. Baid, U., et al.: The RSNA-ASNR-MICCAI BraTS 2021 benchmark on brain tumor segmentation and radiogenomic classification. CoRR, vol. abs/2107.02314 (2021)
9. Sheller, M.J., et al.: Federated learning in medicine: facilitating multi-institutional collaborations without sharing patient data. Sci. Rep. **10**, 12598 (2020)
10. Karargyris, A.: MedPerf: open benchmarking platform for medical artificial intelligence using federated evaluation. Working paper, arXiv, September 2021
11. Khan, M.I., Jafaritadi, M., Alhoniemi, E., Kontio, E., Khan, S.A.: Adaptive weight aggregation in federated learning for brain tumor segmentation. In: Crimi, A., Bakas, S. (eds.) Brainlesion: Glioma, Multiple Sclerosis, Stroke and Traumatic Brain Injuries. LNCS, vol. 12963, pp. 455–469. Springer, Cham (2022). https://doi.org/10.1007/978-3-031-09002-8_40

12. Mächler, L.: FedCostWAvg: a new averaging for better federated learning. In: Crimi, A., Bakas, S. (eds.) Brainlesion: Glioma, Multiple Sclerosis, Stroke and Traumatic Brain Injuries. BrainLes 2021. LNCS, vol. 12963, pp. 383–391. Springer, Cham (2021). https://doi.org/10.1007/978-3-031-09002-8_34

13. Zhang, Z., Liu, Q., Wang, Y.: Road extraction by deep residual U-Net. CoRR, vol. abs/1711.10684 (2017)

14. Ronneberger, O., Fischer, P., Brox, T.: U-Net: convolutional networks for biomedical image segmentation. In: Navab, N., Hornegger, J., Wells, W.M., Frangi, A.F. (eds.) MICCAI 2015. LNCS, vol. 9351, pp. 234–241. Springer, Cham (2015). https://doi.org/10.1007/978-3-319-24574-4_28

Ensemble Outperforms Single Models in Brain Tumor Segmentation

Jianxun Ren[1(✉)], Wei Zhang[2], Ning An[2], Qingyu Hu[2,3], Youjia Zhang[2], and Ying Zhou[2]

[1] School of Aerospace Engineering, Tsinghua University, Beijing, China
davidren555@outlook.com
[2] Neural Galaxy Inc., Beiqing Road, Changping District, Beijing, China
[3] School of Computer Science and Technology, University of Science and Technology of China, Hefei, Anhui, China

Abstract. Brain Tumor Segmentation (BraTS) and Federated Tumor Segmentation (FeTS) are open and popular challenges, for which countless medical image segmentation models have been proposed. Based on the platform that BraTS challenge 2021 provided for researchers, we implemented a battery of cutting-edge deep neural networks, such as nnU-Net, UNet++, CoTr, HRNet, and Swin-Unet to compare performances amongst distinct models directly. To improve segmentation accuracy, we first tried several modification techniques (e.g., data augmentation, region-based training, batch-dice loss function, etc.). Next, the outputs from the five best models were averaged using a final ensemble model, of which four models in the committee were organized in different architectures. As a result, the strengths of every single model were amplified by aggregation. Our model took one of the best performing places in the BraTS 2021 competition amongst over 1200 excellent researchers from all over the world, and robustly produced outstanding segmentation results across different unseen datasets from various institutions in the FeTS 2022 Challenge, which achieved Dice score of 0.9256, 0.8774, 0.8576 and Hausdorff Distances (95%) of 4.36, 14.80, 14.49 for whole tumor, tumor core, and enhancing tumor respectively. Since our model is not successfully evaluated on the test data due to a bug, all the scores stated in this manuscript are based on the validation dataset.

Keywords: Brain Tumor Segmentation · Federated Tumor Segmentation · Ensemble Learning · nnU-Net · UNet++ · CoTr · HRNet

1 Introduction

Glioma is one of the most aggressive and fatal brain tumor. The precise segmentation of glioma based on medical images plays a crucial role in treatment planning, computer-aided surgeries, and health monitoring. However, the ambiguous boundaries of tumors and their variations in shape, size and position, pose difficulties in distinguishing them from brain tissues. It is especially challenging for the traditional medical domain to accurately and automatically segment the glioma tissues.

The Brain Tumor Segmentation (BraTS) Challenge enables researchers to fairly evaluate their state-of-the-art algorithms in segmenting brain glioma. The BraTS challenge has been running since 2012, attracting top research teams around the world each year. In 2021, the challenge was jointly organized by the Radiological Society of North America (RSNA), the American Society of Neuroradiology (ASNR), and the Medical Image Computing and Computer Assisted Interventions (MICCAI) society. Around 1200 researchers participated in the challenge. The number of cases collected by the BraTS committee has drastically risen from 660 to 2000 in 2021, compared to 2020 [19]. The dataset consists of 1251 training, and 219 validation cases, while the test data are not open to the public [3–7]. Multi-parametric magnetic resonance imaging (mpMRI) includes four modalities available for all cases: the native T1-weighted (T1), post-contrast T1-weighted (T1Gd), T2-weighted (T2), and T2-weighted Fluid Attenuated Inversion Recovery (T2-FLAIR) images [17]. BraTS evaluates brain glioma sub-regions segmentation, including the enhancing tumor (ET), the tumor core (TC), and the whole tumor (WT) [18]. To test the generalizability and robustness of models, the Federated Tumor Segmentation (FeTS) Challenge 2022 provides unseen data from various federations, where the training and validation data are borrowed from BraTS with additional data partitioning [1–3, 8, 9].

Due to the rapid development of deep learning, various newly evolved deep neural networks outperformed traditional algorithms. A state-of-the-art medical image segmentation method termed U-Net was first introduced in 2015 [10]. The encoder-decoder based deep neural network with skip-connections achieved an advanced performance. Since then, numerous algorithms have been developed using the U-Net as the backbone. A self-adaptive UNet-like neural network called nnU-Net (no new U-Net) can automatically optimize multiple processes including preprocessing, network architecture, and post-processing without manual interventions [11]. Another recently proposed cutting-edge U-shaped transformer neural network named Swin-Unet has given a demonstrated performance on multi-organ and cardiac segmentation challenges [15]. In addition to the impressive performance of these individual models, ensemble learning aggregating two or more models could achieve better and more generalizable results. The most popular ensemble methods include ensemble mean, ensemble vote, ensemble boosting, and ensemble stacking methods. Ensemble mean is a method that averages predictions across multiple models to make the most of them. Ensemble vote method calculates the votes and accepts the majority votes, which could lower result variances. Ensemble boosting methods train models based on mistakes from previous models, and ensemble stacking methods use a model to combine predictions from different types of models.

In this study, we implemented multiple different models and applied the ensemble learning to collaborate them. We used two metrics, Dice similarity coefficient (Dice) and Hausdor Distance (HD), to evaluate the model performance. Dice ranges from 0 to 1, which indicates the similarity between predictions and ground truth, and HD signifies the largest segmentation error. To promote model accuracy, we have added several modification methods. The final ensemble model gave an unprecedented result based on the selected top-performing models. In Sect. 2, we will briefly introduce the main model architectures that have been utilized on the BraTS 2021 dataset, then further implementation details will be introduced. In Sect. 3, we described the performances of individual models and the ensemble model on both the BraTS 2021 and the FeTS 2022 datasets. Lastly, all the findings of the current research and potential improvements for future studies will be proposed in Sect. 4.

2   Methods

2.1   Ensemble Learning

Ensemble is the most popular fusion method. Not only does it address advantages over various models, but it also improves the overall predictive performances, while increases the robustness and generalization. Ensemble mean averages the unweighted output from multiple models, whereas the ensemble vote takes the unweighted voting results from the majority models. The ensemble mean model showed a convincing performance over most individual models as well as the ensemble vote method. The detailed individual models attempted in the current study are explained as follow:

nnU-Net. F. Isensee et al. proposed a powerful automatic biomedical image segmentation, named nnU-Net (no new net), which can be trained out-of-the-box to segment diverse 3D medical datasets and requires zero manual intervention and expert knowledge. nnU-Net surpasses a broad variety of datasets in many international biomedical image segmentation competitions [12]. Due to the great success of nnU-Net has performed in the medical image segmentation competitions, we applied nnU-Net on the BraTS2021 dataset, the baseline model without any modifications has already achieved an impressive performance on this auxiliary domain. nnU-Net is well-known for its U-Net-like architecture, a symmetric encoder-decoder structure with skip-connections. The encoder completes downsampling, and the decoder upsamples the salient features passed from the bottleneck. Both encoder and decoder have five convolutional layers and are connected by a bottleneck block.

Despite the architecture itself, hyper-parameter is another key determinant in influencing the overall model performance. Data are normalized before being fed into the first layer. The input patch size is $128 \times 128 \times 128$, and uses a batch size of 2, followed by a Leaky ReLU function to handle data nonlinearities. Skip-connections collect high-resolution features from the encoder to reduce the spatial information loss caused by downsampling. At the end of the decoder, a $1 \times 1 \times 1$ filter is applied to guarantee the number of channels is 3, then the output is passed to a softmax function. Loss function sums Dice and Cross-Entropy (CE) loss during 1000 training epochs, consisting of 250 iterations per epoch, and the initial learning rate is 0.001.

U-Net++. U-Net++ is one of the popular variants that uses U-Net as the backbone. U-Net performance is hindered by its suboptimal depth design and the same level feature maps fusion through skip-connections. To overcome the shortcomings listed above, U-Net++ embedded nested U-Nets and redesigned the skip-connections. To this end, pruning is allowed to dispose the burden of unnecessary layers and parameters, while maintaining its outstanding segmenting ability [13].

The initialized input patch size is $96 \times 96 \times 96$ with a batch size of 2 and followed by an Instance Normalization (IN) layer. The 3D model has trained 320 epochs on Dice and HD95 loss and using 0.001 as the learning rate.

High-Resolution Net (HRNet). Unlike many state-of-the-art architectures, HRNet does not encode input images into low-resolution representations and then decode information from the salient features. On the contrary, HRNet keeps high-resolution representations throughout the entire process. Hence, more precised semantic and spatial information are maintained to its architecture. Brain tumor segmentation is a position-sensitive task. Comparing with other model structures, HRNet can improve the ability to capture detailed positional information [14]. Therefore, we further developed a 3D version HRNet to implement on the BraTS dataset.

The model has been trained by $128 \times 128 \times 128$ input images, with a total number of 320 epochs, where 250 iterations were performed per epoch. We adopted a small batch size equals to 2, the initial learning rate is 0.001, and the sum of Dice loss and CE are used for model evaluation.

Swin-Unet. Due to the transformer's convincing performance in the Natural Language Processing (NLP) domain, Swin-Unet is developed to draw its strength in long-term semantic segmentation and transferring to the computer vision domain. Swin-Unet is the first pure transformer-based Unet variant, with a symmetric transformer-based encoder and decoder, which are interconnected by skip-connections. According to H. Cao et al. [15], Swin-Unet effectively solves the over-segmentation problem encountered by Convolutional Neural Network (CNN)-based models.

Comparing with HRNet, it shares similar parameters with the Swin-Unet 2D model. However, its 2D performance is a lot worse than expected. Hence, the 3D model has not been completed.

CoTr. CNN has achieved a competitive performance, but its performance is still inevitably hindered by its limited receptive fields. Since Transformer can effectively address this issue, Xie et al. [16] proposed a novel architecture that combines CNN and Transformer. The introduced architecture in CoTr successfully inherits the advantages of CNN and Transformer.

The patch size of $128 \times 128 \times 128$ is fed into the three-stage-algorithm, each stage consists of one transformer and one convolutional layer. CoTr opt for Dice and CE as the loss function. The model has trained 320 epochs (250 iterations per epoch) with a learning rate of 0.001.

2.2 Data Augmentation (DA)

Limited data can seriously constrain model performance, especially on the unseen dataset. Therefore, data augmentation is necessary, as it expands the limited dataset and supports the models in gaining more insights. Each data has a 20% chance of being scaled, rotated, increased in contrast or mirrored, where the probability is randomized and independent of each other.

2.3 Batch Normalization (BN)

Batch normalization is believed in bringing benefits like faster convergence, more robustness, better generalization and mitigating overfitting [20].

2.4 Batch Dice (BD)

The Batch-wise Dice loss is computed over the batch. This approach avoids large targets dominating the prediction results [21]. BD processes the data as an integral sample, computed over all samples in the batch. Unlike minibatches which assume samples are independent. Hence, the model is less sensitive to the imperfect predictions [22]. However, according to our empirical results, batch dice actually degrades model performance, the implementation details are explained in Sect. 3.1.

2.5 Postprocessing

The predicted enhancing tumor (ET) are sometimes too small to be taken into consideration. In other words, when the predicted enhancing tumor volume is smaller than some thresholds, it can be replaced with necrosis labels [22]. The best threshold is selected via optimizing the ET Dice. Postprocessing may sacrifice the HD95 ET score by a small amount, but ET Dice can be improved by around 2%, or even more.

The performance of three selected models before and after postprocessing on the BraTS training dataset are shown in Table 1 for comparison. Obviously, the ET Dice improvement is attributed to postprocessing.

2.6 Evaluation Metrics

Evaluating model performance is an essential process. The following metrics are the main tools used to measure medical image segmentation qualities.

Dice Similarity Coefficient (Dice). Dice quantifies how closely the prediction matches the ground truth, a perfect prediction results in 1, and 0 vice versa.

Table 1. The performances of each model on the BraTS training data, before and after postprocessing, are presented in the table, the results for individual Dice and HD95 predictions are listed on the left, and the mean values are on the right. Postprocessing is specially designed to improve the Dice scores of enhancing tumors (ET). Although the postprocessing could cause slight sacrifices in the HD95 mean, but the overall results after postprocessing outperform the results original predictions.

Model	Dice			HD95			Dice mean	HD95 mean
	WT	TC	ET	WT	TC	ET		
nnU-Net	0.9322	0.9032	0.8405	4.57	4.66	14.69	0.8919	7.97
nnU-Net(Post)	0.9322	0.9032	**0.8599**	4.57	4.66	**11.47**	**0.8984**	**6.90**
UNet++	0.9292	0.9097	0.8491	4.58	7.54	13.54	0.8960	8.55
UNet++(Post)	0.9292	0.9097	**0.8593**	4.58	7.54	**13.28**	**0.8994**	8.47
CoTr	0.9322	0.9111	0.8501	4.41	5.97	**13.11**	0.8978	**7.83**
CoTr(Post)	0.9322	0.9111	**0.8643**	4.41	5.97	14.24	**0.9025**	8.21

Hausdorff Distance 95 (HD95). HD measures the longest distance between the predictions and the ground truth. HD95 calculates the 95th percentile of the distance, which reduce the impact caused by a small number of outliers.

Cross Entropy (CE). CE is another widely used loss function that aims to alleviate the negative influences caused by an imbalanced dataset. Hence, other class re-balancing methods or weighted class training techniques can be neglected.

Specificity and Sensitivity. Specificity and sensitivity measure how valid a test is. The sensitivity of ET measures whether the model is capable of correctly identifying the enhancing tumor. Specificity of ET measures the model's ability in correctly differentiating the surrounding brain tissues from the enhancing tumor. In other words, sensitivity demonstrates the true-positive rate and specificity demonstrates the true-negative rate of the model in terms of identifying tumors.

3   Results

3.1   Batch Dice (BD) Implementation

In the initial design, the BD modification was expected to improve the segmentation ability, but in practice, it does the opposite. Our results suggest that BD implementation has the tendency of over delineating normal brain tissues as enhancing tumor. Table 2 compares two nnU-Net models tested on the BraTS training dataset that share the same hyperparameters. As seen, the one trained without BD outperforms the others.

Visual predictions are depicted in Fig. 1. Enhancing tumor areas are plotted in red, blue defines the tumor core, and the whole tumor areas are shown in

Table 2. Batch Dice (BD) Implementation on the BraTS training data Comparison: The whole tumor (WT), tumor core (TC), enhancing tumor (ET) Dice and HD95 score of nnU-Net are shown in the first row respectively, where the second row compares the nnU-Net model with the BD modification. Batch dice loss function degrades the nnU-Net model overall performance, especially on HD95 score.

Model	Dice			HD95			Dice mean	HD95 mean
	WT	TC	ET	WT	TC	ET		
nnU-Net	**0.9283**	**0.9074**	0.8466	**4.45**	**7.91**	**11.04**	**0.8941**	**7.80**
nnU-Net + BD	0.9237	0.9025	**0.8472**	6.31	9.43	15.06	0.8911	10.27

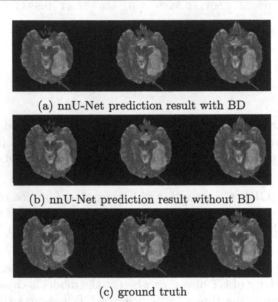

(a) nnU-Net prediction result with BD

(b) nnU-Net prediction result without BD

(c) ground truth

Fig. 1. Comparison of nnU-Net Neural Network performance before and after using Batch Dice (BD). Green indicates the whole tumor, red indicates the enhancing tumor, and blue indicates the tumor core. 1a depicts three tumor regions predicted by nnU-Net with batch dice loss function. 1b depicts three tumor regions predicted by nnU-Net without batch dice loss function. 1c displays the ground truth. As the region pointed by the arrow suggests, model with BD predicts normal brain tissues as enhancing tumor, whereas models without BD do not have this tendency. (Color figure online)

green. Obviously, Fig. 1a shows that BD is prone to over delineate enhancing tumor parts, while Fig. 1b proves that predictions without BD are closer to the ground truth. BD updates Dice more frequently, resulting in its overemphasis on tiny components and neglecting the whole picture.

3.2   Individual Model Comparison

All baseline models implemented on the BraTS training data without hyperparameter tuning are summarized in Table 3, all of which achieved approximately 89% mean of Dice. Slight variations can be seen in the HD95 mean, but all results are around 8.

Table 3. Baseline Models Summary: All baseline models evaluated on the BraTS training dataset with zero hyparemeter tuning have already achieved good performances with approximately Dice mean of 89% and HD95 mean of 8.

Model	Dice			HD95			Dice mean	HD95 mean
	WT	TC	ET	WT	TC	ET		
nnU-Net	**0.9322**	0.9032	0.8405	4.57	**4.66**	14.69	0.8919	7.97
CoTr	0.9321	**0.9108**	**0.8498**	4.42	5.99	**13.16**	**0.8976**	**7.85**
UNet++	0.9292	0.9097	0.8491	4.58	7.54	13.54	0.8960	8.55
HRNet	0.9226	0.8976	0.8404	6.75	11.58	15.44	0.8869	11.25
Swin-Unet (2D)	0.9214	0.8796	0.8370	6.23	9.10	14.47	0.8793	9.93

Since the baseline of nnU-Net already showed a convincing performance in segmenting brain tumors, we fine-tuned the baseline and further compared other combinations of hyperparameters. First, the training epoch was increased from 320 to 500. Ideally, increasing the number of times that the model learns from the training set, allows the model to minimize the error. The experimental findings showed that Dice and HD95 scores were optimized to 0.9056 and 7.69 respectively in 500 training epochs with Adam optimizer after postprocessing. Second, unbalanced data could potentially mislead the model in producing severely biased results. Thus, we replaced Dice loss with Tversky loss function [23], which evolves from Dice specialized to overcome this challenge. The proposed method did not change Dice much but has improved the HD95 by 10%. In addition, brain tumor segmentation can be viewed as a pixel-wise classification task. P. Arbeláez et al. designed a brand-new region-based object detector that classifies every single pixel and aggregates the votes to come up with the final segmentation result [24]. We implemented this method along with multiple DA approaches. However, none of them surpasses the existing models.

3.3   Ensemble Model Comparison

Ensemble is an effective way to make the utmost of the combination of multiple models. To compare the ensemble models in terms of averaging and voting methods, we compare the same models with these two methods. Specifically, ensemble mean and vote models of nnU-Net, CoTr, UNet++, HRNet, and Swin-Unet are developed for comparison. The ensemble mean model slightly outperformed the vote model with 0.9036 Dice mean and 8.13 HD95 mean, whereas ensemble vote ends up with 0.9019 and 8.15 for Dice mean and HD95 mean respectively. Other comparisons are in line with the above findings. In other words, the ensemble mean consistently beats ensemble vote. For this reason, ensemble vote will not be studied further.

3.4 Overall Comparison

Amongst all of the models attempted, five best performing models on the validation set are selected for the aggregation of the final ensemble mean model. The every single model and the ensemble model validation results on the FeTS challenge are presented in Table 4. As elaborated above, the ensemble model produces the highest Dice mean of 0.8783, the best HD95 score of the whole tumor and the tumor core equals to 3.65 and 7.65 respectively.

Table 4. Model Comparison on the FeTS Validation Dataset: The five best-performing individual models are selected to aggregate the ensemble mean model. According to the validation results, the overall ensemble model showed highest Dice mean than each single model and acceptable HD95 mean on the FeTS validation dataset.

Model	Dice			HD95			Dice mean	HD95 mean
	WT	TC	ET	WT	TC	ET		
nnU-Net 500[1]	0.9230	0.8727	0.8349	3.83	7.73	24.18	0.8769	11.91
HRNet 320[2]	0.9234	0.8689	0.8284	3.72	7.85	20.80	0.8734	**10.79**
nnU-Net 320[3]	0.9195	**0.8752**	**0.8372**	5.61	7.70	20.91	0.8773	11.41
UNet++ 320[4]	0.9210	0.8659	0.8217	4.13	8.15	27.65	0.8695	13.31
CoTr 320[5]	0.9207	0.8566	0.8349	4.43	10.06	**19.68**	0.8707	11.39
Ensemble [6]	**0.9258**	0.8747	0.8344	**3.65**	**7.65**	24.14	**0.8783**	11.81

[1]nnU-Net with AdamW optimizer and 500 training epochs, postprocessing using optimal threshold equals to 500.
[2]HRNet with half channel, AdamW optimizer, and 320 training epochs, postprocessing using optimal threshold equals 500.
[3]nnU-Net with AdamW optimizer and 320 training epochs, postprocessing using optimal threshold equals to 500.
[4]UNet++ three stage with AdamW optimizer and 320 training epochs, postprocessing using optimal threshold equals to 500.
[5]CoTr with AdamW optimizer and 320 training epochs, postprocessing using optimal threshold equals to 500.
[6]Ensemble of the above five models, average outputs with equal weights, and postprocessing using the optimal threshold equals to 750.

4 Discussion

In the current research, we have implemented numerous cutting-edge deep neural networks, in terms of individual and ensemble models with various architectures to improve segmentation of brain tumors. We found prediction Dice and HD95 were strengthened using ensemble models and the ensemble mean consistently

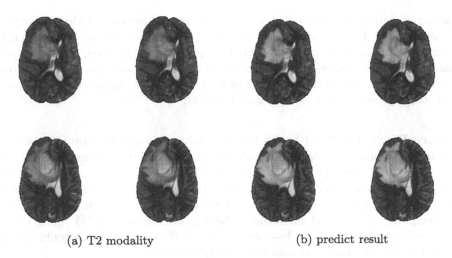

(a) T2 modality   (b) predict result

Fig. 2. A graphical example is demonstrated in this figure. Figure 2a on the left illustrates an example of input T2 modality, the high-signal gray areas are the abnormal regions; Fig. 2b visualised the predicted results by our best model. Green indicates the whole tumor (WT), red refers to the enhancing tumor (ET), and tumor core (CT) is demonstrated in blue. (Color figure online)

outperformed other aggregating models. The final model was obtained from top five models according to their 5-fold cross-validation and postprocessing results. The code is written in PyTorch, and all the models were conducted on AWS p2.xlarge, Tesla K80 (12G GPU RAM), RAM 61G, 4vCPU. These models are trained with AdamW optimizer but with different number of epochs. To be specific, CoTr 320 training eopchs, three-stage unet++ with 320 epochs, nnU-Net with 320 and 500 training epochs, and HRNet with half channel 320 training epochs. The robustness and generalization of our model are demonstrated on the out-of-sample datasets from various FeTS federations, which produces the best predictions with whole tumor, tumor core and enhancing tumor Dice score of 0.9256, 0.8774, 0.8576, and HD95 score of 4.36, 14.80, and 14.49 correspondingly.

By implementing deep neural networks with various architectures, like nnU-Net, UNet++, HRNet, Swin-Unet, and CoTr, our research has addressed different challenges in brain tumor segmentation. In addition, hyperparameters are further fine-tuned to obtain better performance, such as loss function, DA, postprocessing, etc. The advantages of various models are strengthened by aggregating the unweighted averages, which is in line with previously reported findings demonstrated by K. Kamnitsas et al. [25].

According to our research, a few techniques have been tried in an attempt to boost model performance, yet the results were unsatisfactory. First of all, The exemplary results emphasize that BD does not improve the model ability in depicting tiny tumors, but instead depicts the background as part of the enhancing tumor. Since BD failed to capture small tumors, we chose to remove the entire enhancing tumor if it is less than some thresholds. Indeed, postprocessing effectively optimized ET loss, but tiny enhancing tumor recognition is critical in clinical practice. Moreover, the specially designed region-based optimization method and DA are not efficient in enhancing model accuracy. Last but not least, more epochs do not guarantee excellent performance but may cause overfitting problems and bring negative effects.

Future Work. Firstly, although the predominant ensemble approach achieves excellent performance, the individual models still have the potentials to be further developed. According to our research, HRNet is capable of capturing abundant high-resolution information and may thus better handle complex segmentation problems, which underlies the potential of delving into relative studies.

Secondly, as reflected in Table 3, the lowest Dice and HD95 mean scores indicate that CoTr worth an in-depth study, which future research could extend upon the current study to make further exploration.

Finally, the ensemble mean does give reliable predictions, but the prediction accuracy of some models on the committee is slightly worse than others. In this case, reducing the corresponding model weights is expected to get better results.

References

1. Pati, S., et al.: The federated tumor segmentation (FeTS) challenge. arXiv preprint arXiv:2105.05874 (2021)
2. Reina, G.A., et al.: OpenFL: an open-source framework for federated learning. arXiv preprint arXiv: 2105.06413 (2021)
3. Baid, U., et al.: The RSNA-ASNR-MICCAI BraTS 2021 benchmark on brain tumor segmentation and radiogenomic classification. arXiv:2107.02314 (2021)
4. Menze, B.H., et al.: The multimodal brain tumor image segmentation benchmark (BRATS). IEEE Trans. Med. Imaging **34**(10), 1993–2024 (2015). https://doi.org/10.1109/TMI.2014.2377694
5. Bakas, S., et al.: Advancing the cancer genome atlas glioma MRI collections with expert segmentation labels and radiomic features. Nat. Sci. Data **4**, 170117 (2017). https://doi.org/10.1038/sdata.2017.117
6. Bakas, S., et al.: Segmentation labels and radiomic features for the pre-operative scans of the TCGA-GBM collection. The Cancer Imaging Archive (2017). https://doi.org/10.7937/K9/TCIA.2017.KLXWJJ1Q
7. Bakas, S., et al.: Segmentation labels and radiomic features for the pre-operative scans of the TCGA-LGG collection. The Cancer Imaging Archive (2017). https://doi.org/10.7937/K9/TCIA.2017.GJQ7R0EF
8. Sheller, M.J., et al.: Federated learning in medicine: facilitating multi-institutional collaborations without sharing patient data. Nat. Sci. Rep. **10**, 12598 (2020). https://doi.org/10.1038/s41598-020-69250-1
9. Karargyris, A., Umeton, R., Sheller, M., Aristizabal, A., George, J., Bala, S.: MedPerf: open benchmarking platform for medical artificial intelligence using federated evaluation. arXiv preprint arXiv: arXiv:2110.01406 (2021)

10. Ronneberger, O., Fischer, P., Brox, T.: U-Net: convolutional networks for biomedical image segmentation. In: Navab, N., Hornegger, J., Wells, W.M., Frangi, A.F. (eds.) MICCAI 2015. LNCS, vol. 9351, pp. 234–241. Springer, Cham (2015). https://doi.org/10.1007/978-3-319-24574-4_28

11. Isensee, F., Jäger, P.F., Kohl, S.A., Petersen, J., Maier-Hein, K.H.: Automated design of deep learning methods for biomedical image segmentation. arXiv preprint arXiv:1904.08128 (2019)

12. Isensee, F., Jäger, P.F., Kohl, S.A., Petersen, J., Maier-Hein, K.H.: nnU-Net: a self-configuring method for deep learning-based biomedical image segmentation. Nat. Methods 18, 203–211 (2021). https://doi.org/10.1038/s41592-020-01008-z

13. Zhou, Z., Siddiquee, M.M.R., Tajbakhsh, N., Liang, J.: UNet++: redesigning skip connections to exploit multiscale features in image segmentation. arXiv:1912.05074v2 (2020)

14. Wang, J., et al.: Deep high-resolution representation learning for visual recognition. arXiv:1908.07919v2 (2020)

15. Cao, H.: Swin-Unet: Unet-Like pure transformer for medical image segmentation. arXiv:2015.05537v1 (2021)

16. Xie, Y., Zhang, J., Shen, C., Xia, Y.: CoTr: efficiently bridging CNN and transformer for 3D medical image segmentation. arXiv:2013.03024v1 (2021)

17. BraTS Challenge Data. https://www.synapse.org/#!Synapse:syn25829067/wiki/610865. Accessed 2 Aug 2021

18. BraTS Challenge Overview. https://www.synapse.org/#!Synapse:syn25829067/wiki/610863. Accessed 19 Aug 2021

19. Center for Biomedical Image Computing & Analytics. http://braintumorsegmentation.org/. Accessed 23 Dec 2021

20. Ioffe, S., Szegedy, C.: Batch normalization: accelerating deep network training by reducing internal covariate shift. arXiv:1502.03167v3 (2015)

21. Chang, Y., Lin, J., Wu, M., Chen, T., Hsu, W.H.: Batch-wise dice loss: rethinking the data imbalance for medical image segmentation (2019)

22. Isensee, F., Jäger, P.F., Full, P.M., Vollmuth, P., Maier-Hein, K.H.: nnU-net for brain tumor segmentation. arXiv:2011.00848v1 (2020)

23. Salehil, S.S.M., Erdogmus, D., Gholipour, A.: Tversky loss function for image segmentation using 3D fully convolutional deep networks. arXiv:1706.05721v1 (2017)

24. Arbelez, P., Hariharan, B., Gu, C., Gupta, S., Bourdev, L., Malik, J.: Semantic segmentation using regions and parts (2012). https://doi.org/10.1109/CVPR.2012.6248077

25. Kamnitsas, K., et al.: Ensembles of multiple models and architectures for robust brain tumour segmentation. In: Crimi, A., Bakas, S., Kuijf, H., Menze, B., Reyes, M. (eds.) BrainLes 2017. LNCS, vol. 10670, pp. 450–462. Springer, Cham (2018). https://doi.org/10.1007/978-3-319-75238-9_38

FeTS Challenge 2022 Task 1: Implementing FedMGDA + and a New Partitioning

Vasilis Siomos[1](✉), Giacomo Tarroni[1], and Jonathan Passerrat-Palmbach[1,2]

[1] University of London, London, UK
vasilis.siomos@city.ac.uk
[2] Imperial College London, London, UK

Abstract. Federated Learning is becoming ubiquitous in settings where privacy and data ownership make sharing raw data infeasible. Medical imaging presents a prominent such scenario. Despite fervent interest in Federated Learning from the Medical Imaging community, there is a general lack of standardised test-beds, datasets, and challenges that can fast-track progress in the domain. The Federated Tumour Segmentation Challenge attempts to fill that gap for the task of brain tumour segmentation. For this iteration of FeTS, we present two additional dataset splits for prototyping and test how the FedMGDA+ algorithm performs on the problem. Code for this report is provided at https://github.com/siomvas/FeTS_2022.

Keywords: Federated Learning · Tumour Segmentation · Medical Imaging

1 Introduction

In this short study, we take a look at the challenges of the competition, develop two new splits that reduce the idle time and allow us to perform more aggregation calls, and implement the FedMGDA+ [5] algorithm to provide a model that performs well across all institutions.

Federated Learning [6] is a collaborative learning paradigm where clients can jointly train a machine learning model without their local data leaving the premises; instead, only model updates are exchanged, aggregated, and redistributed in an iterative process. This inherent data protection mechanism is appealing in all the scenarios where data privacy and ownership are paramount, such as Medical Imaging. However, despite the momentum that research into Federated Learning has gathered [2, 4, 12–14], there is a distinct lack of standard experiment settings, which are necessary to facilitate fair comparisons [7]. The FeTS initiative [9] is the largest federation of medical institutions, and the FeTS Challenge is one of the first federated learning challenges in the medical imaging community.

Task 1 of the competition concerns the study of robust aggregation methods that leverage the clients' local updates most effectively to produce a global model. For this reason, an infrastructure is provided with only specific modifications allowed in four areas: collaborator sampling, aggregation, hyper-parameter choice, and dataset partitioning. The infrastructure stack consists of OpenFL [11] to handle the federated logic and GaNDLF [10] to handle the deep learning logic.

2 Data

FeTS 2022 is the second iteration of the Federated Tumour Segmentation Challenge. The challenge dataset and format are based on the BraTS Challenge [1], except the data in FeTS cannot leave the local sites. This year's training set contains mpMRI (T1, T1-Gd, T2, T2-FLAIR) brain scans from 1251 patients across 33 institutions. The data has been centrally pre-processed and expertly annotated, as described in the challenge manuscript [9].

2.1 Partitioning

The organisers have provided three splits for the challenge. A split corresponds to the number of clients in the federation, and the patient records at each simulated federated site.

- A small split with a handful of samples for debugging purposes.
- The natural split; each collaborator corresponds to a different physical institution.
- An artificial refinement of the natural split, where the records from the biggest collaborators were split to different artificial collaborators based on each record's tumour size compared to the median tumour size for the original collaborator. More concretely, the 5 biggest collaborators were split into 3 new collaborators each.

Early on in the challenge, we emphasised training using the original split, as it introduces no confounding variables, such as an appropriate metric or threshold to use for splintering a collaborator's samples or aggregating the samples from smaller collaborators. However, the challenge's simulated time limit means the original split is quite restrictive; in the original split, the largest contributor takes 25 simulated hours to complete one epoch of training, capping the maximum possible number of rounds to 6 (using the minimum of 1 local epoch). Moreover, the number of local epochs has to be the same for all collaborators, essentially imposing idle time for every collaborator proportional to the difference between the size of their data and the size of the biggest collaborator's data.

This incentivizes us to fraction the dataset into smaller, more uniformly sized participants to minimise idle time and maximise the number of federated rounds that fit within the simulation threshold.

Additionally, since the total number of records is high, training on the full dataset takes a lot of wall time. For the purposes of prototyping and exploring the potential of different hyperparameters and aggregation methods, we propose the following splits, based on the original method of splitting the largest collaborators according to the tumour size:

- A small split, which includes a total of 117 patients (10% of the original dataset) from 7 collaborators, containing the records of all the physical collaborators that contributed between 10 and 30 records. This ensures no collaborator dominates the split, and that the heterogeneity mimics a realworld scenario (Fig. 1).

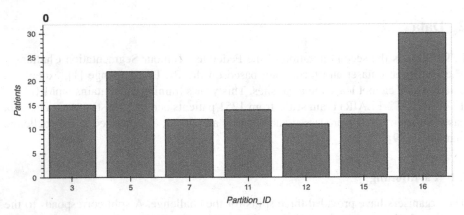

Fig. 1. The small split for prototyping.

– A medium split, which includes all the natural collaborators except the two biggest ones, which we split into 10 bins each, based on tumour volume, then include the middle two bins only. This leads to a dataset with 536 patients (42% of the original size) from 25 collaborators. We find this to present an adequate middle ground between the small and original split, both in imbalance and size (Fig. 2).

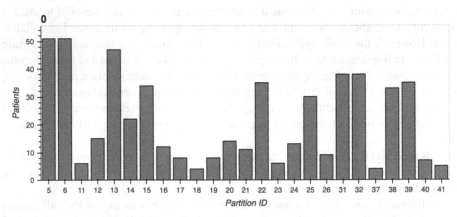

Fig. 2. The medium split for scaling up experiments.

– An alternative split of the full dataset, for which we use the same methodology as the original artificial partitioning, but we splinter the two largest participants into 10 instead of 3 quantiles, based on tumour volume, resulting in 41 collaborators. As shown in Fig. 3, this new split greatly smooths out the imbalance of the original split, alleviating the aforementioned problems of maximum federated rounds and idle time on smaller collaborators.

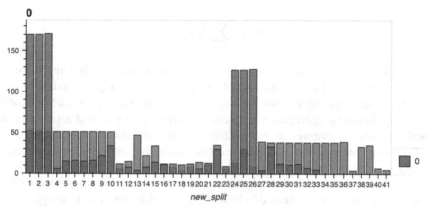

Fig. 3. The full new split compared to the given artificial split.

3 Methods

3.1 Sampling Participants

One crucial dimension of control in federated learning systems is the choice of the participating clients in each round. This choice is especially important in scenarios with millions of possible clients, such as smartphone users. In cross-silo scenarios, like the one for the challenge, where all participants can participate in every round, we argue constant and full participation is needed to allow each local site's characteristics to influence the model, in line with our ultimate goal of personalised FL models, as described in Sect. 1. Hence, we used all the collaborators in every round.

3.2 Hyperparameter Choice

The default available hyperparameters are the learning rate and the number of epochs e. As e had to be an integer, and, as explained in Sect. 2, more local epochs extend the idle time for all collaborators except the largest, we keep e fixed at 1. Regarding the learning rate, we found that doubling the default learning rate to 1e-4 improved performance.

Additionally, while the MGDA algorithm automatically tunes the collaborator weights without any hyperparameters, FedMGDA+ interpolates between that result and a uniform weighing based on a hyper-parameter ϵ. Setting ϵ equal to 0 recovers FedAvg, while setting it equal to 1 recovers MGDA. We used $\epsilon = 0.5$ for our experiments.

3.3 Aggregation Function

Task 1 focuses on aggregation methods that can effectively pool the information from the participants' local updates. The collaborator computes the weights of the global model as the weighted sum of the local weights:

$$w^r = \sum_{i=1}^{N} \lambda_i w_i^r \tag{1}$$

The popular Federated Averaging algorithm [8] sets these coefficients to be the ratio of the clients' local data to the total dataset size, thus biasing the update towards the optima of the contributors with the largest number of records. Instead of treating the Federated Learning aggregation problem as a server trying to find a single model that performs best *on average* across different client distributions, we can attempt to find a Pareto optimal solution, such that no client is disadvantaged by the aggregation. Especially in cross-silo [6] scenarios, where the trained model will be deployed to the institutions that participated in the training, or others with local datasets similar to those of the original participants, instead of a heuristic approach to determine the aggregation weights, we can use the Multiple Gradient Descent Algorithm, borrowed from multi-objective optimisation, to determine the common descent direction for all participants. This ensures optimisation moves only towards areas of the solution space that do not worsen the model's performance on any client. One such method is the FedMGDA+ [5] algorithm, which interpolates between an even weighing of $1/N$ and the common descent direction as produced by the Multiple Gradient Descent Algorithm (MGDA) [3].

For every federated round, every participating client executes an SGD step, in parallel:

$$\mathbf{w}_i^{\tau+1} = \mathbf{w}_i - \eta \nabla f_i(w_i) \tag{2}$$

Instead of Eq. 1, MGDA uses the following update rule:

$$\mathbf{w}_i^{\tau+1} = \mathbf{w}_i - \eta d_t, \ d_t = J_f(wt)\lambda_t^* \ \lambda_t^* = \arg \min_{\lambda \in \Delta} n \left\| J_f(wt)\lambda \right\| \tag{3}$$

Here η is a server learning rate (assumed to be 1 in our case), and the vector of coefficients λ is found by solving a simple quadratic programming problem once per federated round. We note that the MGDA algorithm requires the gradient of the models to compute the Jacobian, and the vector λ. In the case of multiple local epochs, we would instead have to approximate the gradients by the model delta, i.e. the difference between the weight values at the beginning and end of the round, but since we use a single epoch to minimise the idle time as explained in Sect. 1, the delta *is* the model gradient.

FedMGDA+ refines that, by setting the update rule to be:

$$\lambda_t^* = \arg \min_{\lambda \in \Delta, \|\lambda - \lambda_0\|_\infty \le \varepsilon} \left\| J_f(w_t)\lambda \right\| \tag{4}$$

meaning the solution for λ is forced to lie close to the FedAvg solution, with the closeness dictated by ϵ.

4 Results

Despite the theoretical reasoning, we found that FedMGDA+ actually underperformed the FedAvg baseline in the challenge's setting. Our hypothesis is that due to the large number of participants in our split, and the small number of records in some participants, optimising towards the common descent direction performs worse on average than biasing the updates towards the biggest collaborators as FedAvg does (Tables 1, 2 and 3).

Table 1. ET test scores using our new split

ET	Dice	H95	Sensitivity	Specificity
FedMGDA+	0.56	44.13	0.52	0.99
FedAvg	0.67	36.57	0.65	0.99

Table 2. TC test scores using our new split

TC	Dice	H95	Sensitivity	Specificity
FedMGDA+	0.59	30.25	0.57	0.99
FedAvg	0.69	23.63	0.69	0.99

Table 3. WT test scores using our new split

WT	Dice	H95	Sensitivity	Specificity
FedMGDA+	0.67	24.73	0.59	0.99
FedAvg	0.77	35.62	0.81	0.99

5 Discussion

5.1 Memory Requirements

We found training with the full dataset to be very memory demanding, requiring 130 GB of RAM during the preprocessing phase, and increasingly more of it while training continued. After investigation, we found that the culprit is the pin_memory argument in the configuration files, which caused the whole dataset to be pinned to CPU memory during the initial pre-processing. By setting this to false, we find that initial processing only takes 10 GB of RAM, with no negative performance impact on training; on the contrary, training was significantly sped up for a 128 GB RAM system which previously had to use disk swapping to run the experiment. There is an additional memory leak that causes memory to fill proportionally to the number of rounds in an ongoing run, but restoring from a checkpoint can alleviate that.

5.2 Time Constraints

This year, all the collaborators had to use the same number of local epochs regardless of their size. Additionally, there was a fixed time limit calculated based on the time the biggest collaborator needed to complete training.

The combination of these two factors imposed idle/wasted time in all but the biggest collaborators, and perhaps even more importantly, heavily deincentivised training for more than a single local epoch, as the idling/wasted time increases linearly with the number of local epochs.

This limits the solution space, while not mirroring real-world conditions.

References

1. Baid, U., et al.: The rsna-asnr-miccai brats 2021 benchmark on brain tumor segmentation and radiogenomic classification. arXiv preprint arXiv:2107.02314 (2021)
2. Bernecker, T., et al.: Fednorm: modality-based normalization in federated learning for multi-modal liver segmentation. https://doi.org/10.48550/ARXIV.2205.11096, https://arxiv.org/abs/2205.11096 (2022)
3. Désidéri, J.A.: Multiple-gradient descent algorithm (MGDA) for multiobjective optimization. Comptes Rendus Mathematique **350**(5–6), 313–318 (2012)
4. Guo, P., et al.: Auto-fedrl: federated hyperparameter optimization for multi-institutional medical image segmentation. arXiv preprint arXiv:2203.06338 (2022)
5. Hu, Z., Shaloudegi, K., Zhang, G., Yu, Y.: Federated learning meets multiobjective optimization. IEEE Transactions on Network Science and Engineering **9**, 2039–2051 (2022)
6. Kairouz, P., et al.: Advances and open problems in federated learning. Found. Trends® Mach. Learn. **14**(1–2), 1–210 (2021)
7. Karargyris, A., et al.: Medperf: open benchmarking platform for medical artificial intelligence using federated evaluation. https://doi.org/10.48550/ARXIV.2110.01406. https://arxiv.org/abs/2110.01406 (2021)
8. Konečný, J., McMahan, H.B., Yu, F.X., Richtárik, P., Suresh, A.T., Bacon, D.: Federated learning: Strategies for improving communication efficiency. arXiv preprint arXiv:1610.05492 (2016)
9. Pati, S., et al.: The federated tumor segmentation (fets) challenge. arXiv preprint arXiv:2105.05874 (2021)
10. Pati, S., et al.: Gandlf: a generally nuanced deep learning framework for scalable end-to-end clinical workflows in medical imaging. arXiv preprint arXiv:2103.01006 (2021)
11. Reina, G.A., et al.: Openfl: An open-source framework for federated learning. arXiv preprint arXiv:2105.06413 (2021)
12. Sheller, M.J., et al.: Federated learning in medicine: facilitating multi-institutional collaborations without sharing patient data. Sci. Rep. **10**(1), 1–12 (2020)
13. Tedeschini, B.C., et al.: Decentralized federated learning for healthcare networks: a case study on tumor segmentation. IEEE Access **10**, 8693–8708 (2022)
14. Xu, A., et al.: Closing the generalization gap of cross-silo federated medical image segmentation. In: Proceedings of the IEEE/CVF Conference on Computer Vision and Pattern Recognition, pp. 20866–20875 (2022)

Efficient Federated Tumor Segmentation via Parameter Distance Weighted Aggregation and Client Pruning

Meirui Jiang[1], Hongzheng Yang[1], Xiaofan Zhang[2], Shaoting Zhang[2], and Qi Dou[1]([✉])

[1] Department of Computer Science and Engineering, The Chinese University of Hong Kong, Hong Kong, HKSAR, China
qdou@cse.cuhk.edu.hk
[2] Shanghai Artificial Intelligence Laboratory, Shanghai, China

Abstract. Federated learning has become a popular paradigm to enable multiple distributed clients collaboratively train a model, providing a promising privacy-preserving solution without data sharing. To fully make use of federated training efforts, it is critical to promote the global model performance as well as the generalization capability based on diverse data samples provided in the federated cohort. The Federated Tumor Segmentation (FeTS) Challenge 2022 proposes two tasks for participants to improve the federated training and evaluation. Specifically, task 1 seeks effective weight aggregation methods to create the global model given a pre-defined segmentation algorithm. Task 2 aims to find robust segmentation algorithms which perform well on unseen testing data from various remote independent institutions. In federated learning, the data collected from different institutions present heterogeneity, largely affecting the training behavior. The heterogeneous data results in the variation of clients' local optimization, therefore making the local client update not consistent with each other. The vanilla weighted average aggregation only takes the number of samples into account but ignores the differences in clients' updates. As for task 1, we devise a parameter distance-based aggregation algorithm to mitigate the drifts of client updates. On top of this, we further propose a client pruning strategy to reduce the convergence time upon uneven training time among local clients. Our method finally achieves the convergence score of 0.7433 and an average dice score of 71.02% on the validation data, which is split out from the training data. For task 2, we propose to use the nnU-Net as the backbone and utilize the test-time batch normalization, which incorporates test data specific mean and variance to fit the unseen test data distribution during the testing phase.

Keywords: Federated Learning · Brain Tumor Segmentation · nnU-Net · Test-time Adaptation

---

M. Jiang and H. Yang—Contributed equally.

1   Introduction

Glioblastoma (GBM) is an aggressive brain tumor for adults, it is heterogeneous, with less than 10% of patients surviving for over five years [25]. To perform the clinical diagnosis and response assessment in GBM, a routine choice is to use magnetic resonance imaging (MRI). It is widely believed that segmentation for brain MRI images shows benefits to the clinical treatment [27]. Although the Brain Tumor Segmentation (BraTS) challenges [5,6,24] have provided widely-used benchmarking data and state-of-the-art average Dice has reached an uplift-ing score as high as around 85% [9,11] on the test set, applying these algo-rithms in the real world still remains challenging due to regulatory and privacy hurdles [1]. The collection of data among different clinical institutions is very hard to achieve, since institutions usually do not intend to share the local pri-vate data with others. Therefore, models under this scenario cannot be trained with all data centralized together. To enable the model training on distributed data, federated learning (FL) [8,15,16,19,20,22,23,29–33,36] provides a promis-ing solution. In FL, each clinical institution can be treated as a client, and each client trains local models using its own data; then the global aggrega-tion is performed to collect local models' weights to generate the global model. This training paradigm with only model parameters transferred well solves the above-mentioned issues. Following this trend, the Federated Tumor Segmenta-tion (FeTS) Challenge [26] is proposed as the first challenge for FL. The challenge is structured in two explicit tasks, i.e., federated training (weight aggregation) and federated evaluation (generalization in the wild, and we participate in both of the tasks.

Task 1 provides a baseline federated learning algorithm implementation supported by the OpenFL [28]. On top of this, it allows participants to cus-tomize certain core functions to further improve the baseline consensus models. Specifically, there are mainly three functions to be adjusted for participants. (i) Aggregation function: This function defines how model weights collected from different clients will be aggregated to generate the global model. Besides the client weights, this function allows access to other information during the train-ing (e.g., the sample number weight, the metrics saved in previous rounds, etc.) to help design the aggregation weight. (ii) Choose training collaborator func-tion: This function defines which collaborator (client) will be selected to join the next round of federated training. Participants are allowed to select clients based on training information, such as the validation accuracy from the previ-ous round. (iii) Training hyperparameters: This function defines two important hyperparameters for federated training. One is the learning rate for each local client, and the other one is the batches or epochs to be performed locally at each round. Here all local clients share the same hyperparameter settings. Except for the above-mentioned three functions, all other details and methods in the fed-erated learning framework have been prepared and fixed by organizers to keep the same settings for all participants. The final ranking will be determined by considering both the Dice similarity coefficient (for each of the three evaluated regions), Hausdorff distance - 95th percentile (for each of the three evaluated regions), and the communication cost during model training.

Task 2 aims to find algorithms that robustly produce accurate segmentation results across different medical institutions. These institutions can have different imaging acquisition protocols and populations, while the data samples are not presented during the training. That is, after the training, the proposed algorithms will be evaluated in a distributed way on unseen out-of-sample datasets from various institutions that did not contribute data to the training set. The participants will submit the trained model as well as the inference code.

For this task, the most critical challenge lies in improving the generalization capability of the model on unseen data. Since the i.i.d assumption between training and testing distributions may not always hold, the model can suffer a great performance drop when applied to unseen testing data. According to [7,11,21], they observe a depressing performance drop when shifting from the training dataset to the test dataset, which confirms the fact that there is a deviation between the training dataset and the test dataset in the FeTS challenge. To tackle this problem, we propose to use test-time batch normalization (BN) layers to reduce the distance between training and testing data. The test-time BN can help the model to re-estimate and normalize data, thus mitigating the distribution shift. Besides, we further apply the mix-of-expert strategy to make use of training diversities, which can help reduce the bias of models during the testing phase. aining diversities, which can help reduce the bias of models during the testing phase.

2 Solution for Task 1

Task 1 aims to identify effective weight aggregation and client selection methods for real-world federated brain tumor segmentation. More precisely, the focus of this task is on the methodologies specific to federated learning related parts (e.g., aggregation, client selection, and hyperparameters for FL) instead of identifying the best segmentation method. In this regard, an existing infrastructure for federated tumor segmentation using federated averaging is provided to all participants, in which the local network architecture and training logic are pre-defined by organizers. Given the data partition across multiple individual institutions, the job of participants is to develop methods for effective aggregation of model updates, selection criteria for clients at each federated round, and the training hyperparameters, including the learning rate and the local update epochs.

2.1 Efficient Federated Aggregation via Parameter Distance Re-Weighting

Denote $(\mathcal{X}, \mathcal{Y})$ as the joint image and label space over K clients and a data sample is an image-label pair (x, y) with $x \in \mathcal{X}, y \in \mathcal{Y}$. The federated optimization objective can be formulated as follows:

$$arg \min_{w_g^t} f(x; \omega_g^t), \quad \text{where } f(x; \omega_g^t) = \sum_{k=1}^{K} p_k f(x; \omega_k^t), \tag{1}$$

where ω_g^t and ω_k^t denotes the global and local parameters at the t-th communication round and $p_k = \frac{n_k}{\sum_{k=1}^{K} n_k}$ is the relative sample size used for re-weighting. At each round t, the global parameter ω_g^t is updated by aggregating local updated parameters ω_k^{t-1}, which is denoted as:

$$w_g^t = \sum_{k=1}^{K} p_k \cdot \omega_k^{t-1}. \tag{2}$$

The vanilla federated objective function optimizes global parameters by aggregating local parameter updates with the consideration of relative sample size. However, the clients participating in federated optimization are highly heterogeneous, only calculating the sample number is not sufficient to alleviate differences among local client optimization.

To address this problem, a promising solution is to reduce the inconsistency among the local client parameters [37]. By quantifying the distance of local parameter updates, we are allowed to re-weight the client weights in a more flexible way, i.e., some client updates may lie in a different direction from other clients, and we can weigh less for these parameters to aggregate the global consensus parameters. In specific, we use the ℓ_1-norm to measure the parameter distance between ω_k and the averaged parameter $\omega_{avg} = \frac{1}{K} \sum_{k=1}^{K} \omega_k$, and take the inverse of this distance as the new re-weighting factor for the global aggregation. The parameter distance aggregation (PDA) is denoted as:

$$p_k = \frac{1}{Z} \|\omega_{avg} - \omega_k\|^{-1}, \tag{3}$$

where $Z = \sum_{k=1}^{K} \|\omega_{avg} - \omega_k\|^{-1}$ is a normalization factor to ensure the summation of p_k equals to 1. In practice, we add a small term ϵ to both numerator and denominator to avoid the numerical instability.

On top of the PDA, we propose to consider the metrics during the training to further enhance the calculation of aggregation weight factors. Denote the training metric score of each local client as s_k, we can calculate the re-weighting coefficient $p_k' = \frac{S}{s_k}$. Here the S denotes the normalization factor which is calculated as $S = \sum_{k \in K} s_k$. In practice, the training metric score can be chosen as the Dice score or the Hausdorff distance. By using the training score metric, we can penalize the clients that overfit the training data and give more weight to the under-trained models during aggregation to encourage the training. For the final aggregation strategy, a comprehensive way is to combine the sample weight in FedAvg [23] and our proposed PDA and training metric score. The final aggregation weight is obtained by multiplying these three factors and performing the normalization again to make the weight in the range of (0,1].

2.2   Time-Based Client Pruning for Fast Federated Training

In realistic scenarios, federated collaborators also present the heterogeneity at the system level, such as different computing resources and upload and download speeds. In one communication round, some clients need more wall-clock CPU time to complete the local training tasks, causing idle waiting for quicker clients. The speed gap across participating clients hinders the parallel computing efficiency of federated training and incurs a slower convergence rate.

To tackle this problem, we propose an adaptive client pruning strategy to filter out slower clients based on the training time. Specifically, for each client, we measure the simulated time it takes from the previous round and generates the time list $\mathcal{T}$:

$$\mathcal{T} = [h_1^{t-1}, h_2^{t-1}, ..., h_k^{t-1}], \tag{4}$$

where h_k^{t-1} denotes the simulated time for client k at the t-th communication round. Then we calculate a threshold α by averaging the simulated time and multiplying a scale factor β as follows:

$$\alpha = (\frac{1}{K} \sum_{k=1}^{K} h_k^{t-1}) * \beta. \tag{5}$$

The scale factor β is used to control the threshold for time-based selection. We empirically set the value of β to 0.75, which can help filter out top-2 clients which present a significant speed gap compared with other clients. All clients within this threshold are selected to join the next round of federated training. In the meanwhile, to make sure all clients' data contribute to the global model, the pruning mechanism is performed only at odd rounds, and all clients will participate in the training at even rounds.

2.3   Learning Rate Scheduling and Local Update Epochs

Besides the above strategies to improve the federated training, we also investigate the effects of different learning rate scheduling in order to identify the most appropriate hyperparameters. The initial learning rate is set as a constant during training, we propose to apply a dynamic learning rate schedule with the aim of being compatible with our re-weighting and pruning strategy and considering the convergence behavior during training. Specifically, denote the learning rate as η, and the initial learning rate as η_0, we propose to use the polynomial decay of learning rate as below:

$$\eta = \eta_0 * (1 - \frac{t}{T})^\tau, \tag{6}$$

where T refers to the maximum training round number and τ is the polynomial factor. By applying this learning scheduler, the model converges faster at the beginning and gradually becomes stable, which can improve the convergence speed as well as keep the quality of the global model. For the local update epochs, we empirically set the value to 1 with the consideration that this can well balance the convergence performance and speed. As identified in SCAFFOLD and HarmoFL [13,18], with more local update epochs, the local client training tends to fit its own data distribution, which incurs a drift between the client parameter and global parameter. The drift distracts the aggregation stage and makes the global model suffer a performance drop.

3   Solution for Task 2

In this section, the details of our task-2 solution are described. Our method builds on the strong baseline nnUNet, which won the BraTS 2020 Challenge. Several modifications are applied at test time to improve the model performance.

3.1   Backbone NnUNet

We adapt nnUNet as our backbone model. Specifically, a 3D UNet with encoder-decoder architecture is adopted. The input patch is randomly cropped from training cases with size $128 \times 128 \times 128$. The encoder receives the input patch and generates $4 \times 4 \times 4$ feature maps with five levels of strided convolutional layers. The number of encoder convolution filters is initialized as 32 and doubled after each layer. The decoder mirrors the encoder architecture with five transpose convolutions to upsample the feature maps to the input patch size. Leaky ReLU with the slope of 0.01 and batch normalization is utilized as nonlinearity and normalization methods. As discussed in [12] , several BraTS-specific modifications are integrated to complete the baseline. First, the network predicts three overlapping regions of enhancing tumor (ET), tumor core or TC (ET + necrotic tumor), and whole tumor or WT (ET + NT + ED), instead of the three original sub-regions provided in the segmentation labels, ET, ED, and NCR. Second, stronger data augmentations, such as rotation, scaling, elastic deformation, and additive brightness augmentation are used during training. Third, the final prediction results are post-processed by converting the ET class into NT if there are less than 200 positive predictions.

3.2   Test Time Batch Normalization

When deploying models to unseen institutions with domain shifts, the internal activation of a deep model can deviate from the ranges encountered during training. When this happens, the model layers receive out-of-domain inputs, and the prediction accuracy is degraded. To alleviate this issue, we implement a simple yet effective strategy, test-time batch normalization, using test data information to effectively correct internal activation distributions under domain shift.

Specifically, test-time batch normalization re-calculates BN statistics on the batch at prediction time. Typically, the BN statistics are collected during training and frozen after training time. For test time batch normalization, BN statistics are re-computed for each test batch. Assuming we need to predict unlabeled test data $\{x_i\}_{i=1}^{T}$. At prediction time, we can get batches of t examples $\{x_i^b\}_{i=1}^{t}$ and calculate the final predictions for those samples simultaneously.

4   Experiments

4.1   Dataset and Experiment Setup

Based on the previous BraTS and FeTS challenges, the FeTS 2022 challenge provides more routine clinically acquired MRI scans with their source information, indicating the relationship between each case and its original institutions. Task 1 and task 2 share the same training data with 1251 cases [2–5,26,28,31]. All FeTS mpMRI scans are available as NIfTI files (.nii.gz) and describe a) native (T1) and b) post-contrast T1-weighted (T1Gd), c) T2-weighted (T2), and d) T2 Fluid Attenuated Inversion Recovery (T2-FLAIR) volumes. In the dataset, three kinds of regions have been manually segmented as annotations, including the ET, TC, and WT. Two non-imaging csv files are provided to indicate the partitioning relationship according to the acquisition origin and brain tumor size. Participants can also access the unlabeled validation data to evaluate their algorithms before the official testing stage.

We performed experiments using the provided training data, and the training data is further split into training and validation sets with the ratio of 0.8:0.2. As for task 1, both the performance in terms of Dice coefficient (Dice) and Hausdorff distance-95 percent (HD95) of our algorithm will be taken for evaluation. Besides, the convergence score, which is calculated by multiplying the Dice with the algorithm's total running time, is also used to assess convergence speed. For task 2, we also use Dice and HD95 as the evaluation metrics.

4.2   Implementation Details

Task 1. For task 1, we implement the parameter distance based aggregation (PDA), the training metric score re-weighting strategies, and the client pruning mechanism using the open-fl framework [28]. For client pruning, we set the maximum round $T = 20$ and the threshold $\beta = 0.75$. We set the learning rate schedule with an initial learning rate of $5e - 4$ and the polynomial factor of 0.9. All experiments are performed with a fixed seed to alleviate randomness.

Task 2. (i) Training Settings: For task 2, the network is trained with 5-fold cross-validation. The objective function is the sum of dice and cross-entropy loss, calculated at the final output layer and outputs of lower resolution to apply deep supervision. The optimizer is SGD with the initial learning rate of 1e-2 and a Nesterov momentum of 0.99. To stabilize the training process, the batch version of dice loss is used, and the batch size is set to 2. The whole training lasts 1000 epochs, with each epoch consisting of 250 iterations. **(ii) Data Augmentation:** We use the following combination in [12]: (a) Increase the probability of applying rotation and scaling from 0.2 to 0.3. (b) Increase the scale range from (0.85, 1.25) to (0.65, 1.6) (c) Select a scaling factor for each axis individually. (d) Use elastic deformation with a probability of 0.2 and scale range (0, 0.25). (e) Use additive brightness augmentation with a probability of 0.3. (f) Increase the aggressiveness of the gamma augmentation to range (0.5, 1.6).

Table 1. Comparison results for task 1 on split-1

Method			Dice [%]				HD95				C-Score
Aggregation	Pruning	LR	ET	TC	WT	Mean	ET	TC	WT	Mean	
FedAvg	✗	5e-5	65.43	68.43	75.71	69.86	8.81	31.72	13.74	18.09	0.6822
FedAvg	✗	5e-4	67.84	71.13	78.53	72.50	7.59	**13.73**	7.72	**9.68**	0.6960
FedAvg	✗	5e-4(Dyn.)	**69.22**	**73.31**	**79.39**	**73.97**	8.39	15.78	7.39	10.52	**0.7122**
FedAvg	✗	1e-3(Dyn.)	66.60	70.81	77.38	71.59	**6.07**	15.95	8.81	10.28	0.6956
FedAvg	✗	1e-4(Dyn.)	61.53	65.06	74.08	66.89	6.98	31.05	9.08	15.70	0.6711
FedNova	✗	5e-4(Dyn.)	55.99	50.08	72.44	59.50	13.54	52.63	16.33	27.50	0.5226
PDA	✗	5e-4(Dyn.)	55.81	59.46	69.27	61.51	11.49	38.27	15.30	21.69	0.6250
PDA+S_{Dice}	✗	5e-4(Dyn.)	58.98	67.35	73.38	66.57	9.97	22.29	10.42	14.23	0.6516
FedAvg+PDA	✗	5e-4(Dyn.)	64.14	68.20	76.81	69.72	6.34	19.60	8.26	11.40	0.6815
FedAvgM	✗	5e-4(Dyn.)	65.50	67.18	77.19	69.96	6.52	15.42	**7.21**	9.71	0.6952
FedAvgM	75%	5e-4(Dyn.)	56.97	68.72	74.67	66.97	6.66	21.67	13.16	13.83	0.6765

Table 2. Comparison results for task 1 on split-2, last row is results on testing cohort.

Method			Dice [%]				HD95				C-Score
Aggregation	Pruning	LR	ET	TC	WT	Mean	ET	TC	WT	Mean	
FedAvg	✗	5e-5	61.25	63.61	73.59	66.15	8.44	29.22	8.72	15.46	0.6783
FedAvg	✗	5e-4(Dyn.)	62.70	67.51	74.29	68.17	7.73	24.47	8.80	13.67	0.7217
FedAvg	75%	5e-4(Dyn.)	64.59	67.08	77.34	69.67	**6.54**	26.52	9.62	14.23	0.7350
FedNova	✗	5e-4(Dyn.)	60.72	67.38	76.05	68.05	9.63	25.35	9.83	14.94	0.7208
FedAvgM	✗	5e-4(Dyn.)	66.57	65.46	78.58	70.20	11.73	35.74	12.09	19.86	0.7130
PDA	✗	5e-4(Dyn.)	62.29	66.61	75.87	68.26	13.12	30.35	7.02	16.83	0.7109
PDA+S_{Dice}	✗	5e-4(Dyn.)	62.79	68.36	73.17	68.44	9.36	21.13	**6.54**	12.36	0.7121
FedAvg+PDA	✗	5e-4(Dyn.)	63.04	67.93	75.61	68.86	6.70	22.43	8.19	12.45	0.7327
FedAvg+PDA	75%	5e-4(Dyn.)	65.08	68.30	77.62	70.33	7.03	24.35	8.32	13.24	0.7322
FedAvg+PDA+S_{HD}	75%	5e-4(Dyn.)	63.82	**68.92**	74.40	69.04	7.32	**19.56**	7.79	**11.56**	0.7282
FedAvg+PDA+S_{Dice}	75%	5e-4(Dyn.)	**65.15**	68.00	**79.92**	**71.02**	7.16	23.66	7.32	12.71	**0.7433**
FedAvg+PDA+S_{Dice}	75%	5e-4(Dyn.)	73.53	76.26	76.66	75.48	32.51	32.61	24.52	29.88	0.7130

(iii) Test Time Batch Normalization: At prediction time, we re-calculate the BN statistics on each test batch. The test time batch size is set to 1. **(iii) Developed Models:** The following models were developed and validated at the online platform: **BL:** nnunet baseline; **Tent** [34]: nnunet baseline with test time parameters adaptation by entropy minimization; **Test Time BN:** nnunet baseline with test time batch normalization; **IO-PFL** [14]: nnunet baseline with test time dynamic ensembling; **Avg -Ens:** nnunet baseline with test time batch normalization, ensembling results of all 5 folds.

4.3 Results

We compare the proposed method with different baseline methods and state-of-the-art FL methods, including the FedAvg [23] which is the widely used FL algorithm, the FedNova [35] which improves the aggregation by gradients normalization, and the FedAvgM [10] which applies momentum on the server update. We also report the performance on testing cohort released by the organizers [17].

Table 3. Comparison results for task 2, last row is results on testing cohort.

Method	Dice				HD95			
	ET	TC	WT	Average	ET	TC	WT	Average
nnUNet	83.87	86.61	92.28	87.59	**17.50**	12.60	3.72	11.27
+IOP-FL	83.67	88.49	92.73	88.30	20.10	8.75	3.55	10.80
+Tent	83.25	88.14	92.67	88.02	20.75	8.12	3.91	10.93
+Test-specific BN	84.18	87.26	92.53	87.99	19.14	7.70	3.83	10.22
+Test-specific BN + MoE	**84.31**	**88.21**	**92.76**	**88.43**	20.15	**7.24**	**3.50**	**10.29**
+Test-specific BN + MoE	88.28	89.96	92.95	90.40	10.61	10.87	5.88	9.12

Study and Discussion for Task 1. We applied our method and other methods on both split-1 and split-2, the results are shown in Table 1 and 2. It can be observed that our dynamic learning strategy improves the performance on both data splits, showing the effectiveness of our designed learning rate scheduling. However, since different aggregation methods do not outperform baseline methods on the split-1, we further validate our aggregation and pruning methods on the split-2. The PDA denotes the parameter distance based aggregation, and S_{AC} and S_{HD} denote the training metrics scores with Dice and HD95, respectively. By combining different factors together, our final method outperforms other compared methods on most of the Dice scores and the convergence score (C-Score). The aggregation with the help of S_{HD} achieves higher ranks regarding the HD95 metrics while the S_{Dice} ranks higher on Dice metrics. Since the Dice also relates to the convergence score calculation, our final solution chooses to combine the weights of FedAvg, PD, and the S_{Dice}.

Study and Discussion for Task 2. Table 3 shows the Dice score and HD95 computed by the online validation platform. For BL, Tent, and Test Time BN, we use the fixed train and validation split with a ratio of 8:2. It is observed that both Tent and Test Time BN improve the dice score of all three tumor sub-regions. For HD95, Tent and Test Time BN decrease the HD95 of TC by a large margin while slightly increasing the HD95 of ET and WT. Compared with Tent, Test Time BN achieves a comparable dice score and largely decreases the HD95 of ET and TC regions. Thus we choose the **Test Time BN** model as our submission. We also try to ensemble multiple Test Time BN models trained with different seeds and validation split. Two ensemble methods are performed. As shown in Table 3, the vanilla Avg-Ens method slightly outperforms the dynamic ensembling method IO-PFL and achieves an average dice score of 88.43 and HD95 of 10.29 at the online validation platform. So our final solution chooses to ensemble 6 Test Time BN models by directly averaging model predictions.

5 Conclusion

We present two new methods for the federated efficient training and model generalization problem. Our proposed parameter distance aggregation combined with the client pruning strategy significantly improves the training efficiency and model performance. For model generalization, our test time adaptation scheme well mitigates the domain shift and shows significant performance improvements.

Acknowledgement. This work was supported by the Hong Kong Innovation and Technology Fund (Projects No. ITS/238/21).

References

1. Annas, G.J.: Hipaa regulations - a new era of medical-record privacy? N. Engl. J. Med. **348**(15), 1486–1490 (2003)
2. Baid, U., et al.: The RSNA-ASNR-MICCAI brats 2021 benchmark on brain tumor segmentation and radiogenomic classification. arXiv preprint arXiv:2107.02314 (2021)
3. Bakas, S., Akbari, H., Sotiras, A., Bilello, M., Rozycki, M., Kirby, J.: Segmentation labels and radiomic features for the pre-operative scans of the TCGA-GBM collection (brats-TCGA-GBM). The Cancer Imaging Archive (2017)
4. Bakas, S., Akbari, H., Sotiras, A., Bilello, M., Rozycki, M., Kirby, J.: Segmentation labels and radiomic features for the pre-operative scans of the TCGA-LGG collection (brats-TCGA-LGG). The Cancer Imaging Archive (2017)
5. Bakas, S., et al.: Advancing the cancer genome atlas glioma MRI collections with expert segmentation labels and radiomic features. Scientific Data (170117) (2017)
6. Bakas, S., et al.: Identifying the best machine learning algorithms for brain tumor segmentation, progression assessment, and overall survival prediction in the brats challenge (2019)
7. Chen, C., Liu, Q., Jin, Y., Dou, Q., Heng, P.A.: Source-free domain adaptive fundus image segmentation with denoised pseudo-labeling. In: de Bruijne, M., et al. (eds.) MICCAI 2021. LNCS, vol. 12905, pp. 225–235. Springer, Cham (2021). https://doi.org/10.1007/978-3-030-87240-3_22
8. Dou, Q., et al.: Federated deep learning for detecting covid-19 lung abnormalities in CT: a privacy-preserving multinational validation study. NPJ Digit. Med. **4**(1), 1–11 (2021)
9. Isensee, F., Jaeger, P.F., Kohl, S.A.A., Petersen, J., Maier-Hein, K.H.: nnu-net: a self-configuring method for deep learning-based biomedical image segmentation. Nat. Methods **18**, 203–211 (2021)
10. Hsu, T.M.H., Qi, H., Brown, M.: Measuring the effects of non-identical data distribution for federated visual classification. arXiv preprint arXiv:1909.06335 (2019)
11. Isensee, F., Jaeger, P.F., Full, P.M., Vollmuth, P., Maier-Hein, K.H.: nnu-net for brain tumor segmentation (2020)
12. Isensee, F., Jäger, P.F., Full, P.M., Vollmuth, P., Maier-Hein, K.H.: nnU-Net for brain tumor segmentation. In: Crimi, A., Bakas, S. (eds.) Brainlesion: Glioma, Multiple Sclerosis, Stroke and Traumatic Brain Injuries. BrainLes 2020. LNCS, vol. 12659, pp. 118–132. Springer, Cham (2021). https://doi.org/10.1007/978-3-030-72087-2_11
13. Jiang, M., Wang, Z., Dou, Q.: Harmofl: harmonizing local and global drifts in federated learning on heterogeneous medical images. In: AAAI, vol. 36, pp. 1087–1095 (2022)
14. Jiang, M., Yang, H., Cheng, C., Dou, Q.: Iop-fl: inside-outside personalization for federated medical image segmentation. arXiv preprint arXiv:2204.08467 (2022)

15. Jiang, M., Yang, H., Li, X., Liu, Q., Heng, P.A., Dou, Q.: Dynamic bank learning for semi-supervised federated image diagnosis with class imbalance. In: Wang, L., Dou, Q., Fletcher, P.T., Speidel, S., Li, S. (eds.) MICCAI 2022. LNCS, vol. 13433, pp. 196–206. Springer, Cham (2022). https://doi.org/10.1007/978-3-031-16437-8_19

16. Kaissis, G.A., Makowski, M.R., Rückert, D., Braren, R.F.: Secure, privacy-preserving and federated machine learning in medical imaging. Nat. Mach. Intell. 1–7 (2020)

17. Karargyris, A., et al.: Medperf: open benchmarking platform for medical artificial intelligence using federated evaluation. arXiv preprint arXiv:2110.01406 (2021)

18. Karimireddy, S.P., Kale, S., Mohri, M., Reddi, S., Stich, S., Suresh, A.T.: Scaffold: stochastic controlled averaging for federated learning. In: ICML, pp. 5132–5143. PMLR (2020)

19. Li, D., Kar, A., Ravikumar, N., Frangi, A.F., Fidler, S.: Federated simulation for medical imaging. In: Martel, A.L., et al. (eds.) MICCAI 2020. LNCS, vol. 12261, pp. 159–168. Springer, Cham (2020). https://doi.org/10.1007/978-3-030-59710-8_16

20. Li, W., et al.: Privacy-preserving federated brain tumour segmentation. In: Suk, H.I., Liu, M., Yan, P., Lian, C. (eds.) MLMI 2019. LNCS, vol. 11861, pp. 133–141. Springer, Cham (2019). https://doi.org/10.1007/978-3-030-32692-0_16

21. Liu, Q., Chen, C., Qin, J., Dou, Q., Heng, P.A.: Feddg: federated domain generalization on medical image segmentation via episodic learning in continuous frequency space. In: CVPR (2021)

22. Liu, Q., Yang, H., Dou, Q., Heng, P.A.: Federated semi-supervised medical image classification via inter-client relation matching. arXiv preprint arXiv:2106.08600 (2021)

23. McMahan, H.B., Moore, E., Ramage, D., Hampson, S.: Arcas. Communication-efficient learning of deep networks from decentralized data, B.A. (2017)

24. Menze, B.H., et al.: The multimodal brain tumor image segmentation benchmark (brats). IEEE TMI **34**(10), 1993–2024 (2015)

25. Ostrom, Q.T., et al.: Cbtrus statistical report: primary brain and central nervous system tumors diagnosed in the united states in 2008–2012. Neuro-oncology **17**(suppl. 4), iv1–iv62 (2015)

26. Pati, S., et al.: The federated tumor segmentation (FETS) challenge (2021)

27. Pati, S., et al.: Reproducibility analysis of multi-institutional paired expert annotations and radiomic features of the IVY glioblastoma atlas project (IVY gap) dataset. Med. Phys. **12**, 6039–6052 (2020)

28. Reina, G.A., et al.: Openfl: an open-source framework for federated learning (2021)

29. Rieke, N., et al.: The future of digital health with federated learning. NPJ Digit. Med. **1**, 1–7 (2020)

30. Roth, H.R., et al.: Federated learning for beast density classification: a real-world implementation. In: Albarqouni, S., et al. (eds.) DART DCL 2020. LNCS, vol. 12444, pp. 181–191. Springer, Cham (2020). https://doi.org/10.1007/978-3-030-60548-3_18

31. Sheller, M.J., et al.: Federated learning in medicine: facilitating multi-institutional pruning without sharing patient data. Sci. Rep. **1**, 1–12 (2020)

32. Sheller, M.J., Reina, G.A., Edwards, B., Martin, J., Bakas, S.: Multi-institutional deep learning modeling without sharing patient data: a feasibility study on brain tumor segmentation. In: Crimi, A., Bakas, S., Kuijf, H., Keyvan, F., Reyes, M., van Walsum, T. (eds.) BrainLes 2018. LNCS, vol. 11383, pp. 92–104. Springer, Cham (2018). https://doi.org/10.1007/978-3-030-11723-8_9

33. Silva, S., Gutman, B.A., Romero, E., Thompson, P.M., Altmann, A., Lorenzi, M.: Federated learning in distributed medical databases: Meta-analysis of large-scale subcortical brain data. In: ISBI, pp. 270–274. IEEE (2019)
34. Wang, D., Shelhamer, E., Liu, S., Olshausen, B., Darrell, T.: Tent: fully test-time adaptation by entropy minimization (2021)
35. Wang, J., Liu, Q., Liang, H., Joshi, G., Poor, H.V.: Tackling the objective inconsistency problem in heterogeneous federated optimization (2020)
36. Yang, Q., Liu, Y., Chen, T., Tong, Y.: Federated machine learning: concept and applications. ACM TIST **2**, 1–19 (2019)
37. D Yeganeh, Y., Farshad, A., Navab, N., Albarqouni, S.: Inverse distance aggregation for federated learning with non-IID data. In: Albarqouni, S., et al. (eds.) DART DCL 2020. LNCS, vol. 12444, pp. 150–159. Springer, Cham (2020). https://doi.org/10.1007/978-3-030-60548-3_15

Hybrid Window Attention Based Transformer Architecture for Brain Tumor Segmentation

Himashi Peiris[1(✉)], Munawar Hayat[3], Zhaolin Chen[1,2], Gary Egan[2], and Mehrtash Harandi[1]

[1] Department of Electrical and Computer Systems Engineering,
Monash University, Melbourne, Australia
{Edirisinghe.Peiris,Zhaolin.Chen,Mehrtash.Harandi}@monash.edu
[2] Monash Biomedical Imaging (MBI), Monash University, Melbourne, Australia
Gary.Egan@monash.edu
[3] Department of Data Science and AI, Faculty of IT,
Monash University, Melbourne, Australia
Munawar.Hayat@monash.edu

Abstract. As intensities of MRI volumes are inconsistent across institutes, it is essential to extract universal features of multi-modal MRIs to precisely segment brain tumors. In this concept, we propose a volumetric vision transformer that follows two windowing strategies in attention for extracting fine features and local distributional smoothness (LDS) during model training inspired by virtual adversarial training (VAT) to make the model robust. We trained and evaluated network architecture on the FeTS Challenge 2022 dataset. Our performance on the online evaluation is as follows: Dice Similarity Score of 85.70%, 90.59% and 87.27%; Hausdorff Distance (95%) of 10.46 mm, 7.40 mm, 12.66 mm for the enhancing tumor, whole tumor, and tumor core, respectively. Overall, the experimental results verify our method's effectiveness by yielding better performance in segmentation accuracy for each tumor sub-region. Our code implementation is publicly available.

Keywords: Deep Learning · Brain Tumor Segmentation · Medical Image Segmentation · Vision Transformers · Virtual Adversarial Training

1 Introduction

Interpreting clinically acquired, multi-institutional multi-parametric magnetic resonance imaging (mpMRI) scans is a long-standing challenge in medical AI as these medical volumes consist of intrinsically heterogeneous lesions, tumors, or anatomical objects. Accurate segmentation is a prerequisite for clinical diagnosis and treatment planning. Federated Tumor Segmentation (FeTs) challenge has clinically acquired mpMRI, and the task of the challenge is to segment intrinsically heterogeneous brain tumors (gliomas). The objective is to create a consensus segmentation model acquired from various institutions without pooling their data together [1,13,17,19]. Segmenting brain tumors from medical scans is a tedious process requiring expertise and concentration since tumors are heterogeneous. Therefore, implementing a generalized deep learning model that can produce reliable predictions or segmentation masks with distinct regions of interest for patient data from various institutional distributions is highly demanded in scientific research. Traditionally, automated segmentation tools were implemented using manual feature engineering-based learning methods such as decision forest [24], conditional random field (CRF) [22]. However, with the recent progress in Convolutional Neural networks (CNN) and improvements in computational resources (*e.g.*, Graphical Processing Units (GPU)), deep learning models for tumor segmentation have been widely developed and studied by many researchers in medical AI domain [10,15]. The majority of medical image segmentation works [14,15] follow, U-Net [18] and 3D U-Net [3] as their baseline architectures. These U-Shaped architectures enable local feature extraction while maintaining contextual cues. However, what is lacking in these CNN-based methods is their inability to extract long-range dependencies during training. Focusing more on local cues than global cues may sometimes lead to extracting uncertain or imprecise information, which degrades the segmentation performance and reliability.

Transformer architectures were originally proposed to address the above inductive bias issues. These transformer models are designed to extract long-range dependencies for sequence-to-sequence tasks [20]. Inspired by recent progress in Vision Transformers for Volumetric brain tumor segmentation [7, 16,21,23], medical image reconstruction [6] and its unique abilities over Convolutional Neural Network (CNN), based models, we propose a U-shaped encoder-decoder neural network that adapts two-way windowing approach during decoding for fine detail extraction. Vision Transformers [2,4,5] have shown groundbreaking performance improvement in extracting long-range dependencies by maintaining a flexible receptive field. Also, the better robustness against data corruptions and occlusions [12], shown in Transformer based deep learning models, is unarguably the best thing that is ever asked for in a neural network design. Considering these aspects of the Transformer Network, in our proposed method, we used two popular window-based attention mechanisms namely, Cross-Shaped window attention based Swin Transformer block and Shifted window attention based Swin Transformer block to construct a U-shaped Volumetric Transformer (CR-Swin2-VT). In the CR-Swin2-VT model, Swin Transformer blocks [2] and CSWin Transformer blocks [4] are constructed parallel in the encoder side to capture voxel information precisely. At the same time, only Swin Transformer blocks are used on the decoder side.

In summary, our major contributions are, (**1**) We propose a volumetric transformer architecture that can process medical scans as volumes in entirety. (**2**) We design an encoding path with two window-based attention mechanisms to capture local and global features of medical volumes. **(3)** We conduct extensive experiments on FeTS Challenge 2022 dataset for the brain tumor segmentation task.

2   Method

We denote vectors and matrices in bold lower-case $\mathbf{x}$ and bold upper-case $\mathbf{X}$, respectively. Let $\mathbb{X} = \{\mathbf{x}_1, \mathbf{x}_2, \cdots, \mathbf{x}_\tau\}, \mathbf{x}_i \in \mathbb{R}^C$ be a sequence representing the voxel patches of the medical volume (*e.g.*, an MRI volume). Each $\mathbf{x}_i$ is considered a token. Following previous work by Vaswani *et al.* [20], we define Self-Attention (SA) as:

$$\mathrm{SA}(\mathbf{Q}, \mathbf{K}, \mathbf{V}) = \mathrm{SoftMax}\Big(\mathbf{Q}\mathbf{K}^\top / \sqrt{C}\Big)\mathbf{V}, \tag{1}$$

where $\mathbb{R}^{\tau \times C_v} \ni \mathbf{V} = \mathbf{X}\mathbf{W}_{\mathbf{V}}$, by stacking tokens $\mathbf{x}_i$s into the rows of $\mathbf{X}$ (*i.e.*, $\mathbf{X} = [\mathbf{x}_1|\mathbf{x}_2|\cdots\mathbf{x}_\tau]^\top$).

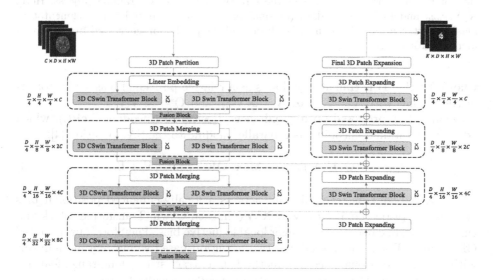

Fig. 1. Proposed CR-Swin2-VT Network Architecture.

In recent transformer-based studies, this conventional SA mechanism is altered in many ways, mainly by including typical positional encoding methods during SA calculation. This allows adding back positional information back in action during model training. One of the most popular methods is Relative Positional Encoding (RPE), which is used in celebrated work Swin Transformer [9]. SA with RPE is defined as:

$$\mathrm{SA}(\mathbf{Q}, \mathbf{K}, \mathbf{V}) = \mathrm{SoftMax}\Big(\mathbf{Q}\mathbf{K}^\top / \sqrt{C} + \mathbf{B}\Big)\mathbf{V}, \tag{2}$$

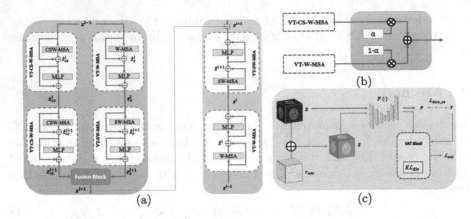

Fig. 2. (a) Illustrates VT-UNet Architecture. Here, k denotes the number of classes. (b) shows the structure of the Fusion Block that aggregates two attention maps generate from the CSwin Transformer block and the Swin Transformer block in the decoder side of the network. (c) illustrates the CR-Swin2-VT model training process. Here, X, Y, r_{adv} and P are input data (original patient data), ground truth segmentation masks, perturbation added on input data, and the prediction generated from the segmentation network.

where, $\mathbb{R}^{\tau \times \tau} \ni \mathbf{B}$ is trainable and acts as a relative positional bias across tokens in the volume with $\mathbf{V} = \mathbf{XW_V}$, $\mathbf{K} = \mathbf{XW_K}$, and $\mathbf{Q} = \mathbf{XW_Q}$.

Dong *et al.* proposed Locally-enhanced Positional Encoding (LePE), which adds the positional encoding as a parallel module to the SA operation [4].

$$\mathrm{SA}(\mathbf{Q}, \mathbf{K}, \mathbf{V}) = \mathrm{SoftMax}\left(\mathbf{QK}^{\top} / \sqrt{C}\right)\mathbf{V} + \mathbf{L}, \tag{3}$$

where $\mathbb{R}^{\tau \times C_v} \ni \mathbf{L}$ is trainable and acts as a locally-enhanced positional bias operates on projected *Values*, $\mathbf{V} = \mathbf{XW_V}$ in each CSwin Transformer block and this mechanism can enforce stronger local inductive bias. Therefore, our proposed CR-Swin2-VT architecture adapts two attention-based windowing mechanisms with distinct positional encoding methods to extract strong long-range features accurately during the contracting path of encoder-decoder design.

2.1 Overall Architecture

The overall architecture of CR-Swin2-VT is illustrated in Fig. 1. The input to the CR-Swin2-VT model is a 3D volume of size $D \times H \times W \times C$. The output is a $D \times H \times W \times K$ dimensional volume. Here, k denotes the number of classes. Similar to [16], the proposed model comprises CR-Swin2-VT Encoder, CR-Swin2-VT Bottleneck, and CR-Swin2-VT Decoder.

CR-Swin2-VT Encoder. CR-Swin2-VT Encoder consists of 3D Patch Partitioning layer combined with a Linear embedding layer, 3D CSwin Transformer blocks, 3D Swin Transformer blocks, a Fusion block, and 3D Patch merging layer. During 3D patch partitioning, the input medical volumes (e.g., T1, T1CE, Flair, T2 MRI sequences) are split into non-overlapping voxel/3D patches and fed to the next linear embedded layer as a set of tokens. Here we used a partitioning kernel $P \times M \times M$ where $P = 2$ and $M = 4$, which results in $2 \times 4 \times 4$ patch partitioning kernel. During linear embedding, the resultant tokens are mapped into a C dimensional vector (Embedded Dimensions). In our experiments, we set $C = 48$. These tokens are then passed through two successive 3D Swin Transformer blocks [9] (**VT-W-MSA-Blk**), which are comprised of **(1)** Window Multi Head SA (W-MSA), **(2)** Shifted Window Multi Head SA (SW-MSA) and two successive CSwin Transformer blocks [4] (**VT-CS-W-MSA-Blk**) which are consisted of Cross-shaped Window SA (CSW-MSA).

VT-W-MSA-Blk. During W-MSA operation, the volume is evenly split into smaller non-overlapping windows, and attention is calculated for those windows. To extract long-range dependencies, shifted window approach is used during SW-MSA operation [9]. Therefore, VT-W-MSA Block's functionality is defined as:

$$\hat{\mathbf{z}}_s^l = \text{W-MSA}\left(\text{LN}\left(\mathbf{z}^{l-1}\right)\right) + \mathbf{z}^{l-1}, \qquad \hat{\mathbf{z}}_s^{l+1} = \text{SW-MSA}\left(\text{LN}\left(\mathbf{z}_s^l\right)\right) + \mathbf{z}_s^l,$$
$$\mathbf{z}_s^l = \text{MLP}\left(\text{LN}\left(\hat{\mathbf{z}}_s^l\right)\right) + \hat{\mathbf{z}}_s^l, \qquad \mathbf{z}_s^{l+1} = \text{MLP}\left(\text{LN}\left(\hat{\mathbf{z}}_s^{l+1}\right)\right) + \hat{\mathbf{z}}_s^{l+1}, \quad (4)$$

where $\hat{\mathbf{z}}_s^l$ and $\mathbf{z}_s^l$ denote the output features of the W-MSA module and the Multi-Layer Perceptron (MLP) module for block l, respectively. A Layer Normalization (LN) is applied before every MSA and MLP, and a residual connection is applied after each module.

VT-CS-W-MSA-Blk. CSW-MSA operation consisted of calculating SA in horizontal and vertical stripes in parallel that form a cross-shaped window [4]. The VT-CS-W-MSA Block's functionality is defined as:

$$\hat{\mathbf{z}}_{cs}^l = \text{CSW-MSA}\left(\text{LN}\left(\mathbf{z}^{l-1}\right)\right) + \mathbf{z}^{l-1}, \qquad \hat{\mathbf{z}}_{cs}^{l+1} = \text{CSW-MSA}\left(\text{LN}\left(\mathbf{z}_{cs}^l\right)\right) + \mathbf{z}_{cs}^l,$$
$$\mathbf{z}_{cs}^l = \text{MLP}\left(\text{LN}\left(\hat{\mathbf{z}}_{cs}^l\right)\right) + \hat{\mathbf{z}}^l, \qquad \mathbf{z}_{cs}^{l+1} = \text{MLP}\left(\text{LN}\left(\hat{\mathbf{z}}_{cs}^{l+1}\right)\right) + \hat{\mathbf{z}}_{cs}^{l+1}, \quad (5)$$

where $\hat{\mathbf{z}}_{cs}^l$ and $\mathbf{z}_{cs}^l$ denote the output features of the CSW-MSA module and the Multi-Layer Perceptron (MLP) module for block l, respectively. A Layer Normalization (LN) is applied before every MSA and MLP, and a residual connection is applied after each module.

Fusion Block. The output tokens generated from each VT-W-MSA-Blk and VT-CS-W-MSA-Blk are then aggregated using fusion function $\mathcal{F}(\cdot)$ which gives $\mathbf{z}^{l+1}$. $\mathcal{F}(\cdot)$ is defined as:

$$\mathcal{F}(\mathbf{z}_s^{l+1}, \mathbf{z}_{cs}^{l+1}) = \alpha \, \mathbf{z}_s^{l+1} + (1 - \alpha) \, \mathbf{z}_{cs}^{l+1}, \quad (6)$$

where we use a linear combination with $\alpha = 0.5$, the aggregated output produced from the fusion block is then passed into the 3D patch merging layer to generate feature hierarchies in the encoder of CR-Swin2-VT.

Bottleneck. The bottleneck consisted of one successive block from VT-W-MSA-Blk and VT-CS-W-MSA-Blk together with 3D Patch Expanding layer.

CR-Swin2-VT Decoder. The CR-Swin2-VT decoder starts with successive VT-W-MSA-Blks together with 3D patch expanding layers and a classifier at the end to generate final volumetric segmentation masks.

2.2   Training Objective

The CR-Swin2-VT model's objective is to segment volumetric medical images, and its model learning process is deeply shared across the loss function we used.

Loss Function. Let $\mathcal{X} = \{(\mathbf{X}_1, \mathbf{Y}_1), \cdots, (\mathbf{X}_n, \mathbf{Y}_n)\}$ denote the labeled data from n patients, where each pair $(\mathbf{X}_i, \mathbf{Y}_i)$ has an image $\mathbf{X}_i \in \mathbb{R}^{D \times H \times W \times C}$ and its associated ground-truth mask $\mathbf{Y}_i \in \mathbb{R}^{D \times H \times W \times K}$. To train CR-Swin2-VT, we jointly minimize the Dice Loss (DL), Cross Entropy (CE) loss, and VAT loss. The three loss terms are modified and computed in a voxel-wise manner. The DL is defined as:

$$\mathcal{L}_{\mathrm{dl}}(\theta; \mathcal{X}) = -\mathbb{E}_{(\mathbf{X}, \mathbf{Y}) \sim \mathcal{X}} \left[\frac{2 \langle \mathbf{Y}, \mathcal{H}(\mathbf{X}) \rangle}{\|\mathbf{Y}\|_1 + \|\mathcal{H}(\mathbf{X})\|_1} \right], \tag{7}$$

where $\mathcal{H}(\cdot)$ and θ denote the transformer model and the model parameters, respectively. The CE loss is defined as:

$$\mathcal{L}_{\mathrm{ce}}(\theta; \mathcal{X}) = \mathbb{E}_{(\mathbf{X}, \mathbf{Y}) \sim \mathcal{X}} \left[-\mathbf{Y} \log \mathcal{H}(\mathbf{X}) \right], \tag{8}$$

During CR-Swin2-VT model training, we make use of VAT to update the model by the weighted sum of the gradient and consider the loss introduced during VAT as a regularization term for our full objective function. Inspired by the VAT method by Miyato *et al.* [11], $\mathcal{L}_{vat}$ is calculated as Kullback-Leibler (KL) divergence loss which measures the divergence between ground truth distribution and perturbed prediction distribution. The VAT block improves the CR-Swin2-VT model's robustness against adversarial samples that violates the virtual adversarial direction. Therefore, the VAT loss term is defined as a divergence-based Local Distributional Smoothness (LDS):

$$\mathcal{L}_{\mathrm{vat}}(\theta_G; \mathcal{X}; r_{adv}) = \mathbb{E}_{(\mathbf{X}, \mathbf{Y}) \sim \mathcal{X}} \left[\mathcal{D}_{KL}(\mathbf{Y} \| \mathcal{F}(\theta_G, \mathbf{X} + r_{adv})) \right]. \tag{9}$$

Therefore, the full objective function is:

$$\mathcal{L}_{\mathrm{seg}}(\theta; \mathcal{X}) = \mathcal{L}_{\mathrm{dl}}(\theta; \mathcal{X}) + \mathcal{L}_{\mathrm{ce}}(\theta; \mathcal{X}) + \lambda \mathcal{L}_{vat}(\theta; \mathcal{X}; r_{adv}) \tag{10}$$

where λ is a hyper-parameter that controls the contribution of the VAT loss term.

3 Experiments

Dataset. We use mpMRI from the FeTS Challenge 2022 [1,13,17,19] for CR-Swin2-VT model training and evaluation. The training dataset has 1251 MR volumes of shape $240 \times 240 \times 155$ from four MRI sequences that are conventionally used for glioma detection: T1 weighted sequence (T1), T1-weighted contrast-enhanced sequence using gadolinium contrast agents (T1Gd) (T1CE), T2 weighted sequence (T2), and Fluid attenuated inversion recovery (FLAIR) sequence. These sequences are then used to identify four distinct tumor sub-regions as: The Enhancing Tumor (ET), which corresponds to the area of relative hyper-intensity in the T1CE with respect to the T1 sequence, Non-Enhancing Tumor (NET), Necrotic Tumor (NCR), which are both hypo-intense in T1-Gd when compared to T1, Peritumoral Edema (ED) which is hyper-intense in FLAIR sequence. These almost homogeneous sub-regions are then converted into three semantically meaningful tumor classes Enhancing Tumor (ET), the addition of ET, NET, and NCR represents the Tumor Core (TC) region, and the addition of ED to TC represents the Whole Tumor (WT).

Image Pre-processing. MRI volumes' intensity is inconsistent due to various factors such as patients' motions during the examination, different manufacturers of acquisition devices, sequences, and parameters used during image acquisition. To standardize all volumes, min-max scaling was performed, followed by clipping intensity values. Images were then cropped to a fixed patch size of $128 \times 128 \times 128$ by removing unnecessary background pixels.

Implementation Details. The proposed CR-Swin2-VT model is implemented in PyTorch with a single Nvidia RTX 3090 GPU with 24GB. The weights of Swin-T [9] pre-trained on ImageNet-22K are used to initialize the model. To train CR-Swin2-VT, we use Adam optimizer with the learning rate of 1e-04 with a batch size of 1, 1000 epochs and ploy decay for the learning rate schedule. We split the original FeTS 2022 training dataset into a training set (80%) and a validation set (20%). Therefore, 1000 MR volumes are used to train the model, while 251 MR volumes are used as a validation set to evaluate the model's performance on unseen patient data during training. The best-performing model for the validation set is saved as the best model for official validation and testing phase evaluation. The FeTS 2022 validation dataset contains 219 MR volumes, and the synapse portal conducts the evaluation. In the inference phase, the original volume re-scaled using min-max scaling and fed forward through the CR-Swin2-VT model. We use the sliding window approach with the patch size of $128 \times 128 \times 128$ to generate predictions from the CR-Swin2-VT model. During inference, the CR-Swin2-VT model is used without the VAT block.

Experimental Results. Segmentation accuracy of three classes (*i.e.*, ET, TC and WT) are evaluated during training and inference. Both qualitative and quantitative analysis is performed to evaluate the model's accuracy. The proposed CR-Swin2-VT model is evaluated using two matrices (1) Dice Sørensen coefficient (DSC) and (2) Hausdorff Distance (HD). The quantitative and qualitative results of the online validation phase evaluation for the proposed approach are shown in Table 1, Fig. 4 and Fig. 3. From the quantitative results shown in Table 1, it can be seen that the proposed method outperforms when it comes to Hausdorff Distance measurements. Table 2 shows the quantitative results in the testing phase for the unseen patient data on 30 different sites.

Table 1. Validation Phase Results.

Method	Average		WT		ET		TC	
	HD	DSC	HD	DSC	HD	DSC	HD	DSC
nnUNet [8]	12.18	87.94	3.55	92.63	22.44	83.73	10.56	87.45
CNN VAT based Method [15]	11.92	85.85	5.37	90.77	21.83	81.40	8.56	85.39
CR-Swin2-VT	9.97	86.16	3.93	91.38	14.81	81.71	11.19	85.40

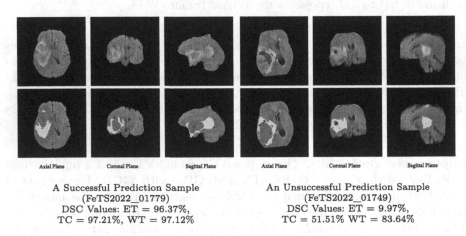

A Successful Prediction Sample
(FeTS2022_01779)
DSC Values: ET = 96.37%,
TC = 97.21%, WT = 97.12%

An Unsuccessful Prediction Sample
(FeTS2022_01749)
DSC Values: ET = 9.97%,
TC = 51.51% WT = 83.64%

Fig. 3. Validation Phase Qualitative Results for Prediction Samples. Here, yellow, red, and blue represent the peritumoral edema (ED), Enhancing Tumor (ET) and necrotic tumor (NCR), respectively.

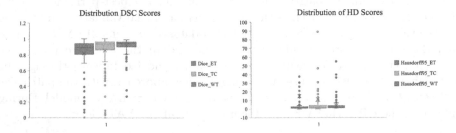

Fig. 4. The box and whisker plots of the distribution of the segmentation metrics for Validation Phase Results. The box-plot shows each tumor class's minimum, lower quartile, median, upper quartile, and maximum. Outliers are shown away from the lower quartile.

Table 2. Testing Phase Results.

Method	Average		WT		ET		TC	
	HD	DSC	HD	DSC	HD	DSC	HD	DSC
CR-Swin2-VT	10.17	87.85	7.40	90.59	10.46	85.70	12.66	87.27

4 Conclusion

We proposed a Transformer-based method that has adapted two windowing strategies in the encoder to extract the long-range dependencies both within and across different modalities of mpMRI. We validated our method on brain tumor segmentation using FeTS Challenge 2022 dataset and the results demonstrate the effectiveness of the proposed method.

References

1. Baid, U., et al.: The RSNA-ASNR-MICCAI brats 2021 benchmark on brain tumor segmentation and radiogenomic classification. arXiv preprint arXiv:2107.02314 (2021)
2. Cao, H., et al.: Swin-unet: Unet-like pure transformer for medical image segmentation. arXiv preprint arXiv:2105.05537 (2021)
3. Çiçek, Ö., Abdulkadir, A., Lienkamp, S.S., Brox, T., Ronneberger, O.: 3D U-Net: learning dense volumetric segmentation from sparse annotation. In: Ourselin, S., Joskowicz, L., Sabuncu, M., Unal, G., Wells, W. (eds.) MICCAI 2016. LNCS, vol. 9901, pp. 424–432. Springer, Cham (2016). https://doi.org/10.1007/978-3-319-46723-8_49
4. Dong, X., et al.: Cswin transformer: a general vision transformer backbone with cross-shaped windows. arXiv preprint arXiv:2107.00652 (2021)
5. Dosovitskiy, A., et al.: An image is worth 16x16 words: transformers for image recognition at scale. arXiv preprint arXiv:2010.11929 (2020)
6. Ekanayake, M., Pawar, K., Harandi, M., Egan, G., Chen, Z.: Multi-head cascaded swin transformers with attention to k-space sampling pattern for accelerated MRI reconstruction. arXiv preprint arXiv:2207.08412 (2022)
7. Hatamizadeh, A., et al.: Unetr: transformers for 3d medical image segmentation. In: Proceedings of the IEEE/CVF Winter Conference on Applications of Computer Vision, pp. 574–584 (2022)
8. Isensee, F., Maier-Hein, K.H.: nnU-Net for brain tumor segmentation. In: Crimi, A., Bakas, S. (eds.) BrainLes 2020. LNCS, vol. 12659, pp. 118–132. Springer, Cham (2021). https://doi.org/10.1007/978-3-030-72087-2_11
9. Liu, Z., et al.: Swin transformer: hierarchical vision transformer using shifted windows. arXiv preprint arXiv:2103.14030 (2021)
10. Luu, H.M., Park, S.H.: Extending nn-unet for brain tumor segmentation. arXiv preprint arXiv:2112.04653 (2021)
11. Miyato, T., Maeda, S.I., Koyama, M., Ishii, S.: Virtual adversarial training: a regularization method for supervised and semi-supervised learning. IEEE Trans. Pattern Anal. Mach. Intell. 41(8), 1979–1993 (2018)

12. Naseer, M., Ranasinghe, K., Khan, S., Hayat, M., Khan, F.S., Yang, M.H.: Intriguing properties of vision transformers. arXiv preprint arXiv:2105.10497 (2021)
13. Pati, S., et al.: The federated tumor segmentation (FETS) challenge. arXiv preprint arXiv:2105.05874 (2021)
14. Peiris, H., Chen, Z., Egan, G., Harandi, M.: Duo-SegNet: adversarial dual-views for semi-supervised medical image segmentation. In: de Bruijne, M., et al. (eds.) MICCAI 2021. LNCS, vol. 12902, pp. 428–438. Springer, Cham (2021). https://doi.org/10.1007/978-3-030-87196-3_40
15. Peiris, H., Chen, Z., Egan, G., Harandi, M.: Reciprocal adversarial learning for brain tumor segmentation: a solution to brats challenge 2021 segmentation task. arXiv preprint arXiv:2201.03777 (2022)
16. Peiris, H., Hayat, M., Chen, Z., Egan, G., Harandi, M.: A robust volumetric transformer for accurate 3D tumor segmentation. In: Wang, L., Dou, Q., Fletcher, P.T., Speidel, S., Li, S. (eds.) MICCAI 2022. LNCS, 13435, pp. 162–172. Springer, Cham (2022). https://doi.org/10.1007/978-3-031-16443-9_16
17. Reina, G.A., et al.: Openfl: an open-source framework for federated learning. arXiv preprint arXiv:2105.06413 (2021)
18. Ronneberger, O., Fischer, P., Brox, T.: U-net: convolutional networks for biomedical image segmentation. In: Navab, N., Hornegger, J., Wells, W.M., Frangi, A.F. (eds.) MICCAI 2015, LNCS, vol. 9351, pp. 234–241. Springer, Cham (2015). https://doi.org/10.1007/978-3-319-24574-4_28
19. Sheller, M.J., et al.: Federated learning in medicine: facilitating multi-institutional collaborations without sharing patient data. Sci. Rep. 10(1), 1–12 (2020)
20. Vaswani, A., et al.: Attention is all you need. Adv. Neural Inf. Process. Syst. 5998–6008 (2017)
21. Wang, W., Chen, C., Ding, M., Yu, H., Zha, S., Li, J.: TransBTS: multimodal brain tumor segmentation using transformer. In: de Bruijne, M., et al. (eds.) MICCAI 2021. LNCS, vol. 12901, pp. 109–119. Springer, Cham (2021). https://doi.org/10.1007/978-3-030-87193-2_11
22. Wu, W., Chen, A.Y., Zhao, L., Corso, J.J.: Brain tumor detection and segmentation in a CRF (conditional random fields) framework with pixel-pairwise affinity and superpixel-level features. Int. J. Comput. Assist. Radiol. Surg. 9(2), 241–253 (2014)
23. Zhou, H.Y., Guo, J., Zhang, Y., Yu, L., Wang, L., Yu, Y.: nnformer: interleaved transformer for volumetric segmentation. arXiv preprint arXiv:2109.03201 (2021)
24. Zikic, D., et al.: Decision forests for tissue-specific segmentation of high-grade gliomas in multi-channel MR. In: Ayache, N., Delingette, H., Golland, P., Mori, K. (eds.) MICCAI 2012. LNCS, vol. 7512, pp. 369–376. Springer, Heidelberg (2012). https://doi.org/10.1007/978-3-642-33454-2_46

Robust Learning Protocol for Federated Tumor Segmentation Challenge

Ambrish Rawat[1]($\boxtimes$), Giulio Zizzo[1], Swanand Kadhe[2], Jonathan P. Epperlein[1], and Stefano Braghin[1]

[1] IBM Research Europe, Dublin, Ireland
{ambrish.rawat,jpepperlein,stefanob}@ie.ibm.com, giulio.zizzo2@ibm.com
[2] IBM Research, Almaden, San Jose, USA
swanand.kadhe@ibm.com

Abstract. In this work, we devise robust and efficient learning protocols for orchestrating a Federated Learning (FL) process for the Federated Tumor Segmentation Challenge (FeTS 2022). Enabling FL for FeTS setup is challenging mainly due to data heterogeneity among collaborators and communication cost of training. To tackle these challenges, we propose a **Ro**bust **Le**arning **Pro**tocol (RoLePRO) which is a combination of server-side adaptive optimisation (e.g., server-side Adam) and judicious parameter (weights) aggregation schemes (e.g., adaptive weighted aggregation). RoLePRO takes a two-phase approach, where the first phase consists of vanilla Federated Averaging, while the second phase consists of a judicious aggregation scheme that uses a sophisticated re-weighting, all in the presence of an adaptive optimisation algorithm at the server. We draw insights from extensive experimentation to tune learning rates for the two phases.

Keywords: Federated Learning · Adaptive Optimisation · Brain Tumor Segmentation

1 Introduction

In this work we investigate a federated learning system for Brain Tumor Segmentation as presented in the Federated Tumor Segmentation Challenge (FeTS) [1–3]. Brain Tumor Segmentation is a medical imaging task where given a an MRI scan a model is tasked to produce the segmentation demarcating the regions corresponding to a tumor namely, enhancing tumor (ET), tumor core (TC) and whole tumor (WT). Traditionally, a deep learning model with a U-Net architecture [4] is trained for this task. The data for training such models often resides with different institutions which prohibits the use of classical Machine Learning (ML) pipelines that require the data to be available centrally at one location. Therefore, in such situations one may resort to the privacy-preserving paradigm of FL [5] for training the model, which is the focus of FeTS. This challenge presents two tasks - the first involves algorithms for FL orchestration for

© The Author(s), under exclusive license to Springer Nature Switzerland AG 2023
S. Bakas et al. (Eds.): BrainLes 2022, LNCS 14092, pp. 183–195, 2023.
https://doi.org/10.1007/978-3-031-44153-0_18

improved model convergence, and the second is testing the generalisability of a model in the "wild" on the data of clients who did not participate in the original federation. We primarily focus on the first task and investigate a combination of approaches for client- and server-side optimisation schedules, parameter aggregation and fine tuning to help with model convergence.

2 FeTS Setup

The federation consists of 23 different institutions [1–3] seeking to collaboratively learn a U-Net model [4] for brain tumor segmentation. Each participating institution owns a variably sized data partition which resides privately with the host. The details of the partitioning are specified in `partitioning1.csv` where one can notice a skewed distribution with two collaborators, namely and together hold a major chunk of the total data. On top of this, the classical iid assumption of machine learning often goes for a toss and the respective partitions may have highly non-iid characteristics. Such skewed distributions are not foreign for federated setups and often the learning protocols are appropriately modified to account for the heterogeneity. In order to moderate the heterogeneity, the challenge also presents an additional partitioning where some institutions are further split based on the tumour size, resulting in a more balanced distribution across 33 clients as specified in `partitioning2.csv`.

More generally, such cross-silo FL setups consists of M clients, where m^{th} client owns data $D_m = \{(x_i, y_i)\}_{i=1}^{n_m}$ with n_m samples. The training is performed iteratively across multiple FL rounds. In round t, first the central server or aggregator selects a set $C_{(t)}$ of clients, referred to as a collaboration, for training. Second it broadcasts the current set of parameter vector $W = \{w_{t,j}\}$ to all N clients for computing a set of validation metrics (for brevity, we will often drop the dependence on j and refer to a single parameter as w). Third the clients in the collaboration $C_{(t)}$ train the model on their local data partitions to obtain the updated parameter w_{t+1}^c along with a set of post-training validation metrics, both of which they share with the aggregator. Finally the aggregator combines the weight vectors from different clients typically with weighted averaging (FedAvg) as, $w_{t+1} = \sum_{c \in C_{(t)}} n_c w_{t+1}^c / N_{C_{(t)}}$ where $N_{C_{(t)}} = \sum_{c \in C_{(t)}} n_c$ is the sum of samples across clients in collaboration $C_{(t)}$. The federation is performed for a total of T rounds with suitable measures like early stopping to help reduce the generalisation error.

Metrics. There are two metrics tracked as part of FeTS setup - Dice similarity score (DSC) which measures the overlap between predicted and ground truth segmentations and Hausdroff distance (HD) which accounts for the distance between segmentation boundaries. The details for these metrics are described in [1]. During the FL training, FeTS maintains the checkpoint of model which achieves the best DSC on the validation set which itself is set locally by each client with a classical 80–20 split.

Modelling Challenges. There are two key challenges in enabling federated learning for such settings. The first stems from the data distributions across different clients which are typically not iid. This often leads to diverging updates during training rounds which hamper model convergence. And second is the communication cost of training rounds and the presence of stragglers in the federation, both of which add an overhead for the learning process.

Typically FL setups either belong to a cross-silo or a cross-device setting. The former comprises of a clientele of the order of 100 participants each holding a relatively large data set while the latter could have as many as a billion clients with only few data samples associated with each participant. A synchronous orchestration with all clients participating in every round adds a massive communication overhead which can adversarially affect the rate of convergence. On the other hand, ignoring certain clients could bias the resultant model towards specific modes thereby deteriorating their generalisation capability.

Practical Challenges. While FeTS presents an interesting setup for exploring a combination of schemes for FL orchestration, it is worth noting that there are inherent assumptions in the system. An understanding of these assumptions helps in scoping out the playing field and shaping strategies for algorithm design and experimentation. For instance, the APIs for Task 1 limit access to local training protocols of participating clients which limits the applicability of approaches like FedProx [6] and Scaffold [7] to tackle the non-iidness in the system. Similarly, the available deployment of FeTS requires relatively large compute, of the order of 300 GB of CPU RAM optionally with at least 16 GB of GPU memory. Additionally, each training rounds can take up to 7 h which can delay the feedback often required for rapid prototyping, hyperparameter optimisation and prohibit re-runs for marginalising the experimentation noise. Finally, it should be mentioned that the orchestration maintains a counter for total simulated time which accounts for the different costs in a typical FL process including communication cost, training time and cost related to computation of validation metrics. The script exits when the total simulated time reaches one week. It is also worth mentioning that the specified FL plan for FeTS involves global computation of metrics, i.e. each client, irrespective of their participation in the collaboration, computes the set of validation metrics on the latest aggregated model. This, as we discuss in Sect. 3, can be beneficial for devising both client selection and parameter aggregation strategies. In summary, we work within these constraints and devise schemes that can help improve the rate of model convergence within the permissible simulated time.

FeTS 2021. The challenge was also hosted in 2021 [1] with some notable differences. To our understanding this year's challenge includes data from additional institutions potentially exacerbating the non-iidness in the system. We also note that Cost Weighted Averaging [8] and Adaptive Weight Averaging [9] resulted in winning solutions for the posed challenge which we explore within our overall FL plan as described in Sect. 3.

3   Our Approach

Summary of Our Approach. We propose to use a combination of server-side adaptive optimisation and judicious parameter aggregation in a two-phase process with all clients participating in every round. In the first phase, the server aggregates the weights with vanilla FedAvg and in the second it employs a judicious aggregation scheme which uses a more sophisticated re-weighting (we discuss several judicious aggregation schemes later). In both phases, server-side adaptive optimisation (e.g., server-side Adam described later) is used. The learning rates are appropriately adjusted for the two phases. We summarise our approach in Fig. 1. In the remaining section, we describe our thinking behind the proposed approach and provide details of its various components.

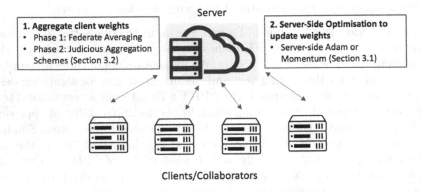

Fig. 1. Summary of our approach: a combination of server-side adaptive optimisation and judicious parameter aggregation in a two-phase process with all clients participating in every round.

FeTS presents a highly constrained and challenging scenario where both modelling and experimentation challenges need to be addressed simultaneously. These constraints limit the use of brute-force approaches for algorithm design, experimentation, and validation as well as hyperparameter optimisation. We therefore break the overall task into smaller components with a seat-of-the-pants strategy. First, we run the vanilla FedAvg algorithm with the default settings and make some observations. This involves every client participating in every round of the collaboration. Based on these observations we conjecture a working theory for this setup and use it to devise experiments. In particular, we note the behaviour of the optimisation and adopt a suitable learning rate schedule to fit this scenario. Additionally, we also adopt the server-side optimisation with adaptive schemes to help speed up convergence. We then look at a set of different aggregation schemes which are inspired from the successful solutions of FeTS 2021. Finally, we consider a two-phase process where we consider aggregation schemes as part of a fine tuning strategy. In this approach we first obtain a reasonable initialisation within first few FL rounds with vanilla FedAvg and follow it up with *fine-tuning* phase for the remaining time. For all of these experiments we only adopt the strategies for weights and biases in the U-Net. All other parameters are aggregated with weights proportional to sample size. It is worth noting that, even though we primarily focus on all clients participating in every round, our approach can in general be adapted to include client selection.

Default Setup. We first run the experiment with the default setting which consist of: all clients participating in every round, vanilla federated averaging, and fixed hyperparameters of learning rate and epochs per round across all rounds. We note the following observations from this experiment - 1) while there are two different partitions available we note that `partitioning2.csv` naturally provides a better fit with data parallelism, 2) the optimisation is not stable with an oscillating objective during the optimisation, 3) we experiment with local epochs of 1 and 3 and do not note any remarkable difference in DICE scores. We also note that it takes an average of 700 min (of simulated time) per round with all clients participating. Thus, with all 33 clients training for one local epoch in each round, one can perform a federation for up to 16 training rounds within the 1 week limit specified in the setup.

3.1   Server-Side Optimisation

In order to dampen the oscillations we explore the use of adaptive optimisation strategies. An FL setup consists of two different rates - a client side learning rate λ_c and a server side learning rate λ_s. In general, at round t the server first computes an aggregate of obtained updates $\hat{w}_{t+1}$ from the clients using the specified aggregation scheme, which is used to form a proxy $\Delta_t = w_t - \hat{w}_{t+1}$ for the gradient from the server's perspective. It then uses an optimisation strategy to modify its parameter state with the obtained delta. Thus, vanilla FedAvg can be thought of as performing a server side Stochastic Gradient Descent (SGD) $w_{t+1} = w_t - \lambda_s \Delta_t$ with $\lambda_s = 1.0$. However, adaptive strategies like momentum-based aggregation or even server-side Adam can be used to accelerate the convergence and dampen the oscillations [10,11]. It is worth pointing out that in FeTS the client-side optimisation is fixed as Adam [12]. The works of [10] and [11] provide an in-depth analysis of optimisation schemes for federated setup with some useful insights. We focus on two key takeaways from this work - they recommend jointly tuning λ_c and λ_s as they observe that the accuracy often follows a staircase pattern for adaptive schemes, and to decay the client-side learning rates when clients take more than a few gradient steps in their local optimisation. Finally, they also note that momentum-based adaption is more sensitive to choice of learning rates, while FedAdam and FedYogi [10] are more stable with respect to these choices.

For this experiment we stick with the classical sample-size-based weighting for aggregation and explore the use of adaptive optimisation strategies at the server end. We later adopt the learning from this experiment across other aggregation schemes. For convenience we refer to this intermediate parameter state as $\hat{w}_t$ which refers to the parameter obtained after using an aggregation scheme at the server end. This is subsequently used in combination with different optimisation approaches

- **OptAlgo A:** server-side SGD with $\lambda_s = 1.0$ combined with step-wise constant learning rates for clients across different rounds where $\lambda_c = 5 \cdot 10^{-5}$ for first 7 rounds followed by $\lambda_c = 5 \cdot 10^{-6}$ for the remaining rounds.
- **OptAlgo B:** server-side momentum where a moving average is maintained with respect to change in Δ_t which is in turn used to update the parameter state. The update can be summarised as,

$$
\begin{aligned}
\Delta_t &= w_t - \hat{w}_{t+1} \\
m_t &= \beta m_{t-1} + \Delta_t \\
w_{t+1} &= w_t - \lambda_s m_t
\end{aligned}
\tag{1}
$$

This has been explored in [13] and an implementation is available in FeTS. We use a β of 0.9 for this approach and fix λ_s as 0.1 and $\lambda_c = 5 \cdot 10^{-4}$ for first 7 rounds followed by $\lambda_c = 5 \cdot 10^{-5}$ for the remaining rounds.

- **OptAlgo C:** server-side Adam adopts a parameter-specific update by upweighting updates for parameters which receive sparse updates

$$
\begin{aligned}
\Delta_t &= w_t - \hat{w}_{t+1} \\
m_t &= \beta_1 m_{t-1} + (1 - \beta_1) \Delta_t \\
v_t &= \beta_2 v_{t-1} + (1 - \beta_2) \Delta_t^2 \\
w_{t+1} &= w_t - \lambda_s \frac{m_t}{\sqrt{v_t} + \tau}
\end{aligned}
\tag{2}
$$

FedAdam has previously been investigated in [10] where the authors fix τ as 0.001 and β_1 and β_2 as 0.9 and 0.99 respectively. They further experiment with a range of values for λ_c and λ_s and note that it often follows a staircase pattern. Following some initial experiments we note that λ_s of 0.001 and λ_c of $5 \cdot 10^{-4}$ provides stable updates. While this scheme differs slightly from the original Adam implementation where the τ is added as part of the square root and m_t and v_t are scaled with a decay for every new update, we didn't find an empirical impact on the algorithm when ran for few rounds.

It was clear in our experimentation and as is shown in Fig. 2 that adaptive schemes of OptAlgo B and OptAlgo C help dampen the oscillations observed for OptAlgo A. We would like to emphasise that we experimented in an ad-hoc fashion with manual intervention at different stages. For example, in some experiment runs that lower the λ_c further by a factor of 10 also helped with convergence. We suspect that normalising the number of updates across clients or reducing the local epochs across rounds with a decay factor can further help with the convergence. In general, our observations were consistent with those made in [10] and [11] - both OptAlgo B and OptAlgo C improved convergence, and OptAlgo C was the most stable with respect to choice of λ_c resulting in similar convergence behaviour across a range of different values for λ_c and λ_s.

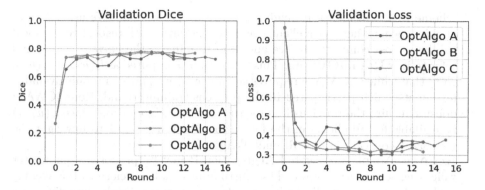

Fig. 2. Performance of Optimisation Algorithms with FedAvg for weight aggregation.

However, the absence of rigorous experimentation with hyperparameters can potentially result in an apples-vs-oranges comparison. We therefore take the teachings with a pinch of salt and only draw some high level conclusions as in the absence of rigorous testing they only serve as guiding approaches for our subsequent experiments.

3.2 Parameter Aggregation Methods

Inspired from the approaches in FeTS 2021, we also experiment with a few different parameter aggregation schemes. These refer to the set of algorithms that are used to obtain $\hat{w}_{t+1}$ from a set of client updates $\{w_t^c\}_{c\in C_{(t)}}$ received in round t. We replicate the setup of [8,9] to the best of our understanding and experiment with some modifications which are described below.

- **CostWAgg:** Cost Weighted Aggregation (CostWAgg) [8] uses the change in the validation loss across different rounds to guide the weighting during parameter aggregation. More specifically, for each client $c \in C_{(t)}$ it first computes the normalised ratio $r_c = l_c(w_{t-1}^c)/l_c(w_t^c)$ of the local validation loss (after training) from the previous round $l_c(w_{t-1}^c)$ with the one obtained for the current round $l_c(w_t^c)$, thereby giving larger weight to updates which resulted in larger decrease in loss. They further take a convex combination of the cost-based weight and sample-size-based weight to obtain the final parameter vector. In their scheme all clients participate in every round, i.e. $C_{(t)} = \{1,\ldots,M\}$ $\forall t$, and train for 10 epochs locally before sharing the updates. The update in round t is obtained as

$$\hat{w}_{t+1} = \sum_{c\in C_{(t)}} \left(\alpha \frac{n_c}{N_{C_{(t)}}} + (1-\alpha)\frac{r_c}{R_{C_{(t)}}} \right) w_t^c, \qquad (3)$$

where $R_{C_{(t)}} = \sum_{c\in C_{(t)}} r_c$ and α is a hyperparameter for balancing the two terms. The authors recommend $\alpha = 0.5$ while remarking that the optimisation wasn't particularly sensitive to the choice of α. Also, note that this scheme results in identical weighting across all parameters. We use a variant of this scheme where each client computes the ratio with respect to the local validation loss computed before and after training in the *current* round, and refer to it as **RoundCWAgg**. This ratio can be computed as $l_c(w_{t-1})/l_c(w_t^c)$. Note that while CostWAgg requires the use of $l_c(w_{t-1}^c)$ which is only available for clients which participated in the previous training round, RoundCWAgg doesn't require the previous loss for the current collaboration, since $l_c(w_{t-1})$ is available for all clients in the federation. We use $\alpha = 0.1$ to upweight the loss based contribution for RoundCWAgg.

- **RegAgg:** Adaptive Weighted Aggregation Policy [9] proposes a parameter weighting scheme that upweights contributions that are close to the average update. First, for each client c it computes an inverse of the absolute difference between client parameter w_t^c and the mean of the collaboration. These are normalised across clients to obtain the client-specific weighting factor u_c^w for the parameter w where clients whose updates are close to the average are assigned larger weights. This is then used in combination with sample-size-based weights $\nu_c = n_c/N_{C_{(t)}}$ to form the final weights with either an additive operator $u_c^w + \nu_c$ or a multiplicative operator $u_c^w \cdot \nu_c$. The former is referred to as Similarity Aggregation Policy (SimAgg) and the latter as Regularised Aggregation Policy (RegAgg) Policy. The authors use random sampling for selecting clients for collaboration (while ensuring fair selection of all clients) and remark that RegAgg with 5 local epochs provided them the best results during their experimentation. RegAgg updates every scalar weight in the weight vector $\hat{w}_{t+1}$ individually. We use $\omega = \hat{w}_{t+1}$ to reduce clutter.

$$\omega_{\text{mean}} = \frac{1}{\#C_{(t)}} \sum_{c \in C_{(t)}} w_t^c$$

$$u_c^w = \frac{1/\left|w_t^c - \omega_{\text{mean}}\right|_\tau}{\sum_{i \in C_{(t)}} 1/\left|w_{t,j}^i - \omega_{\text{mean}}\right|_\tau} \tag{4}$$

$$\omega = \frac{\sum_{c \in C_{(t)}} \left(u_c^w \cdot \nu_c \cdot w_t^c\right)}{\sum_{c \in C_{(t)}} \left(u_c^w \cdot \nu_c\right)},$$

where $|x|_\epsilon := |x| + \epsilon$ avoids divisions by zero; we use $\epsilon = 1 \cdot 10^{-5}$ as specified in [9]. This aggregation scheme results in different weights for different parameters, since u_c^w for every parameter w. We also experiment with a modification to this algorithm **RegMedAgg** which uses median (ω_{median}) for computing u_c^w as opposed to the arithmetic mean.

- **RegCostAgg:** This approach combines the approaches of CostWAgg and RegAgg where the loss ratio r_c is combined with the sample-size weight in a multiplicative way. This results in,

$$\hat{w}_{t+1} = \frac{\sum_{c \in C_{(t)}} \left(r_c \cdot \nu_c \cdot w_t^c\right)}{\sum_{c \in C_{(t)}} \left(r_c \cdot \nu_c\right)} \tag{5}$$

We run 13 rounds of FL training and use OptAlgoB while comparing these different parameter aggregation scheme. We specifically monitor four metrics -

best validation Dice across all labels till round 13, best validation loss till round 13 as well as average validation DICE and validation loss for last five rounds. The results are summarised in Table 1. While in terms of Best Dice (or loss) values many methods are comparable, the Avg Dice (or loss) tells a more relevant story as it sheds light on the stability of the overall optimisation protocol. Mindful of the fact that these numbers weren't obtained over multiple runs, we tentatively conclude that the parameter aggregation schemes provide marginal benefits over vanilla FedAvg (with generally smaller avg loss and higher avg Dice).

Table 1. Performance of different parameter aggregation schemes with OptAlgoB for optimisation. Average values show the stability of the FL process near convergence.

	Best Dice	Avg Dice	Best loss	Avg loss
FedAvg	0.7771	0.7417	0.3008	0.3522
CostWAgg	0.7738	0.7578	0.2984	0.3157
RoundCWAgg	0.7718	0.7022	0.3074	0.4095
RegAgg	0.7783	0.7310	0.2920	0.3608
RegMedAgg	0.7569	0.7448	0.3254	0.3478
RegCostAgg	0.7848	0.7595	0.2900	0.3272

3.3 Fine Tuning Approaches

In Sect. 3.1 we noted that OptAlgoB and OptAlgoC help dampen the oscillations and stabilise the server-side optimisation, and in Sect. 3.2 we noted some benefits in the use of different parameter aggregation schemes over FedAvg. With these two lessons and the proverbial knowledge among practitioners that the benefits of domain specific adaption are more suitable as fine tuning, we conjecture an FL plan - **Ro**bust **Le**arning **Pro**tocol (RoLePRO) that consists of two stages: First, we run vanilla FedAvg for a few initial rounds with all clients participating in each round with either OptAlgoB or OptAlgoC and appropriate choices of learning rates λ_s and λ_c. Then, we fine-tune the obtained model with the one of the following aggregation schemes - CostWAgg, RegAgg, TrimmedMean and TopKRegCost, and preferably a reduced set of learning rates. The use of TrimmedMean and TopKRegCost is motivated by an intent to reduce the effect of variance within client updates during aggregation which we explain below.

As described in Sect. 2 the data split across the different participating institutions is highly imbalanced. Naturally, such scenarios lead to large variance among the client updates in each round. It is worth remarking that within FeTS the institutions share updates after a fixed number of epochs which is common for all clients. Thus, clients perform a varying number of local gradient updates which can exacerbate client drift and result in disparate client updates. The success of CostWAgg and RegAgg in FeTS also bears a mention here. CostWAgg effectively prefers updates with more stable loss changes across different rounds and combines it with sample weights thereby giving a high weight to smoothed updates from large-data clients. Similarly, RegAgg enables preferential weighting by exploiting the geometry of updates in combination with the sample weighting. Effectively, updates which are close the mean-update and correspond to clients with large data receive the largest weights during aggregation. Such weighting for FeTS has also been explored in [14] where they categorised the participating institutions as internal and external depending on their sample contribution and developed different weighting schemes for the two groups. TrimmedMean provides an alternative way to alleviate the variance by only accounting for the geometry where first the set of updates are trimmed by discounting the ones that are too far from the median, and the remaining fraction of filtered updates are averaged (without any weighting). This has been explored in the context of byzantine behaviour in Federated Learning [15, 16]. While this approach can be beneficial for softening the aggregation, it often slows down convergence. Also worth noting that for TrimmedMean, the filtering of updates across different clients before the aggregation step is different for different parameters. In TopKRegCost we account for loss values and sample size for this filtering step by first sorting the clients as per their loss-ratio and sample contribution with the score, $n_c/N_{C(t)} \cdot l_c(w_{t-1}^c)/l_c(w_t^c)$, similar to RegCostAgg, and then averaging (without weighting) the k best updates with the largest scores. We use a filtering factor of 20% for both TrimmedMean and TopKRegCost. Note that TopKRegCost can be thought of as an aggressive or harder version of its soft counterparts RegCostAgg and CostWAgg where instead of down-weighting fruitless contributors one simply discards them and is democratic in its consideration of filtered contributors. Contrary to TrimmedMean, the filtering in TopKRegCost is common across all parameters during a training round.

All of the aforementioned aggregation schemes can result in biased models. For instance, TopKRegCost can lead to a preferential treatment of a select few clients, especially with a high filtering factor. The hyperparameter α controls a similar trade-off for CostWAgg. Such loss-based aggregation has also been explored in other contexts for FL. One example is the Federated Adversarial Training [17] protocol which suffers from highly disparate updates during the training rounds and modifying the weighting scheme helped improve convergence [18]. Similarly, best-k sparsification has been used to combat model poisoning in FL [19].

In Table 2 and 3 we present the results for RoLePro with OptAlgoB and OptAlgoC across different aggregation schemes. We observe that both RegAgg and TopKRegCost lead to high-performing models across both OptAlgoB and OptAlgoC. It should be mentioned that apart from aggregation schemes, the optimisation protocols of OptAlgoB and OptAlgoC also enable parameter specific learning rates, therefore it can be challenging to pin-point the source of the observed gains within the complex orchestration of an FL plan.

Table 2. Performance of different aggregation schemes with OptAlgoB in the fine-tuning phase of the two-phase learning protocol of RoLePro

	Best Dice	Avg. Dice	Best loss	Avg. loss
RegAgg	0.8067	0.7921	0.2639	0.2821
CostWAgg	0.7788	0.7681	0.3107	0.3207
TrimmedMean	0.7928	0.7834	0.2764	0.2958
TopKRegCost	0.7965	0.7806	0.2718	0.2957

Table 3. Performance of different aggregation schemes with OptAlgoC in the fine-tuning phase of the two-phase learning protocol of RoLePro

	Best Dice	Avg. Dice	Best loss	Avg. loss
RegAgg	0.7958	0.7851	0.2709	0.2905
CostWAgg	0.7888	0.7712	0.2880	0.3060
TrimmedMean	0.7588	0.7517	0.3218	0.3314
TopKRegCost	0.7963	0.7700	0.2799	0.3086

3.4 Submission

We used the insights from above for our final submission, which was specifically:

Rounds 1–3 used vanilla WAvg, with the Adam optimiser on both sides. The server-side learning rate was 0.003, and on the client-side it was 0.0005.

For rounds 4–16, we switched to RegAgg, with Adam optimiser on both sides and reduced learning rates of 0.002 on the server side 0.00005 on the client side. The results on the held-out FeTS 2022 test set are reported in Table 4.

Adam's parameters were set to the aforementioned values of $\beta_1 = 0.9$, $\beta_2 = 0.99$ and $\tau = 0.001$ in all rounds and on the server and all clients.

Table 4. Segmentation performance of the submitted algorithm on the FeTS 2022 test set, by label (WT: Whole Tumour, TC: Tumour Core, ET: Expanding Tumour). The reported Communications Cost was 0.702.

	Dice		Hausdorff 95	
	Mean (Std.)	Median (Quartiles)	Mean (Std.)	Median (Quartiles)
WT	0.7752 (0.1753)	0.8316 ([0.7105,0.8975])	28.93 (30.02)	14.88 ([6.428,48.51])
TC	0.7785 (0.2769)	0.9041 ([0.7609,0.9449])	28.81 (80.48)	4.123 ([2.236,10.1])
ET	0.747 (0.2625)	0.8492 ([0.7224,0.9114])	29.59 (85.79)	2.236 ([1.414,7.45])

4   Conclusions

It is well known that an FL system has many moving parts from the numerous components within its system design to the set of hyperparameters in the learning algorithm. These can often result in intractable experimentation strategies. In this work we focused on the cross-silo or enterprise setup of FeTS and developed an FL plan to orchestrate the learning over the data residing with 23 participating institutions. We achieved this by studying two different aspects of FL namely, server-side optimisation and judicious parameter aggregation schemes, which we then used to develop a robust learning protocol for the FeTS setup. This protocol prescribes a two phase process where vanilla FedAvg is followed by a fine-tuning phase that is enabled with sophisticated parameter aggregation schemes, all in the presence of an adaptive optimisation algorithm at the server end (such as server-side Adam). While we found the choice of learning rates for the two phases to be crucial for our FL plan, we acknowledge that these hyperparameter choices require thorough analysis. Finally, we hope that this empirical investigation can serve as a guiding document for tackling the underlying challenge of FeTS.

Acknowledgements. This work has been partially supported by the MORE project (grant agreement 957345), funded by the EU Horizon 2020 program.

References

1. Pati, S.: The federated tumor segmentation (FeTS) challenge. CoRR, abs/2105.05874 (2021)
2. Anthony Reina, G.: OpenFL: an open-source framework for federated learning. CoRR, abs/2105.06413 (2021)
3. Baid, U.: The RSNA-ASNR-MICCAI BraTS 2021 benchmark on brain tumor segmentation and radiogenomic classification. CoRR, abs/2107.02314 (2021)
4. Ronneberger, O., Fischer, P., Brox, T.: U-Net: convolutional networks for biomedical image segmentation. In: Navab, N., Hornegger, J., Wells, W.M., Frangi, A.F. (eds.) MICCAI 2015. LNCS, vol. 9351, pp. 234–241. Springer, Cham (2015). https://doi.org/10.1007/978-3-319-24574-4_28
5. McMahan, B., Moore, E., Ramage, D., Hampson, S., Arcas, B.A.: Communication-efficient learning of deep networks from decentralized data. In: Singh, A., (Jerry) Zhu, X. (eds.) Proceedings of the 20th International Conference on Artificial Intelligence and Statistics, AISTATS 2017, Fort Lauderdale, FL, USA, 20–22 April 2017. Proceedings of Machine Learning Research, vol. 54, pp. 1273–1282. PMLR (2017)
6. Li, T., Sahu, A.K., Zaheer, M., Sanjabi, M., Talwalkar, A., Smith, V.: Federated optimization in heterogeneous networks. In: Dhillon, I.S., Papailiopoulos, D.S., Sze, V. (eds.) Proceedings of Machine Learning and Systems 2020, MLSys 2020, Austin, TX, USA, 2–4 March 2020. mlsys.org (2020)

7. Karimireddy, S.P., Kale, S., Mohri, M., Reddi, S.J., Stich, S.U., Suresh, A.T.: SCAFFOLD: stochastic controlled averaging for federated learning. In: Proceedings of the 37th International Conference on Machine Learning, ICML 2020, 13–18 July 2020, Virtual Event. Proceedings of Machine Learning Research, vol. 119, pp. 5132–5143. PMLR (2020)
8. Mächler, L., et al.: FedCostWAvg: a new averaging for better federated learning. In: Crimi, A., Bakas, S. (eds.) BrainLes 2021. LNCS, vol. 12963, pp. 383–391. Springer, Cham (2021). https://doi.org/10.1007/978-3-031-09002-8_34
9. Khan, M.I., Jafaritadi, M., Alhoniemi, E., Kontio, E., Khan, S.A.: Adaptive weight aggregation in federated learning for brain tumor segmentation. In: Crimi, A., Bakas, S. (eds.) Brainlesion: Glioma, Multiple Sclerosis, Stroke and Traumatic Brain Injuries. BrainLes 2021. LNCS, vol. 12963, pp. 455–469. Springer, Cham (2021). https://doi.org/10.1007/978-3-031-09002-8_40
10. Reddi, S.J.: Adaptive federated optimization. In: 9th International Conference on Learning Representations, ICLR 2021, Virtual Event, Austria, 3–7 May 2021. OpenReview.net (2021)
11. Wang, J., et al.: A field guide to federated optimization. CoRR, abs/2107.06917 (2021)
12. Kingma, D.P., Ba, J.: Adam: a method for stochastic optimization. In: Bengio, Y., LeCun, Y. (eds.) 3rd International Conference on Learning Representations, ICLR 2015, San Diego, CA, USA, 7–9 May 2015, Conference Track Proceedings (2015)
13. Isik-Polat, E., Polat, G., Kocyigit, A., Temizel, A.: Federated brain tumor segmentation: multi-institutional privacy-preserving collaborative learning (2021)
14. Luo, R., Hu, S., Yu, L.: Rethinking client reweighting for selfish federated learning (2022)
15. Mhamdi, E.M.E., Guerraoui, R., Rouault, S.: The hidden vulnerability of distributed learning in Byzantium. In: Dy, J.G., Krause, A. (eds.) Proceedings of the 35th International Conference on Machine Learning, ICML 2018, Stockholmsmässan, Stockholm, Sweden, 10–15 July 2018. Proceedings of Machine Learning Research, vol. 80, pp. 3518–3527. PMLR (2018)
16. Baruch, G., Baruch, M., Goldberg, Y.: A little is enough: circumventing defenses for distributed learning. In: Wallach, H.M., Larochelle, H., Beygelzimer, A., d'Alché-Buc, F., Fox, E.B., Garnett, R. (eds.) Advances in Neural Information Processing Systems 32: Annual Conference on Neural Information Processing Systems 2019, NeurIPS 2019, Vancouver, BC, Canada, 8–14 December 2019, pp. 8632–8642 (2019)
17. Zizzo, G., Rawat, A., Sinn, M., Buesser, B.: FAT: federated adversarial training. CoRR, abs/2012.01791 (2020)
18. Zhu, J.: α-weighted federated adversarial training (2022)
19. Panda, A., Mahloujifar, S., Bhagoji, A.N., Chakraborty, S., Mittal, P.: SparseFed: mitigating model poisoning attacks in federated learning with sparsification. In: Camps-Valls, G., Ruiz, F.J.R., Valera, I. (eds.) International Conference on Artificial Intelligence and Statistics, AISTATS 2022, 28–30 March 2022, Virtual Event. Proceedings of Machine Learning Research, vol. 151, pp. 7587–7624. PMLR (2022)

Model Aggregation for Federated Learning Considering Non-IID and Imbalanced Data Distribution

Yuan Wang[✉], Renuga Kanagavelu, Qingsong Wei, Yechao Yang,
and Yong Liu

Institute of High Performance Computing, Singapore, Singapore
{wang_yuan,renuga_k,wei_qingsong,yang_yechao,liuyong}@ihpc.a-star.edu.sg

Abstract. With the ever increasing importance and requirements to ensure data privacy, federated learning emerges as an promising technology for training deep learning models without having hospitals to share the raw data. MICCAI Federated Tumor Segmentation Challenge 2021 is the first international challenge on federated learning to strengthen the understanding of real-world challenges and create practical solutions in the related area. In the challenge of this year, we proposed a series of new aggregation strategies towards improving the learning performance in the context of non-IID and imbalanced data distribution. We also designed a simple collaborator selection scheme to shorten the training time while achieving a good level of model performance for brain tumor segmentation.

Keywords: Federated Learning · Multi-institutional Collaboration · Medical Imaging · Brain Tumor Segmentation

1 Introduction

Artificial intelligence (AI) techniques find applications in healthcare such as medical imaging, patient care, diagnostics, and predictions of diseases. In computational radiology, AI plays a key role in helping diagnostic radiologists to characterise and interpret the disease like cancers and tumors and save their time to achieve goals with minimal errors [1,2] and make better decisions. Such AI models require large amount of medical data for training to achieve improved performance and thus the user experience. Though multi-institutional multi-parametric magnetic resonance imaging (MRI) scans are publicly available for the analysis of brain tumor by Brain Tumor Segmentation (BraTS) challenge, it is unlikely to scale well as many hospitals are reluctant to share the details due to data privacy regulations and data ownership [3,4] as patients' diagnosis data are privacy-sensitive, making it unrealistic to collect raw data from different hospitals into centralized location for model training.

Federated learning (FL) [5] has emerged as a reference architecture for collaborative machine learning, dealing with data privacy. It allows the medical

S. Bakas et al. (Eds.): BrainLes 2022, LNCS 14092, pp. 196–208, 2023.
https://doi.org/10.1007/978-3-031-44153-0_19

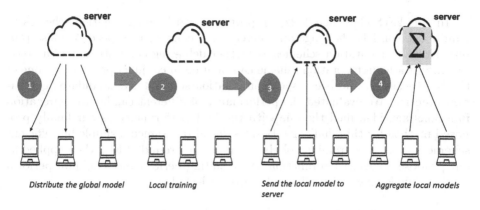

Fig. 1. Federated learning workflow.

institutions/hospitals to model their sensitive data in a collaborative manner without any actual exchange of their clinical data sets. This allows the hospitals to maintain the privacy of their data as well as the usability of the data. Model training in FL is an iterative process with four steps in each iteration as shown in Fig. 1. The steps are as follows: 1) The server sends the initial global model to the selected parties; 2) Each of the selected parties (i.e., the collaborators) updates the received model with their local data. 3) The model updates are sent to the server; 4) The server aggregates all the received model updates and then update the global model. This process is repeated until the underlying global model manages to perform acceptably in a test environment.

Currently FedAvg [5] is the most popular model aggregation algorithm that uses coordinate-wise averaging of the model parameters. However, this it is not suitable for non-Independent and Identically Distributed (non-IID) scenarios [6] which are usually encountered in real world as the aggregation of divergent models that are locally trained on non-IID data can significantly reduce the model accuracy and hurt the convergence speed, which requires more communication rounds and time to reach an acceptable level of performance.

To address the above issue, Federated Tumor Segmentation (FeTS) challenge [7] provides the participants with the patient records of which the distribution is in non-IID fashion, the participants are tasked to pursue an improved learning performance for the model trained via FL by developing techniques in the following aspects:

1. Custom aggregation logic (i.e., aggregation functions),
2. Strategy of selecting training hyper-parameters for each round of FL,
3. Strategy of selecting training collaborators participated in each round of FL.

The first FeTS challenge was conducted in 2021 [12,13], using MRI scans (i.e., th patient records) from various remote independent institutions as well as from the BraTS 2020 challenge [14]. An existing infrastructure (referred to as the base package) based on OpenFL [15] is provided to every challenge participants to implement and validate the proposed new federated aggregation and segmentation algorithms.

In this FeTS challenge 2022, we proposed two base aggregation schemes to handle the non-IID challenge and increase the convergence speed. We also proposed two augmentation schemes as further debiasing calibrations for the base schemes. Each augmentation scheme can be used in conjunction with any one of the base schemes, and every such combination stands for a candidate aggregation function. We evaluated the performance of different candidate aggregation functions and identified the one with the best performance as our finally proposed method for this challenge. Besides, we also designed a simple but efficient scheme for selecting training collaborators in each round of FL, when applied to our proposed aggregation function, the resulting performance could outperform the baseline FedAvg with all collaborators selected.

2   Related Work

Sheller et al. [8] proposed FL framework for healthcare applications, which allows the utilization of distributed clinical data sets without direct sharing, allowing institutions to collaborate on distributed training. Each institute trains a global model on their local data, sharing only the model updates to an aggregating server, completely circumventing the need of sharing sensitive medical data. Li et al. [9] proposed federated brain tumor segmentation using a deep neural network (DNN) on the BraTS dataset and applied differential privacy as a privacy protection technique to protect patient data. protection costs. Yi L. et al. focused on enhancing the model to facilitate federated brain tumour segmentation [10]. They combine the inception module and a dense block into standard U-Net to enhance multi-scale receptive fields and information reuse. Guo et al. [11] proposed a FL platform to reconstruct the MR images from multiple institutions.

2.1   Model Aggregation

FedAvg is the widely used model aggregation method in FL due to its simplicity, communication efficiency and acceptable performance in weakly non-IID scenarios. After performing local training Collaborators send their updated model parameters to central aggregator/server. Upon receiving updated weights from collaborators, server calculates the average of the collaborators' model updates as the global model following the equation below,

$$w^t = \sum_{i \in \mathcal{C}} p_i w_i^t, \tag{1}$$

where w_i^t is the model updates contributed by collaborator i at t-th round of FL, w^t is the global model, $\{p_i\}$ are aggregation weighting factors for the set of selected collaborators which is denoted by $\mathcal{C}$. These $\{p_i\}$ are usually calculated as the normalized number of data of each collaborator, see the equation below as a reference where $\mathcal{D}_i$ denotes the local data set of i-th collaborator,

$$p_i = \frac{|\mathcal{D}_i|}{\sum_{i \in \mathcal{C}} |\mathcal{D}_i|}. \tag{2}$$

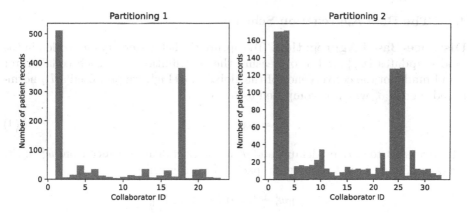

Fig. 2. Training data sets splits data distribution

Though FedAvg is currently the default model aggregation algorithm for FL, its performance degrades when the collaborators have strongly non-iid data distribution, so FedAvgM [17] is proposed to mitigate the performance degradation in this context. Simply enough, FedAvgM retains the basic logic of FedAvg and includes an additional server momentum. It updates the global model by

$$w \leftarrow w - \gamma v; v \leftarrow \beta v + \Delta w, \tag{3}$$

where v is the exponentially weighted moving average of the model updates with powers of β, γ is the server learning rate. This update rule is relatively stable when degree of non-idd increases in collaborators data distribution.

3   Data

The data set provided in FeTS challenge 2022 consists of multi-institutional MRI scans from the BraTS challenge and other institutions that are participated in the FeTS initiative [7,12,16]. The training set contains 1251 patient records, and has two partitioning: 1) a natural partitioning by institution denoted by partitioning 1 where the data are partitioned 23 originating institutions; and 2) an artificial partitioning denoted by partitioning 2 which is largely same as the institution split, but further partitions each of the 5 largest institutions according to the information extracted from the images, so that it contains data from 33 artificial institutions [7]. The validation set contains 219 patients records. In either partitioning 1 or 2, each institution plays the role of a collaborator in FL, they have non-IID data distribution as shown in Fig. 2.

4   The Proposed Methods

During this Challenge, due to time and resource constraints, we have been primarily focused on developing custom aggregation functions and tentatively designed a simple yet efficient training collaborator selection scheme.

4.1   The Base Aggregation Schemes

Distance-Based Aggregation. To capture the heterogeneity embedded in the model updates $\{w_i^t\}$ and also measure the contribution that each collaborator could made for the convergence of the global model w^t, we proposed a L_2 norm-based metric β_i^t which is computed as below

$$\beta_i^t = \exp\left(-\gamma \times d_i^t\right), \tag{4}$$

where γ is set to 0.01 by default and d_i^t is the Euclidean distance from w_i^t to the average of $\{w_i^t\}$ in the parameter space, which is given by

$$d_i^t = \|w_i^t - \mathbf{mean}(w_i^t; \forall i \in \mathcal{C})\|. \tag{5}$$

We then normalize all these $\{\beta_i^t\}$ to obtain the distance-based aggregation weighting factors as,

$$\beta_i^t \leftarrow \frac{\beta_i^t}{\sum_{i \in \mathcal{C}} \beta_i^t}, \tag{6}$$

and the new aggregation function is as follows,

$$w^t = \sum_{i \in \mathcal{C}} \beta_i^t w_i^t. \tag{7}$$

Validation-Based Aggregation. In this challenge, the organizer provides a base package for simulating the FL process where the loss generated by validating the local model updates w_i^t over local validation data (20% of $\mathcal{D}_i$) is stored in each round. The local validation loss of each collaborator will be uploaded to the server/aggregator together with the corresponding local model update. Therefore, the server can evaluate the quality of $\{w_i^t\}$ according to how small the local validation loss that every w_i^t leads to. Following the above reasoning, we also proposed a metric based on the local validation loss to measure how good a model updates can potentially be:

$$\beta_i^t = \mathcal{L}_{\mathcal{D}_i}(w_i^t), \tag{8}$$

where $\mathcal{L}$ is the loss function, the subscript $\mathcal{D}_i$ denotes the loss evaluated over local data $\mathcal{D}_i$.

Similar to the distance-based approach, we then normalize all these $\{\beta_i^t\}$ to obtain the aggregation weighting factors by (6) and establish the validation-based aggregation by (7). Note that we have abused a little bit the notation β_i^t to denote our proposed metrics either for distance- or validation-based approach.

4.2   The Augmentation Schemes

In addition to the two base aggregation schemes, i.e., the distance- and validation-based approaches, we also developed two augmentation schemes, in order to calibrate the potential bias in the custom aggregation weighting factors $\{\beta_i^t\}$.

The biased weighting factors are likely to be found in a scenario where the collaborator only has very limited number of data. For example, although the distance between w_i^t and the mean parameters of all model updates may happen to be small in certain round, the local training performed by i-th collaborator may have a relatively high gradient noise which could harm the convergence in the long term. Another example of such bias can be resulted from a situation where the local validation loss is relatively small but the underlying model might not be generalizable enough due to the collaborator only has limited amount of data (so that the amount of validation data is also limited). On the other hand, the standard aggregation weighting factors used in FedAvg, i.e., (2) can be a good indicator to capture the contribution based on the amount of data. Therefore, combining the custom aggregator weighting factors with the standard ones can be helpful to mitigate the bias described above, so that we were motivated to develop the following augmentation approaches.

Debiasing by Multiplication. The first method for debiasing the custom aggregation weight factors is simply to multiply the standard weighting factors p_i with the custom weighting factor β_i^t that is computed from either distance- or validation-based base aggregation schemes, i.e.,

$$s_i = p_i \beta_i^t, \tag{9}$$

where s_i is thus the new augmented metric. We then normalize these $\{s_i; \forall i \in \mathcal{C}\}$ by applying a procedure similar to (6),

$$s_i \leftarrow \frac{s_i}{\sum_{i \in \mathcal{C}} s_i}, \tag{10}$$

so that the augmented aggregation scheme is given by

$$w^t = \sum_{i \in \mathcal{C}} s_i w_i^t \tag{11}$$

Table 1. List of the proposed candidate aggregation functions

Method	Descriptions
Dist	Distance-based aggregation without any debiasing
Dist-Mul	Distance-based aggregation with multiplication debiasing (9)
Dist-Avg	Distance-based aggregation with weighted averaging debiasing (12)
Val	Validation-based aggregation without any debiasing
Val-Mul	Validation-based aggregation with multiplication debiasing (9)
Val-Avg	Validation-based aggregation with weighted averaging debiasing (12)

Debiasing by Weighted Average. In addition to the previously described multiplication-based method, we also proposed another method for debiasing the custom aggregation weighting factors using a weighted average as below,

$$s_i = \alpha p_i + (1 - \alpha)\beta_i^t, \tag{12}$$

where hyper-parameter α takes a default value of 0.5. Then applying (10) we arrive at (11).

4.3   The Candidate Aggregation Functions

Combining the base aggregation schemes and the augmentation schemes leads to six different candidate aggregation schemes summarized in Table 1. Therefore, we selected the most promising one among these candidate methods for our final submission to the challenge. To do so, we first ran a series of preliminary verification tests on the small-scale scenario provided in the base package (i.e., using smallsplits.csv as the partitioning profile), and we found that Dist perform considerably worse than the other five, then we conducted further verification and benchmark with the rest five candidate aggregation functions. The related results and the finally selected custom aggregation function are presented later in Sect. 5.

4.4   Selections of Training Hyper-parameter and Collaborator

Learning Rate and Number of Epoch. Due to constraints on available computing resources and limited allowed time, we were not able to attempt extensive experiments to optimize for learning rate, the number of local epoch per rounds. Instead, we used the default learning rate of 5.0×10^{-5} and the default one-epoch-per-round setup for all the results reported in this article.

Training Collaborator Selection. We used partitioning 2 as the data partitioning profile. During our initial trial experiments, we found that including all the collaborators leads to inferior performance in terms of mean Dice score[1] of the global model obtained at the aggregator.

Table 2. Descriptions of three random collaborator selection schemes

Method	Descriptions
Rand-Sel8	Randomly select 8 collaborators from all collaborators
Rand-Sel8-Subset	Randomly select 8 collaborators from the subset of collaborators who have more than 10 data samples
Rand-Sel6-Subset	Randomly select 6 collaborators from the subset of collaborators who have more than 10 data samples

---

[1] The mean Dice score refers to the metric 'valid_dice' computed by the base package, which denotes the average dice across the dice of all the four label 0, 1, 2 and 4.

It can be observed from Fig. 2 that the underlying data distribution is highly imbalanced in data volume. Indeed, while most of the collaborators have no more than 35 data samples[2] (some only have less than 10 samples), approximately 71.4% of the entire data is held at only six collaborators. Considering that collaborators have limited data are less likely to contribute good model updates due to possible overfitting, including these collaborators during the FL process may end up with a deteriorated performance and convergence speed. Therefore, we adopted a fixed collaborator selection scheme: while all the collaborators will still be able to receive global model from the aggregator and conduct local validation, only those six collaborators with more than 120 data samples will participate the local training and model aggregation. We refer to this selection scheme as Sel-Top6 in the sequel.

Besides, we also compared Sel-Top6 with three random selection schemes listed in Table 2 where the probability of being selected for each collaborator is computed as the normalized number of data samples, which means collaborators have more the data samples also have higher chances to be selected. Detailed numerical results regarding this comparison and the determination of the training collaborator selection scheme can be found in the next section.

5 Results

In this section we report the details of the numerical studies regarding our final choice of the custom aggregation function and the training collaborator selection scheme. We used partitioning 2 for all the experiments, for each collaborator, the training data and validation data are split from the entire local data as per

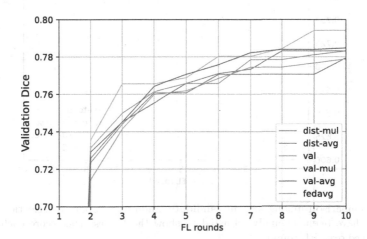

Fig. 3. Comparison among candidate custom aggregation functions. The curves have been manually adjusted to show the highest Dice score each method has achieved over FL rounds.

---

[2] We refer to the records of one patient as one data sample.

Table 3. Comparison among different candidate aggregation functions

Metric	Dist-Mul	Dist-Avg	Val	Val-Mul	Val-Avg	FedAvg
Highest mean Dice	0.7831	0.7795	0.7860	**0.7941**	0.7861	0.7789
Convergence score	0.7402	0.7368	0.7430	**0.7501**	0.7437	0.7368

partitioning 2 by a ratio of 80% : 20%. The base package runs validation function for the resulting model and compute the mean Dice score in each round of FL, a convergence score is also calculated by the base package once the experiment completes. Due to constraints on resource and time, we did not opt for validating Hausdorff metric since this can take significantly longer time than only validating Dice score. Note that, the comparisons reported should be regarded only as a visualization of how different methods may behave, also due to time and resource constraints, we ran two trials for each methods and average the results to generate figures and numbers in this section.

5.1   Identifying the Best Candidate Aggregation Function

We evaluated and compared the performance of shortlisted candidate aggregation function, i.e., Dist-Mul, Dist-Avg, Val, Val-Mul, and Val-Avg, in terms of mean Dice score and convergence score[3]. We ran 10 rounds of FL for each

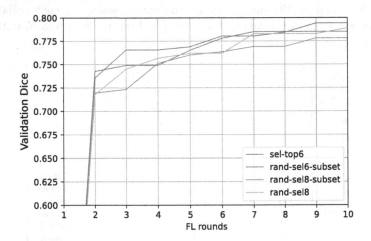

Fig. 4. Comparison among several candidate training collaborator selection scheme. he curves have been manually adjusted to show the highest Dice score each method has achieved over FL rounds.

---

[3] The convergence score is calculated as the area under the curve of validation Dice where the horizontal axis is the runtime, so a higher convergence score indicates a better convergence performance.

Table 4. Comparison among different training collaborator selection schemes

Metric	Sel-Top6	Rand-Sel6-Subset	Rand-Sel8-Subset	Rand-Sel8
Highest mean Dice	**0.7941**	0.7856	0.7800	0.7889
Convergence score	**0.7501**	0.7439	0.7359	0.7419

method[4], and applied Sel-Top6 for selecting training collaborators for each candidate method whereas we used default strategy of selecting all the collaborators (i.e., the function all_collaborators_train) for FedAvg as a baseline. From Fig. 3, we can see that Val-Mul clearly outperforms the other methods, having a higher peak Dice score and the learning curve is almost always above those of the other methods. Therefore, we choose val-mul as our proposed custom aggregation function.

5.2   Determining the Training Collaborator Selection

After identified Val-Mul as our final choice of custom aggregation function, we also implemented a series of tests to evaluate the performance of Val-Mul under different training collaborator selection schemes (refer to Sect. 4.4 for details). From Fig. 4, it is clear that Sel-Top6 outperforms the other training collaborator selection scheme, therefore we stick to combine Val-Mul with Sel-Top6 as our finally proposed FL algorithm for this challenge.

We also conducted comparison between Sel-Top6 and all_collaborators_train for the same aggregation function like Dist-Mul and Val, and the results show that Sel-Top6 obviously outperformed the default counterpart, due to time limit of the challenge we were not able to do more experiments to compare Sel-Top6 and all_collaborators_train for Val-Mul, so we only report the comparison among several selection strategies we designed. Table 4 summarizes the highest mean Dice score and convergence score of each methods. It is interesting that by

Table 5. Final performance of submitted method: Dice and Sensitivity

Label	Dice ET	Dice WT	Dice TC	Sens. ET	Sens. WT	Sens. TC
Mean	0.7282	0.7577	0.7513	0.7202	0.7615	0.7224
StdDev	0.2664	0.1798	0.2862	0.2870	0.1968	0.3024
Median	0.8337	0.8082	0.8825	0.8229	0.8212	0.8504
25 quantile	0.6750	0.6841	0.6895	0.6164	0.6757	0.6121
75 quantile	0.9048	0.8874	0.9408	0.9291	0.9099	0.9458

---

[4] We tried 20 rounds once but the test run ended up with termination at 15-th rounds due to simulation time limit, so 10 rounds should be sufficient for comparison among different methods.

Table 6. Final performance of submitted method: Specificity, Hausdorff95 Distance, and Communication Cost

Label	Spec. ET	Spec. WT	Spec. TC	H95 ET	H95 WT	H95 TC	Comm. cost
Mean	0.9997	0.9985	0.9998	29.0635	31.2901	29.8782	0.7270
StdDev	0.0006	0.0019	0.0006	85.5684	29.9703	82.6631	0.7270
Median	0.9999	0.9992	0.9999	3.0000	18.4115	5.0990	0.7270
25 quantile	0.9997	0.9980	0.9998	1.4142	7.8262	2.2361	0.7270
75 quantile	1.0000	0.9998	1.0000	8.4674	51.8769	11.9666	0.7270

including more collaborators per round, Rand-Sel8-Subset did not improve over Rand-Sel6-Subset, which is inline with our intuition of choosing only the six collaborator with most of the data.

5.3   Final Test Results

The final performance on the testing cohort of our submitted method, namely the combination of custom aggregation function Val-Mul and collaborator selection scheme Sel-Top6, is summarized in Table 5 and Table 6 where the sensitivity, specificity, Hausdorff where also included.

6   Discussion

6.1   More Design Possibilities

In this challenge, although we have developed several aggregation functions for the underlying FL system in the context of non-IID and highly imbalanced data distribution, due to resource and time constraints we have experienced, we have yet to have a chance to explore more possibilities in design space and verify the potentials of some promising alternatives:

1. For the custom aggregation function, we originally proposed four base aggregation schemes, but we could only afford to test and evaluate two of them.
2. For training collaborator selection, although the adopted Sel-Top6 can provide reasonable performance on the validation data set which is split from partitioning 2, only including a fixed choice of collaborators and ignoring the data distributed at the other collaborators may lead to limited generalizability in some cases where the distribution of the testing data considerably differs from the distribution of the data held by those six collaborators. Indeed, comparing the Dice scores in Table 3 and Table 5 indicates that the limited performance on the final testing cohort could be caused by ignoring the majority of the collaborators. Moreover, as Fig. 2 exhibits a long-tail distribution, so that selecting a different amount of clients for different training stages might be interesting.

3. For the training hyper-parameter optimization, we have only tried the default setting.
4. AI community usually uses cross-validation or multiple trials to rule out randomness or outliers, and obtain more trustworthy performance statistics. Even for obtaining more reliable validation results for a single experiment, we were unable to fully utilize the validation platform provided by the organizer which can only generate two sets of validation results per day. Due to the limited time budget, we only took the make-do approaches as best as we could.

6.2 Resource and Infrastructure

We have used an Nvidia DGX A100 workstation with four GPU units each of which has 40 GB memory and the whole system has 500 GB RAM. But when we ran experiments using the provided base package with partitioning 1 or 2, a single test run could consume nearly 200 GB of RAM, which means only two experiments can be performed in parallel every one to two days[5]. Understood that this year the Challenge provides much more data than last year, which essentially requires considerable amount of time to train the model. However, the author still sincerely wish that the organizer could consider over the above issue and optimize for a more efficient python infrastructure to allow the participants to make more contributions.

7 Conclusion

In this FeTS Challenge 2022, we have proposed six candidate aggregation methods to handle the non-IID and imbalanced data distribution for FL. We evaluated the performance of these aggregation methods and benchmark with the baseline FedAvg using the infrastructure provided by the challenge and finally selected the one with best performance potential (i.e., Val-Mul) as our submitted aggregation function. Due to time and resource constraint, we attempted a simple training collaborator selection scheme where we only allow the collaborators with sufficient training data to participate the training and aggregation in each round of FL, combined with the custom aggregation Val-Mul, we have achieved an improved performance against the baseline FedAvg-based approach on validation sets that are split from the training data.

References

1. Modern Medicine. https://www.cnbc.com/2018/02/22/medical-errors-third-leading-cause-of-death-in-america.html
2. Diagnostic Errors. https://psnet.ahrq.gov/primers/primer/12

---

[5] For example, ten FL rounds over partitioning 2 using FedAvg with all collaborator selected can take roughly 40 h to complete on our DGX workstation.

3. Tresp, V., Marc Overhage, J., Bundschus, M., Rabizadeh, S., Fasching, P.A., Yu, S.: Going digital: a survey on digitalization and large-scale data analytics in healthcare. Proc. IEEE **104**(11), 2180–2206 (2016)

4. Chen, M., Qian, Y., Chen, J., Hwang, K., Mao, S., Hu, L.: Privacy protection and intrusion avoidance for cloudlet-based medical data sharing. IEEE Trans. Cloud Comput. **8**(4), 1274–1283 (2020)

5. Mcmahan, H.B., Moore, E., Ramage, D., Hampson, S., Arcas, B.A.A.: Communication-efficient learning of deep networks from decentralized data. In: International Conference on Artificial Intelligence and Statistics, vol. 54, pp. 1273–1282 (2017)

6. Li, X., Huang, K., et al.: On the convergence of FedAvg on non-IID data. In: International Conference on Learning Representations (ICLR) (2020)

7. FeTS 2022 Challenge. https://www.synapse.org/#!Synapse:syn28546456/wiki/617246

8. Sheller, M.J., Reina, G.A., Edwards, B., Martin, J., Bakas, S.: Multi-institutional deep learning modeling without sharing patient data: a feasibility study on brain tumor segmentation. In: Crimi, A., Bakas, S., Kuijf, H., Keyvan, F., Reyes, M., van Walsum, T. (eds.) BrainLes 2018. LNCS, vol. 11383, pp. 92–104. Springer, Cham (2019). https://doi.org/10.1007/978-3-030-11723-8_9

9. Li, W., Milletarì, F., et al.: Privacy-preserving federated brain tumour segmentation. In: Proceedings of the International Workshop on Machine Learning in Medical Imaging, pp. 133–141 (2019)

10. Yi, L., Zhang, J., Zhang, R., et al.: SU-Net: an efficient encoder-decoder model of federated learning for brain tumor segmentation. In: International Conference on Artificial Neural Networks, pp. 761–773 (2020)

11. Guo, P., Wang, P., Zhou, J., Jiang, S., Patel, V.M.: Multi-institutional collaborations for improving deep learning-based magnetic resonance image reconstruction using federated learning. In: IEEE/CVF Conference on Computer Vision and Pattern Recognition (CVPR), pp. 2423–2432 (2021)

12. Pati, S., et al.: The federated tumor segmentation (FeTS) challenge. arXiv preprint arXiv:2105.05874 (2021)

13. Sheller, M.J., et al.: Federated learning in medicine: facilitating multi-institutional collaborations without sharing patient data. Nat. Sci. Rep. **10**, 12598 (2020). https://doi.org/10.1038/s41598-020-69250-1

14. Baid, U., et al.: The RSNA-ASNR-MICCAI BraTS 2021 benchmark on brain tumor segmentation and radiogenomic classification. arXiv preprint arXiv: 2107.02314 (2021)

15. Reina, G.A., et al.: OpenFL: an open-source framework for federated learning. arXiv preprint arXiv: 2105.06413 (2021)

16. Karargyris, A., Umeton, R., Sheller, M., Aristizabal, A., George, J., Bala, S.: MedPerf: open benchmarking platform for medical artificial intelligence using federated evaluation. arXiv preprint arXiv: arXiv:2110.01406 (2021)

17. Hsu, T.M.H., Qi, H., Brown, M.: Measuring the effects of non-identical data distribution for federated visual classification. arXiv preprint arXiv:1909.06335 (2019)

FedPIDAvg: A PID Controller Inspired Aggregation Method for Federated Learning

Leon Mächler[4(✉)], Ivan Ezhov[1,2], Suprosanna Shit[1,2], and Johannes C. Paetzold[1,2,3]

[1] Department of Informatics, Technical University Munich, Munich, Germany
[2] TranslaTUM - Central Institute for Translational Cancer Research, Technical University of Munich, Munich, Germany
[3] ITERM Institute Helmholtz Zentrum Muenchen, Neuherberg, Germany
[4] Département d'Informatique de l'ENS (DI ENS), École Normale Supérieure, PSL University, Paris, France
`leon-philipp.machler@ens.fr`

Abstract. This paper presents FedPIDAvg, the winning submission to the Federated Tumor Segmentation Challenge 2022 (FETS22). Inspired by FedCostWAvg, our winning contribution to FETS21, we contribute an improved aggregation strategy for federated and collaborative learning. FedCostWAvg is a weighted averaging method that not only considers the number of training samples of each cluster but also the size of the drop of the respective cost function in the last federated round. This can be interpreted as the derivative part of a PID controller (proportional-integral-derivative controller). In FedPIDAvg, we further add the missing integral term. Another key challenge was the vastly varying size of data samples per center. We addressed this by modeling the data center sizes as following a Poisson distribution and choosing the training iterations per center accordingly. Our method outperformed all other submissions.

Keywords: Federated Learning · Brain Tumor Segmentation · Control · Multi-Modal Medical Imaging · MRI · MICCAI Challenges · Machine Learning

1 Introduction

Federated learning is a highly promising approach for privacy, and confidential learning across multiple data locations [1]. A vast set of applications exist, ranging from power grids to medicine [2]. Evidently, such approaches are of paramount importance for medical images, because patient information can be highly sensitive [3] and the distribution of medical expertise, as well as the prevalence of certain diseases, is extremely uneven. More practically, medical imaging data is extremely large in size, making the frequent transfer of data from a local

S. Bakas et al. (Eds.): BrainLes 2022, LNCS 14092, pp. 209–217, 2023.
https://doi.org/10.1007/978-3-031-44153-0_20

210   L. Mächler et al.

clinic to a central server location very expensive [3]. Privacy and safety of patient data is even more emphasized when we consider the large illegal leaks of private medical records to the *dark web* [4].

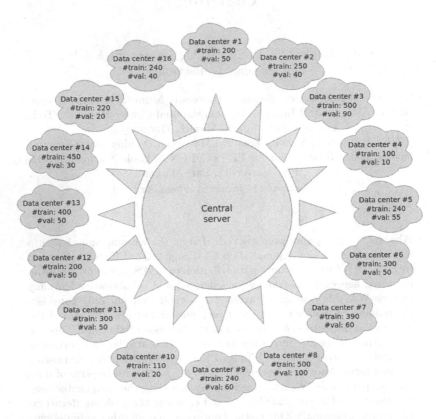

Fig. 1. Schematic illustration of the federated learning concept. One can see how multiple data centers make up one big federation. The training data is stored exclusively at the local centers, where the same model is trained locally for a defined task. E.g., brain tumor segmentation as in our case. In the aggregation step, the model weights are sent and collected at a central server location. Here, the model aggregation is performed and later broadcasted back to the local centers. This procedure is repeated until convergence or another stopping criteria is reached.

1.1 FETS Challenge

The FETS challenge [5–9] is an initiative trying to address the main research question of federated learning: optimal aggregation of network weights coming from various data centers. In this paper, we try to address this issue by proposing a PID and classical statistics-inspired solution.

2 Prior Work

2.1 Federated Averaging (FedAvg)

The traditional federated averaging (FedAvg) approach [10] employs an averaging strategy on the local model weights to update the global model, weighted by the training data set sizes of the local models. A model M_{i+1} is updated as follows:

$$M_{i+1} = \frac{1}{S} \sum_{j=1}^{n} s_j M_i^j.$$

(1)

Here, s_j is the number of samples that model M^j was trained on in round i and $S = \sum_j s_j$. The definition is adapted from [11].

2.2 Federated Cost Weighted Averaging (FedCostWAvg)

Last year, we proposed a new weighting strategy, which won the FETS21 challenge. It not only weighs by data center sizes but also by the amount by which the cost function decreased during the last step [11]. We termed this method FedCostWAvg, where the new model M_{i+1} is calculated in the following manner:

$$M_{i+1} = \sum_{j=1}^{n} (\alpha \frac{s_j}{S} + (1 - \alpha) \frac{k_j}{K}) M_i^j.$$

(2)

with:

$$k_j = \frac{c(M_{i-1}^j)}{c(M_i^j)}, K = \sum_j k_j.$$

(3)

Here, $c(M_i^j)$ is the cost of the model j at time-step i, which is calculated from the local cost function [11]. Moreover, α ranges between $[0, 1]$ and is chosen to balance the impact of the cost improvements and the data set sizes. Last year, we won the challenge with an alpha value of $\alpha = 0.5$. We discussed that this weighting strategy adjusted for the training dataset size and also for local improvements in the last training round.

3 Methodology

In the following chapter, we will first introduce and formalize our novel averaging concept named *FedPIDAvg*. Next, we will quickly describe the neural network architecture for brain tumor segmentation that was given by the challenge organizers and finally discuss our strategy regarding when to train and aggregate from which specific centers, depending on their training samples modeled using a simple Poisson distribution.

3.1 Federated PID Weighted Averaging (FedPIDAvg)

As was already mentioned in [11] David Nacacche offered the observation that the idea of FedCostAvg is similar to that of a PID controller. Only the integral term is missing. The methodology of our new averaging method is novel in two ways: the PID-inspired added integral term, and a different way to calculate the differential term. Our method calculates the new model M_{i+1} in the following manner:

$$M_{i+1} = \sum_{j=1}^{n} (\alpha \frac{s_j}{S} + \beta \frac{k_j}{K} + \gamma \frac{m_j}{I}) M_i^j. \tag{4}$$

with:

$$k_j = c(M_{i-1}^j) - c(M_i^j), K = \sum_j k_j. \tag{5}$$

and:

$$m_j = \sum_{l=0}^{5} c(M_{i-l}), I = \sum_j m_j. \tag{6}$$

$$\alpha + \beta + \gamma = 1 \tag{7}$$

Note that this time we use the absolute difference between the last cost and the new cost and no longer the ratio. The new strategy is still a weighted averaging strategy, where the weights are themselves weighted averages of three factors: the drop of the cost in the last round, the sum over the cost in the last rounds and the size of the training data set. These three factors are weighted by α, β and γ. Their choice needs to be optimized based on the use case, we chose $0.45, 0.45, 0.1$ although we did not have the resources to cross validate them.

3.2 U-Net for Brain Tumor Segmentation

As a segmentation architecture, we were given by the organizers the 3D-Unet, a vastly successful neural network architecture in medical image analysis [12]. No modifications to the architecture were allowed in the challenge, we quickly depict it in Fig. 1 for completeness. U-Nets constitute the state of the art for a vast set of applications, for example, brain tumor segmentation [5,13], vessel segmentation [14,15] and many more (Fig. 2).

3.3   Poisson-Distribution Modeling of the Data Samples per Center

In order to optimize the training speed over several federated rounds, it was possible to only select a subset of data centers for each federated round. In our last year's submission, we simply selected all centers every time. Another part of our submission this year is a novel way to select participating data centers at each federated round. To do so, we resorted to classical statistics means, namely, under the assumption that the dataset sizes follow a Poisson distribution:

$$p(x; \lambda) = \frac{e^{-\lambda}\lambda^x}{x!}$$

(8)

$$\text{with } x = 0, 1, 2, \cdots$$

we made the natural choice of dropping out outliers in most rounds, where outliers were defined as having $x > 2\lambda$.

4   Results

The methods were evaluated on the data of the Fets challenge. It is described as: "FeTS borrows its data from the BraTS Continuous Evaluation, but additionally providing a data partitioning according to the acquisition origin for the training data. Ample multi-institutional, routine clinically-acquired, pre-operative baseline, multi-parametric Magnetic Resonance Imaging (mpMRI) scans of radiographically appearing glioblastoma (GBM) are provided as the training and validation data for the FeTS 2022 challenge. Specifically, the datasets used in the FeTS 2022 challenge are the subset of GBM cases from the BraTS Continuous Evaluation. Ground truth reference annotations are created and approved by expert board-certified neuroradiologists for every subject included in the training, validation, and testing datasets to quantitatively evaluate the performance of the participating algorithms." Amongst all submitted methods, FedPIDAvg performed best and won the challenge.

In Tables 1 and 2 we give last years results of FedCostWAvg in the last challenge and in Tables 3 and 4 the results of FedPIDAvg in FETS22. Note that the data was different this year as well as the limits on available federated rounds.

Table 1. Final performance of FedCostWAvg in the 2021 FETS Challenge, DICE and Sensitivity

Label	Dice WT	Dice ET	Dice TC	Sens. WT	Sens. ET	Sens. TC
Mean	0,8248	0,7476	0,7932	0,8957	0,8246	0,8269
StdDev	0,1849	0,2444	0,2643	0,1738	0,2598	0,2721
Median	0,8936	0,8259	0,9014	0,948	0,9258	0,9422
25th quantile	0,8116	0,7086	0,8046	0,9027	0,7975	0,8258
75th quantile	0,9222	0,8909	0,942	0,9787	0,9772	0,9785

Table 2. Final performance of FedCostWAvg in the 2021 FETS Challenge, Specificity, Hausdorff95 Distance and Communication Cost

Label	Spec WT	Spec ET	Spec TC	H95 WT	H95 ET	H95 TC	Comm. Cost
Mean	0,9981	0,9994	0,9994	11,618	27,2745	28,4825	0,723
StdDev	0,0024	0,0011	0,0014	31,758	88,566	88,2921	0,723
Median	0,9986	0,9996	0,9998	5	2,2361	3,0811	0,723
25th quantile	0,9977	0,9993	0,9995	2,8284	1,4142	1,7856	0,723
75th quantile	0,9994	0,9999	0,9999	8,6023	3,5628	7,0533	0,723

Table 3. Final performance of FedPIDAvg in the 2022 FETS Challenge, DICE and Sensitivity

Label	Dice WT	Dice ET	Dice TC	Sens WT	Sens ET	Sens TC
Mean	0,76773526	0,741627265	0,769244434	0,749757737	0,770377324	0,765940502
StdDev	0,183035406	0,266310234	0,284212379	0,208271565	0,280923214	0,297081407
Median	0,826114563	0,848784494	0,896213442	0,819457864	0,886857246	0,893165349
25quant	0,700757354	0,700955694	0,739356651	0,637996476	0,728202272	0,73357786
75quant	0,897816734	0,910451814	0,943718628	0,905620122	0,956570051	0,964129538

Table 4. Final performance of FedPIDAvg in the 2022 FETS Challenge, Specificity, Hausdorff95 Distance and Communication Cost

Label	Spec WT	Spec ET	Spec TC	H95 WT	H95 ET	H95 TC	Comm. Cost
Mean	0,9989230	0,9995742	0,999692	24,367549	32,796706	32,466108	0,300
StdDev	0,0016332	0,0007856	0,0006998	32,007897	89,31835	85,440174	0,300
Median	0,9994479	0,9997990	0,999868	11,57583	2,4494897	4,5825756	0,300
25th quant	0,998690	0,9995254	0,999695	5,4081799	1,4142135	2,2360679	0,300
75th quant	0,9998540	0,9999292	0,9999584	36,454261	10,805072	12,359194	0,300

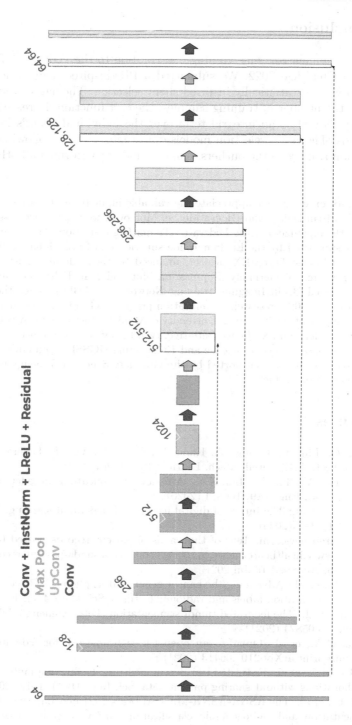

Fig. 2. The common 3D U-net architecture, which is used in many medical imaging tasks. It was provided as such by the FETS challenge, modifications were not allowed [6,12].

5   Conclusion

This paper summarizes our winning contribution to the Federated Tumor Segmentation Challenge 2022. We submitted a PID-inspired aggregation strategy combined with a statistically inspired client selection. The aggregation function considers the number of training samples, the cost function decrease in the previous step as well as an integral term over the individual client's losses in the last rounds. The client selection models data center sizes as following a Poisson distribution and drops the outliers. Our method outperformed all other submissions.

Acknowledgements. We appreciate the valuable input from our supervisors, David Naccache, Adrian Dalca, and Bjoern Menze. Moreover, we want to express our appreciation to the organizers of the Federated Tumor Segmentation Challenge 2022. Leon Mächler is supported by the École normale supérieure in Paris. Johannes C. Paetzold is supported by the DCoMEX project, financed by the Federal Ministry of Education and Research of Germany. Suprosanna Shit and Ivan Ezhov are supported by the Translational Brain Imaging Training Network (TRABIT) under the European Union's 'Horizon 2020' research & innovation program (Grant agreement ID: 765148). With the support of the Technical University of Munich - Institute for Advanced Study, funded by the German Excellence Initiative. Ivan Ezhov is also supported by the International Graduate School of Science and Engineering (IGSSE). Johannes C. Paetzold and Suprosanna Shit are supported by the Graduate School of Bioengineering, Technical University of Munich.

References

1. Yang, Q., Liu, Y., Cheng, Y., Kang, Y., Chen, T., Yu, H.: Federated learning. Synth. Lect. Artif. Intell. Mach. Learn. **13**(3), 1–207 (2019)
2. Li, L., Fan, Y., Tse, M., Lin, K.Y.: A review of applications in federated learning. Comput. Ind. Eng. **149**, 106854 (2020)
3. Rieke, N., et al.: The future of digital health with federated learning. NPJ Digital Med. **3**(1), 1–7 (2020)
4. Healthcareitnews.com: Tens of thousands of patient records posted to dark web. https://www.healthcareitnews.com/news/tens-thousands-patient-records-posted-dark-web. Accessed 16 Jul 2021
5. Bakas, S., et al.: Advancing the cancer genome atlas glioma MRI collections with expert segmentation labels and radiomic features. Sci. Data **4**(1), 1–13 (2017)
6. Pati, S., et al.: The federated tumor segmentation (Fets) challenge. arXiv preprint arXiv:2105.05874 (2021)
7. Reina, G.A., et al.: OpenFL: an open-source framework for federated learning. arXiv preprint arXiv:2105.06413 (2021)
8. Sheller, M.J., et al.: Federated learning in medicine: facilitating multi-institutional collaborations without sharing patient data. Sci. Rep. **10**(1), 1–12 (2020)
9. Baid, U., et al.: The RSNA-ASNR-MICCAI brats 2021 benchmark on brain tumor segmentation and radiogenomic classification. arXiv preprint arXiv:2107.02314 (2021)

10. McMahan, B., Moore, E., Ramage, D., Hampson, S., Arcas, B.A.: Communication-efficient learning of deep networks from decentralized data. In: Artificial intelligence and statistics, pp. 1273–1282. PMLR (2017)
11. Mächler, L., et al.: FedCostWAvg: a new averaging for better federated learning. arXiv preprint arXiv:2111.08649 (2021)
12. Ronneberger, O., Fischer, P., Brox, T.: U-net: convolutional networks for biomedical image segmentation. In: Navab, N., Hornegger, J., Wells, W.M., Frangi, A.F. (eds.) MICCAI 2015. LNCS, vol. 9351, pp. 234–241. Springer, Cham (2015). https://doi.org/10.1007/978-3-319-24574-4_28
13. Menze, B.H., et al.: The multimodal brain tumor image segmentation benchmark (BRATS). IEEE Trans. Med. Imaging 34(10), 1993–2024 (2014)
14. Todorov, M.I., et al.: Machine learning analysis of whole mouse brain vasculature. Nat. Methods 17(4), 442–449 (2020)
15. Shit, S., et al.: clDice - a topology-preserving loss function for tubular structure segmentation. CoRR abs/2003.07311 (2020)

Federated Evaluation of nnU-Nets Enhanced with Domain Knowledge for Brain Tumor Segmentation

Krzysztof Kotowski[1], Szymon Adamski[1], Bartosz Machura[1], Wojciech Malara[1], Lukasz Zarudzki[3], and Jakub Nalepa[1,2(✉)]

[1] Graylight Imaging, Gliwice, Poland
{kkotowski,sadamski,bmachura,wmalara}@graylight-imaging.com,
jnalepa@ieee.org
[2] Silesian University of Technology, Gliwice, Poland
[3] Maria Sklodowska-Curie Memorial Cancer Center and Institute of Oncology,
Gliwice, Poland

Abstract. Accurate and reproducible segmentation of brain tumors from multi-modal magnetic resonance (MR) scans is a pivotal step in practice. In this BraTS Continuous Evaluation initiative, we exploit a 3D nnU-Net for this task which was ranked at the 6th place (out of 1600 participants) in the BraTS'21 Challenge. We benefit from an ensemble of deep models enhanced with the expert knowledge of a senior radiologist captured in a form of several post-processing routines. The experimental study showed that infusing the domain knowledge into the algorithm can enhance their performance, and we obtained the average Dice score of 0.81977 (enhancing tumor), 0.87837 (tumor core), and 0.92723 (whole tumor) over the validation set. For the test data, we had the average Dice score of 0.86317, 0.87987, and 0.92838 for the enhancing tumor, tumor core and whole tumor. To validate the generalization capabilities of the nnU-Nets enhanced with domain knowledge, we performed their federated evaluation within the Federated Tumor Segmentation (FeTS) 2022 Challenge over the datasets captured across 30 institutions. Our technique was ranked 2nd across all participating teams, proving its generalization capabilities over unseen out-of-sample datasets.

Keywords: Brain Tumor · Segmentation · Deep Learning · U-Net · Expert Knowledge

1 Introduction

Brain tumor segmentation from multi-modal MR scans is an important step in oncology care. Accurate delineation of tumorous tissue is pivotal for further diagnosis, prognosis and treatment, and it can directly affect the treatment pathway. Hence, ensuring the reproducibility, robustness, e.g., against different scanners, and quality of an automated segmentation process are critical to design personalized patient care. The state-of-the-art brain tumor segmentation algorithms

S. Bakas et al. (Eds.): BrainLes 2022, LNCS 14092, pp. 218–227, 2023.
https://doi.org/10.1007/978-3-031-44153-0_21

are commonly divided into the *atlas-based, unsupervised, supervised,* and *hybrid* techniques. In the *atlas-based* algorithms, manually segmented atlases are used to segment the unseen scans [21]. *Unsupervised* approaches elaborate intrinsic characteristics of the *unlabeled* data [7,12,24]. Once the labeled data is available, we can use the *supervised* techniques [9,26,27]. Deep learning models span across various networks architectures [16] and include ensembles of deep nets [13], U-Net architectures [11,17,19], encoder-decoder approaches [6], and more [8,18]. Although the classic machine and deep learning are emerging at a steady pace, capturing large and heterogeneous data coupled with high-quality ground-truth information is extremely costly, time-consuming, and suffers from significant inter- and intra-rater variability. However, due to a variety of privacy and ownership hurdles, collecting vast multi-institutional datasets that would help our models better generalize over unseen data is infeasible in practice [20]. Therefore, practical federated learning and federated evaluation challenges have emerged recently [22,23]. In the former case, we are aimed at training well-generalizing models without pooling the data together from different institutions through elaborating a consensus machine learning model that has gained knowledge from data of multiple institutions. On the other hand, federated evaluation allows us to assess such segmentation models in a federated configuration (i.e., "in the wild"), in order to to assess their robustness to dataset shifts in multi-institutional data. Here, we follow this research paper within the Federated Tumor Segmentation (FeTS) 2022 Challenge which focuses on benchmarking methods for federated learning, and particularly we investigate the algorithmic generalizability on out-of-sample data based on federated evaluation in the brain tumor segmentation task.

We use a 3D nnU-Net architecture (Sect. 3) operating over multi-modal MR scans [10], in which brain tumors are segmented into the enhancing tumor (ET), peritumoral edema (ED), and necrotic core (NCR). We utilize five-fold ensembling with stratification based on the distribution of NCR, ET, and ED, together with the post-processing routines that capture the expert knowledge of a senior radiologist. The experiments performed over the BraTS'21 training, validation, and test datasets showed that our architecture delivers accurate multi-class segmentation, and that enhancing the deep models with the expert knowledge may significantly improve their abilities nnU-Nets (Sect. 4).

2   Data

The 2021 release of the Brain Tumor Segmentation (BraTS) set [1–4,15] includes MRI training data of 1251 patients with gliomas. Each study was contoured by one to four experienced and trained readers. The data captures four co-registered MRI modalities, being the native pre-contrast (T1), post-contrast T1-weighted (T1Gd), T2-weighted (T2), and T2 Fluid Attenuated Inversion Recovery (T2-FLAIR) sequences. All pixels are labeled, and the following labels are considered: healthy tissue, Gd-enhancing tumor (ET), peritumoral edema/invaded tissue (ED) and the necrotic tumor core (NCR) [5].

| T1 | T1Gd | T2 | T2-FLAIR |

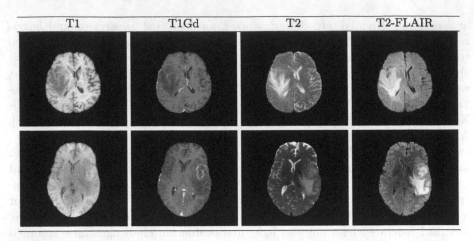

Fig. 1. Example scans of two patients (separate rows) included in the validation set.

The data was acquired with different protocols and scanners at multiple institutions. The studies were interpolated to the same shape ($240 \times 240 \times 155$, hence there are 155 images of 240×240 size, with voxel size of $1\,\text{mm}^3$), and they were skull-stripped. Finally, there are 219 patients in the validation set V (see examples in Fig. 1), for which the manual annotations are not provided.

3   Methods

We built upon the nnU-Net framework [10], which automatically configures itself, including preprocessing, basic post-processing, architecture and training configurations. We train the network over the BraTS'21 training data with the averaged (across all target classes) cross-entropy and soft Dice as the loss function. A patch size of $128 \times 128 \times 128$ with a batch size of 2 was selected.

In our recent BraTS paper [14], we investigated 15 combinations of an array of post-processing routines that capture the expert knowledge, and showed that utilizing the FillTC method (Table 1) allows us to statistically significantly improve the results for Dice obtained for TC and WT ($p < 0.005$, according to the Wilcoxon signed-rank test).

Table 1. The post-processing approach utilized to infuse the expert knowledge into the nnU-Net segmentation framework.

Method's short name	Algorithm	Expert knowledge
FillTC	Any voxels surrounded by TC in 2D in any slice on any plane are iteratively relabeled to NCR. The planes are filled in the following order: axial, coronal, sagittal	Edema cannot be surrounded by necrosis only. Necrosis cannot have "holes" (tissue not labeled by model to any class) inside it. If enhancing tumor is "closed" (ring-shaped) in 2D everything inside it which is not enhancing has to be necrosis. Large tumors usually do not contain "holes" of healthy tissue

4 Experiments

4.1 Experimental Setup

The DNN models were implemented using `Python3` with `Keras` and `PyTorch`. The experiments were run on a high-performance computer equipped with an NVIDIA Tesla V100 GPU (32 GB) and 6 Intel Xeon E5-2680 (2.50 GHz) CPUs.

4.2 Training Process

The metric for training was a sum of the Dice score and cross-entropy. Training was performed on ET, ED, and NCR classes, with the maximum number of epochs set to 500. The optimizer was the stochastic gradient descent with the Nesterov momentum with the initial learning rate of 10^{-2}. The learning rate is decayed gradually to a value close to zero in the last epoch [10].

The training set was split into five non-overlapping stratified folds (each base model is trained over four folds, and one fold is used for validation during the training process; see Table 2). We stratify the dataset at the patient level with respect to the distribution of the size of the NCR, ED, and ET examples. The fold sizes were equal to 251, 253, 250, 248, and 249 patients.

Table 2. Characteristics of the training folds (average volume of the corresponding tumor subregion is reported in cm^3) used for training our model.

	WT vol.	NCR vol.	ED vol.	ET vol.
Fold 1	95.16	14.21	59.85	21.10
Fold 2	96.63	15.38	60.42	20.82
Fold 3	93.97	13.77	57.74	22.47
Fold 4	97.18	14.65	60.72	21.82
Fold 5	96.80	13.43	62.36	21.00

For the purpose of the FeTS 2022 Challenge, we present a distribution of the studies from different institutions between the training folds in Table 3. It turns out that our stratification (in which the volume is utilized as the stratification factor) provided also reasonably well partitioning across the participating institutions that captured the available training data.

Table 3. Characteristics of the training folds: number of studies from each institution.

Institution→	1	2	3	4	5	6	7	8	9	10	11	12
Fold 1	114	2	4	7	4	5	4	1	0	1	2	2
Fold 2	98	2	5	5	2	8	1	1	1	1	4	2
Fold 3	100	0	2	11	5	9	4	0	2	2	2	2
Fold 4	100	2	3	15	3	3	2	2	1	3	3	3
Fold 5	99	0	1	9	8	9	1	4	0	1	3	2
Institution→	13	14	15	16	17	18	19	20	21	22	23	
Fold 1	6	0	3	7	0	76	0	7	4	1	1	
Fold 2	11	1	3	6	4	84	0	5	6	3	0	
Fold 3	4	2	2	7	1	77	1	7	9	0	1	
Fold 4	8	1	4	7	3	65	1	7	9	1	2	
Fold 5	6	2	1	3	1	80	2	7	7	2	1	

4.3   Experimental Results

In this section, we present the results obtained over the BraTS'21 validation and test sets (as returned by the Synapse portal)[1]. The quantitative results are gathered in Table 4—they confirm that our approach delivers accurate segmentation of all regions of interest. Also, our model allowed us to take the 6th place in the BraTS'21 Challenge (across 1600 participants from all over the globe). In Fig. 2, we can appreciate the example of an MRI scan from the validation set which was segmented without and with infusing the expert knowledge into the algorithm (for this patient, we observed the largest improvement in TC Dice). Although there are cases for which the segmentation quality (as quantified by Dice) was around 0.50 (ET), 0.67 (TC) and 0.79 (WT), the qualitative analysis reveals that they are still sensible (Fig. 3). Such cases could be further investigated manually, within a semi-automated clinical process—hence, quantifying the confidence of the segmentation returned by the deep model is of high practical importance, and it constitutes our current research efforts.

In Table 5, we present the segmentation performance quantified by Dice and Hausdorff (95%) distance over the unseen data from 30 institutions—here, the metrics are computed for each center (mean) and then they are aggregated (mean, standard deviation, and so forth) between the 30 sites. The goal was to find algorithms that robustly produce accurate brain tumor segmentations across different medical institutions, MRI scanners, image acquisition protocols,

---

[1] Our team name is Graylight Imaging.

Table 4. Segmentation performance quantified by Dice, sensitivity, specificity, and Hausdorff (95%) distance over the BraTS'21 **validation** and **test** sets obtained using our approach (as returned by the validation server). The scores (average μ, standard deviation s, median m, and the 25 and 75 quantile) are presented for the whole tumor (WT), tumor core (TC), and enhancing tumor (ET).

	Dice ET	Dice TC	Dice WT	Haus. ET	Haus. TC	Haus. WT	Sens. ET	Sens. TC	Sens. WT	Spec. ET	Spec. TC	Spec. WT
Validation set												
μ	0.81977	0.87841	0.92724	17.85334	7.59729	3.63677	0.82215	0.85937	0.92891	0.99979	0.99983	0.99938
s	0.24619	0.17866	0.07349	73.68160	36.04524	5.73084	0.26009	0.19914	0.07878	0.00038	0.00030	0.00082
m	0.89787	0.94117	0.94569	1.41421	1.73205	2.08262	0.91475	0.93699	0.95565	0.99991	0.99993	0.99964
25q	0.82421	0.87842	0.90324	1.00000	1.00000	1.41421	0.83038	0.85134	0.91218	0.99975	0.99983	0.99919
75q	0.95197	0.96874	0.96890	2.44949	3.87083	3.62116	0.96640	0.97357	0.97867	0.99997	0.99998	0.99985
Test set												
μ	0.86317	0.87987	0.92838	13.08531	15.87305	4.77240	0.87607	0.88921	0.92916	0.99979	0.99973	0.99951
s	0.20375	0.23422	0.08992	61.45773	66.68659	17.01573	0.21473	0.21898	0.09462	0.00030	0.00083	0.00077
m	0.93506	0.96346	0.95725	1.00000	1.41421	1.73205	0.95226	0.96930	0.95837	0.99990	0.99992	0.99976
25q	0.85164	0.91752	0.91297	1.00000	1.00000	1.00000	0.88749	0.90947	0.91760	0.99973	0.99979	0.99947
75q	0.96600	0.98219	0.97765	2.00000	3.00000	4.00000	0.97877	0.98760	0.98119	0.99996	0.99997	0.99991

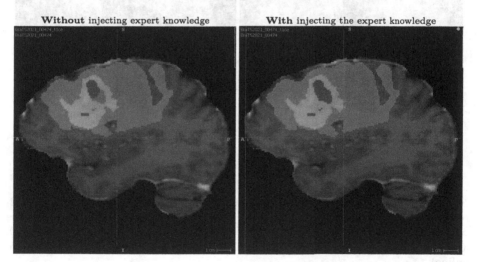

Without injecting expert knowledge   **With** injecting the expert knowledge

Fig. 2. The prediction for a patient with ID: 474 from the BraTS'21 validation data for which the largest improvement of TC Dice was achieved after infusing the expert knowledge into the post-processing routine (green—ED, yellow—ET, red—NCR). (Color figure online)

and patient populations, and the authors of the challenge utilized a real-world federated evaluation environment to achieve it. The results show that our method can indeed generalize well over such out-of-sample datasets—it was ranked 2nd across all participating teams.

Patient 1780   Patient 1752

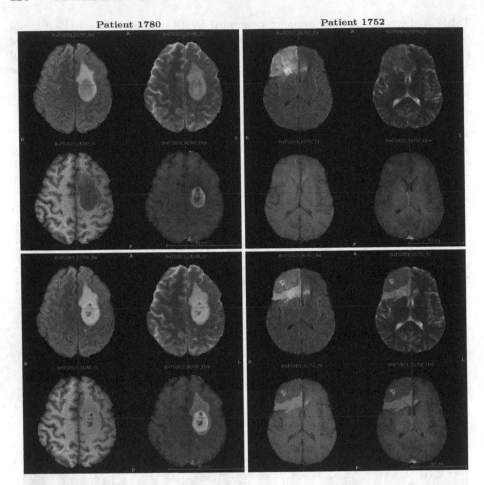

Fig. 3. Examples of high- and low-quality contouring (patients with ID: 1780 and 1752, respectively) from the validation set (green—ED, yellow—ET, red—NCR). The Dice values amounted to 0.98990 (ET), 0.99232 (TC), and 0.98318 (WT) for patient 1780, and to 0.49577 (ET), 0.67378 (TC), and 0.78600 (WT) for patient 1752. (Color figure online)

Table 5. Segmentation performance quantified by Dice and Hausdorff (95%) distance over the unseen data from 30 institutions. The metrics are computed for each center (mean) and then they are aggregated (mean, standard deviation, and so forth) between the 30 sites.

	Dice ET	Dice TC	Dice WT	Haus. ET	Haus. TC	Haus. WT
μ	0.8629	0.9001	0.9314	14.6041	8.4383	4.9561
s	0.0876	0.0724	0.0452	24.7378	12.7456	3.5123
min	0.6317	0.6678	0.7918	1.0568	1.1066	1.2315
25q	0.7997	0.8606	0.9224	2.0987	2.4178	2.8119
50q	0.8803	0.9249	0.9381	3.4765	4.2642	3.9615
75q	0.9302	0.9546	0.9654	18.1168	7.4957	6.0068
max	0.9707	0.9815	0.9783	118.1976	65.0932	19.3530

5   Conclusion

We utilized an ensemble of five nnU-Net models with our custom stratification based on the distribution of NCR, ET, and ED volumes for accurate brain tumor segmentation. To further improve the segmentation capabilities of the nnU-Nets, we infused the expert knowledge into the framework through introducing a post-processing routine. It significantly improves TC and WT Dice, without deteriorating any other metric. It is robust to specific cases with missing classes in ground truth, because it extends the TC volume with additional voxels instead of removing any voxels. Our algorithm allowed us to take the 6th place in the BraTS'21 Challenge over the hidden test data (out of 1600 teams). Finally, our technique was validated in the federated settings over the unseen datasets from 30 institutions—we were ranked 2nd across all participating teams, which clearly shows the generalization capabilities of our method over the unseen out-of-sample datasets.

The research undertaken in this paper constitutes an interesting departure point for further efforts. We currently focus on improving the segmentation quality of ET and TC by creating specialized models that could deal better with the aforementioned specific cases. Additionally, we believe that exploiting the expert knowledge which could be captured as various forms of pre- and post-processing routines (and as the elements of the deep learning model's training strategies) could help us improve the segmentation quality even further, also in other modalities and segmentation tasks. Such methods should be, however, thoroughly validated (as in BraTS and FeTS), in order to objectively understand their generalization capabilities in a fully reproducible and unbiased way [25].

Acknowledgments. JN was supported by the Silesian University of Technology funds through the grant for maintaining and developing research potential. This work was supported by the Polish National Centre for Research and Development grant:

POIR.01.01.01-00-0092/20 (*Methods and algorithms for automatic coronary artery calcium scoring on cardiac computed tomography scans*).

This paper is in memory of Dr. Grzegorz Nalepa, an extraordinary scientist and pediatric hematologist/oncologist at Riley Hospital for Children, Indianapolis, USA, who helped countless patients and their families through some of the most challenging moments of their lives.

References

1. Baid, U., et al.: The RSNA-ASNR-MICCAI brats 2021 benchmark on brain tumor segmentation and radiogenomic classification (2021)
2. Bakas, S., et al.: Advancing the cancer genome atlas glioma MRI collections with expert segmentation labels and radiomic features. Nat. Sci. Data. **4**, 1–13 (2017). https://doi.org/10.1038/sdata.2017.117
3. Bakas, S., et al.: Segmentation labels and radiomic features for the pre-operative scans of the TCGA-GBM collection (2017). The Cancer Imaging Archive. https://doi.org/10.7937/K9/TCIA.2017.KLXWJJ1Q
4. Bakas, S., et al.: Segmentation labels and radiomic features for the pre-operative scans of the TCGA-LGG collection (2017). The Cancer Imaging Archive. https://doi.org/10.7937/K9/TCIA.2017.GJQ7R0EF
5. Bakas, S., et al.: Identifying the bestmachine learning algorithms for brain tumor segmentation, progression assessment, and overall survival prediction in the BRATS challenge. CoRR abs/1811.02629 (2018). arXiv.org:1811.02629
6. Bontempi, D., Benini, S., Signoroni, A., Svanera, M., Muckli, L.: Cerebrum: a fast and fully-volumetric convolutional encoder-decoder for weakly-supervised segmentation of brain structures from out-of-the-scanner MRI. Med. Image Anal. **62**, 101688 (2020)
7. Chander, A., Chatterjee, A., Siarry, P.: A new social and momentum component adaptive PSO algorithm for image segmentation. Expert Syst. Appl. **38**(5), 4998–5004 (2011)
8. Estienne, T., et al.: Deep learning-based concurrent brain registration and tumor segmentation. Front. Comput. Neurosci. **14**, 17 (2020)
9. Geremia, E., Clatz, O., Menze, B.H., Konukoglu, E., Criminisi, A., Ayache, N.: Spatial decision forests for MS lesion segmentation in multi-channel magnetic resonance images. Neuroimage **57**(2), 378–390 (2011)
10. Isensee, F., Jaeger, P., Kohl, S., Petersen, J., Maier-Hein, K.: nnU-net: a self-configuring method for deep learning-based biomedical image segmentation. Nat. Methods **18**, 1–9 (2021). https://doi.org/10.1038/s41592-020-01008-z
11. Isensee, F., Kickingereder, P., Wick, W., Bendszus, M., Maier-Hein, K.H.: No new-net. In: Crimi, A., Bakas, S., Kuijf, H., Keyvan, F., Reyes, M., van Walsum, T. (eds.) BrainLes 2018. LNCS, vol. 11384, pp. 234–244. Springer, Cham (2019). https://doi.org/10.1007/978-3-030-11726-9_21
12. Ji, S., Wei, B., Yu, Z., Yang, G., Yin, Y.: A new multistage medical segmentation method based on SuperPixel and fuzzy clustering. Comput. Math. Methods Med. **2014**, 747549:1-747549:13 (2014)
13. Kamnitsas, K., et al.: Ensembles of multiple models and architectures for robust brain tumour segmentation. In: Crimi, A., Bakas, S., Kuijf, H., Menze, B., Reyes, M. (eds.) BrainLes 2017. LNCS, vol. 10670, pp. 450–462. Springer, Cham (2018). https://doi.org/10.1007/978-3-319-75238-9_38

14. Kotowski, K., Adamski, S., Machura, B., Zarudzki, L., Nalepa, J.: Coupling nnU-nets with expert knowledge for accurate brain tumor segmentation from MRI. In: Crimi, A., Bakas, S. (eds.) Brainlesion: Glioma, Multiple Sclerosis, Stroke and Traumatic Brain Injuries, pp. 197–209. Springer International Publishing, Cham (2022). https://doi.org/10.1007/978-3-031-09002-8_18

15. Menze, B.H., et al.: The multimodal brain tumor image segmentation benchmark (BRATS). IEEE Trans. Med. Imaging **34**(10), 1993–2024 (2015)

16. Myronenko, A.: 3D MRI brain tumor segmentation using autoencoder regularization. In: Crimi, A., Bakas, S., Kuijf, H., Keyvan, F., Reyes, M., van Walsum, T. (eds.) BrainLes 2018. LNCS, vol. 11384, pp. 311–320. Springer, Cham (2019). https://doi.org/10.1007/978-3-030-11726-9_28

17. Nalepa, J., et al.: Data augmentation via image registration. In: 2019 IEEE International Conference on Image Processing (ICIP), pp. 4250–4254, September 2019. https://doi.org/10.1109/ICIP.2019.8803423

18. Nalepa, J., Marcinkiewicz, M., Kawulok, M.: Data augmentation for brain-tumor segmentation: a review. Front. Comput. Neurosci. **13**, 83 (2019)

19. Nalepa, J., et al.: Fully-automated deep learning-powered system for DCE-MRI analysis of brain tumors. Artif. Intell. Med. **102**, 101769 (2020)

20. Pati, S., et al.: The Federated Tumor Segmentation (FeTS) Challenge (2021). https://doi.org/10.48550/ARXIV.2105.05874, arXiv.org:2105.05874

21. Pipitone, J., et al.: Multi-atlas segmentation of the whole hippocampus and subfields using multiple automatically generated templates. Neuroimage **101**, 494–512 (2014)

22. Reina, G.A., et al.: OpenFL: an open-source framework for Federated Learning (2021). https://doi.org/10.48550/ARXIV.2105.06413, arXiv.org:2105.06413

23. Sheller, M.J., et al.: Federated learning in medicine: facilitating multi-institutional collaborations without sharing patient data. Sci. Rep. **10**(1), 12598 (2020)

24. Simi, V., Joseph, J.: Segmentation of glioblastoma multiforme from MR images - a comprehensive review. Egypt. J. Radiol. Nucl. Med. **46**(4), 1105–1110 (2015)

25. Wijata, A.M., Nalepa, J.: Unbiased validation of the algorithms for automatic needle localization in ultrasound-guided breast biopsies. In: 2022 IEEE International Conference on Image Processing (ICIP), pp. 3571–3575 (2022). https://doi.org/10.1109/ICIP46576.2022.9897449

26. Wu, W., Chen, A.Y.C., Zhao, L., Corso, J.J.: Brain tumor detection and segmentation in a CRF (conditional random fields) framework with pixel-pairwise affinity and superpixel-level features. Int. J. Comput. Assist. Radiol. Surg. **9**(2), 241–253 (2014)

27. Zikic, D., et al.: Decision forests for tissue-specific segmentation of high-grade gliomas in multi-channel MR. In: Ayache, N., Delingette, H., Golland, P., Mori, K. (eds.) MICCAI 2012. LNCS, vol. 7512, pp. 369–376. Springer, Heidelberg (2012). https://doi.org/10.1007/978-3-642-33454-2_46

Experimenting FedML and NVFLARE for Federated Tumor Segmentation Challenge

Yaying Shi[1]([✉]), Hongjian Gao[2], Salman Avestimehr[2], and Yonghong Yan[1]

[1] University of North Carolina at Charlotte, North Caroline, USA
yshi10@uncc.edu
[2] University of Southern California, California, USA

Abstract. It has been well accepted that artificial intelligence, machine learning, and deep learning (AI/ML/DL) techniques are on the path to making a revolutionary impact on health care. However, applying AI/MD/DL for clinical use is still challenging for reasons such as the concerns of security and privacy for sharing patient data among medical institutions, and medical data being heterogeneous. To solve those challenges, Federated learning (FL), which enables distributed training of DL networks without sharing data, could be a feasible solution as shown by the successful demonstration of FL in computer vision tasks. In the medical domain, Federated Tumor Segmentation(FeTS) challenge is the first challenge to address image segmentation using federated learning. In this paper, we evaluated and compared two FL frameworks, FedML and NVIDIA FLARE (NVFLARE), for FeTS 2022 challenge dataset in both distributed and centralized training methods. Using UNet as a baseline network, both FedML and NVFLARE are able to train the UNet models, and the accuracies of the two models are close to the accuracy of the model trained from centralized training. Models trained by NVFLARE performs a little better than models trained by FedML.

Keywords: Medical Image Segmentation · FeTS Challenge · Machine Learning · Federated Learning · FedML · NVFLARE

1 Introduction

Brain tumor segmentation is one of the most difficult segmentation challenges in the medical image domain. It is hard to find a uniform pattern to segment tumors since tumors vary in size, type, and shape. In medical institutions, physicians use magnetic resonance imaging (MRI) to locate, track, diagnose and treat the tumor. However, physicians still need to manually contour the boundary of tumor to conduct a high-quality treatment plan. For a 3D MRI, it is time consuming for physicians to manually segment tumor slides by slides. Recently, the RSNA-ASNR-MICCAI Brain Tumor Segmentation Challenge (BraTS) is one of the competitions which provides a well-labeled brain tumor dataset for competitors

© The Author(s), under exclusive license to Springer Nature Switzerland AG 2023
S. Bakas et al. (Eds.): BrainLes 2022, LNCS 14092, pp. 228–240, 2023.
https://doi.org/10.1007/978-3-031-44153-0_22

to find out the best segmentation method for brain tumor [2]. It shows great quality segmentation results of CNN based deep learning method. Meanwhile, it also provided various state-of-art brain tumor segmentation algorithms and demonstrated the potential of deep learning methods.

Recent post-challenge proceedings in BraTS challenge shows that most of the methods are based on UNet [20]. UNet, one of the famous methods in the medical image segmentation domain, is an encoder-decoder based deep neural network. It is wildly used as a baseline architecture for most segmentation in other image segmentation methods. Many variants of UNet were proposed to be used for brain tumor segmentation by adding additional blocks. Residual 3D UNet was implemented by adding residual block on 3D UNet [26]. Densely connected UNet introduces a new densely connected layer [7]. Vnet is another approach to improvement UNet by introducing Dice Coefficient loss which is an innovation loss function broadly used in the segmentation method! [13]. Other approaches combined UNet with self-attention mechanisms, such as TranBTS [25] and TransUNet [4].

However, while existing works show great potential and demonstrate their capability for medical image segmentation in research and experiment studies, there are still challenges in how to effectively harness the distributed medical data and apply ML/DL in clinical applications due to data privacy [17] and data scarcity [11]. Federated learning (FL) for healthcare [27] has recently been recognized as a promising solution to address privacy and data governance challenges by enabling ML from non-co-located data. Federated learning (also known as collaborative learning) was introduced in 2017 as a deep learning technique that trains an algorithm across multiple decentralized edge devices or servers holding local data samples without exchanging them [12]. the Federated Tumor Segmentation (FeTS) 2022 challenge which is the first challenge to ever be proposed to address brain tumor segmentation by using federated learning.

In this work, we implement the training and evaluation of UNet for FeTS 2022 challenge using two federated learning frameworks, FedML [6] and NVIDIA FLARE (NVFLARE) [15]. The UNet baseline got mean dice scores of 0.734, 0.763, and 0.827 of Enhanced Tumor (ET), Tumor Core (TC), and Whole Tumor (WT) of the FeTS validation data. The FedML with FedOPT policy got 0.724, 0.701, and 0.760 of ET, TC, and WT respectively. NVFLARE with FedAVG policy got 0.724, 0.723, and 0.784 of ET, TC, and WT respectively. To compare with the best network and model, we have optimized the UNet network and training hyperparameters, with centralized training, the model of the optimized 3D UNet achieved mean dice scores of 0.811, 0.848, and 0.910 on ET, TC, and WT respectively. We however were not able to use either FedML or NVFLARE to train the models from the optimized network and hyperparameters because both FedML and NVFLARE requires much more computing resources to train this network. This indicates the limitations of the current FL framework of handling complicated network structures and more computation-intensive training tasks.

The remainder of the paper is organized as follows: Sect. 2 discusses related work. Section 3 presents network structure of 3D UNet, how we modify it, and the detailed setting for both federated learning frameworks. Section 4 includes evaluation of the models with FeTS 2022 Challenge dataset. Section 5 discusses the result and future improvements of our work.

2   Related Work

Convolutional neural networks (CNNs) are a type of artificial neural network designed for image recognition and processing tasks [21]. They have been the primary model architecture for computer vision tasks for many years and have shown great success in a variety of applications, including brain tumor image segmentation [3]. One of the most influential models in this area is the UNet [20], which introduced the successful "U-shaped" paradigm for medical image segmentation. Since its introduction, several variants of the UNet have been developed, including V-Net [13], Residual UNet [28], UNet++ [29], and nnUNet [8], which have modified and improved the CNN-based U-shaped network architecture and continue to demonstrate strong performance on many image segmentation tasks [1].

3   Methods

In this section, we will first introduce the baseline UNet model and discuss various optimization and modification techniques. As mentioned in Sect. 1, we will use FedML and NVFLARE for federated training. We will present each federated framework, along with its training details, in the following subsections. We will also provide detailed descriptions of the spilled methods, training parameters, and aggregation policies used for the two different federated learning frameworks.

3.1   3D UNet

To begin with, we implemented a baseline UNet model that is based on the original UNet architecture [20] and extended to 3 dimensions. The network architecture, shown in Fig. 1, has a typical "U" shape with a decoder, encoder part, and a bottom layer. No additional variant blocks, such as dense blocks, residual blocks, or self-attention blocks, were included to extract features. The encoder part consists of three down-sampling blocks, each of which uses a 3D convolution operation with a ReLu activation function. The decoder part has an up-sampling block that uses transposed convolution.

The input consists of four 3D MRI images, each with a size of $128\times128\times128$. We applied three down-sampling operations, each of which includes a convolution operation to obtain a low-resolution feature map. After each convolution operation, we applied a ReLU activation function, normalization, and zero padding. The initial filter size was set to 32. At the bottleneck, we mirrored the feature maps from the encoder to the decoder part. With three up-sampling operations, we restored the segmentation output into four class labels. The initial learning rate was set to 2e-4 and was reduced according to the formula below:

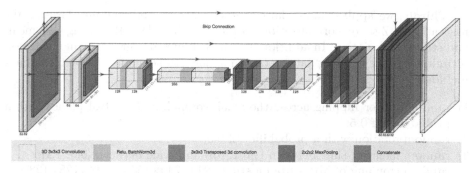

Fig. 1. 3D UNet Network Architecture. For FeTS 2022, we used an input patch size of 128×128×128 and four MRIs as four modalities. The network has a U-shaped architecture with three down blocks for down-sampling. Each down block uses 3D convolution with a 3 × 3x3 filter for each modality. Up-sampling is performed using convolution transpose. The size of the feature map is shown in the encoder part. At the bottom of the U shape, the feature maps are directly copied into the encoder part.

$$a = a * \left(1 - \frac{e}{es}\right)^{0.9} \qquad (1)$$

where e is current epochs, es is total number of epochs. We used L2 norm regularization on the convolutional kernel parameters with a weight of 1e−5. The learning rate is decayed with a schedule at 2e−4. We ran the training for a total of 1000 epochs, with each epoch having 52 iterations. We also applied pre-processing and data augmentation to the training data.

3.2 Optimization and Modifications

We optimized and modified the baseline UNet according to the guideline from nnUNet [9].

Firstly, we applied region-based training optimization. The training dataset has three labels: edema (label 2), necrosis (label 1), and enhancing tumor (label 4). However, the evaluation of the segmentation results is based on three regions: enhancing tumor, tumor core (enhancing tumor with necrosis), and whole tumor (enhancing tumor, necrosis, and edema). According to previous BraTS challenge methods [8,10,14,24], performance can be improved if we optimized the region rather than optimized the label. Therefore, we used a sigmoid function on the three tumor regions at the last layer of the 3D UNet in order to obtain a better segmentation result.

Secondly, we increased the batch size from 2 to 24. According to previous BraTS challenge conclusions, using a lower batch size on a larger dataset can produce noisier gradients, which may reduce the over-fitting issue while also influencing performance. This is a bias-variance trade-off when choosing the batch size [23].

Thirdly, we applied more data augmentation to the training dataset. We first applied Z-score normalization to all modality 3D MRIs using the mean and standard deviation. In addition, we applied several aggressive augmentation techniques to the training data to obtain a more stable model. These techniques included:

1) random mirror flipping across the axial, coronal, and sagittal planes with a probability of 0.5;
2) random rotation with a probability of 0.5;
3) random intensity shift between $[-0.1, 0.1]$ and scale between $[0.9, 1.1]$;
4) random cropping of MRIs from a size of $240\times240\times155$ to $128\times128\times128$;

Lastly, we used batch normalization instead of instance normalization. Based on previous experiences in the BraTS challenge, the performance of the test dataset in terms of dice score was significantly lower than that of the training and validation datasets, likely due to existing domain gaps [8]. To reduce these gaps, we applied more data augmentation techniques and used batch normalization.

3.3 FedML

FedML is an open-source research library and benchmark for federated machine learning [6]. It provides a federated learning framework that covers several domain topics such as computer vision, natural language processing, medical image processing, finance, and more. FedML supports various different computing paradigms: on-device training, distributed training, standalone simulation, and so on. The overview architecture of FedML is shown in Fig. 2.

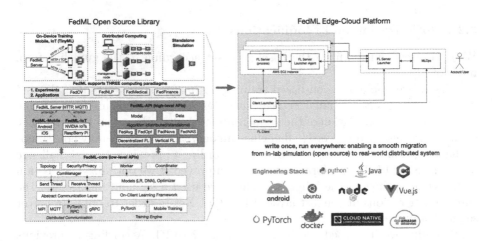

Fig. 2. FedML Core Architecture Design [5]

In this work, we adapted FedML to train FeTS 2022 challenge data on one computer for a standalone federated learning simulation. To use FedML, we split the challenge dataset into several sites based on the medical institution ID provided by the official FeTS training dataset. Each site represents a distinct medical institution during the simulation training process. We also randomly spilt the dataset into train and test at a ratio of 0.8. Then we applied the same pre-process to the training dataset that is the same as centralized training on 3D UNet. We applied two aggregation policies (FedAvg [12] and FedOPT [18]) for two training. We ran the training for 1000 rounds. The learning rate was set as 1e−4. All the other training parameters were consistent with those used in centralized UNet training.

3.4   NVFLARE

NVFLARE is an open-source Federated Learning framework that allows researchers to adapt their ML/DL methods to a federated paradigm and build a distributed collaboration [15]. It provides a robust SDK for users to deploy a real-world federated learning framework with high privacy security and supports federated training simulations on a standalone computer. However, users must assign one site per GPU, which means the number of sites is limited to the number of GPUs when compared to FedML. The overall architecture of NVFLARE is shown in Fig. 3

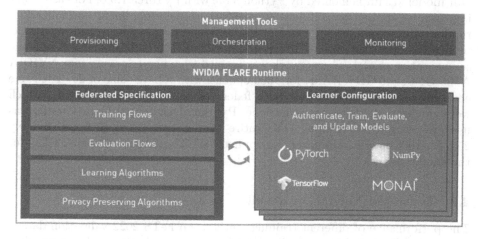

Fig. 3. Overall Core Architecture Design of NVFLARE [15]

In this work, we made several changes to NVFLARE for one computer standalone federated learning simulation on the FeTS 2022 challenge data. Similar to FedML, we randomly split the challenge dataset according to the number of GPUs on their machine, which is 4. Thus, the number of sites for NVFLARE training is 4. We also applied the same pre-processing and augmentation to the training data, used FedAvg [12] as the aggregation policy for training, and ran the training with the same round number as FedML. The learning rate was set as 1e−4 and the rest of the training parameters were the same as centralized UNet training.

4   Result

4.1   FeTS Datasets

We used the FeTS 2022 challenge datasets for evaluation [2,16,19,22]. The FeTS 2022 training dataset comprises of 1251 cases. Each training case includes one segmentation ground truth, and four modalities of 3D MRIs namely T1-weighted, T2-weighted, T1 contrast-enhanced, and T2 FLAIR. Our model was trained solely with the FeTS training dataset, without incorporating any other public or private datasets. In this work, we treated four 3D MRIs as four input channels in the computer vision tasks, and each volume has dimensions of $240 \times 240 \times 155$. The ground truth labels have 4 classes: label 0 represents the background, label 1 represents enhancing tumor, label 4 represents necrosis, and label 2 represents edema. The validation dataset consists of 219 cases with no ground truth provided. For the evaluation metrics, we use Dice score and Hausdorff distances as required by the challenge.

4.2   Implementation Details

Our model was implemented by Python 3.8.5 with PyTorch 1.9.0. For each training case, we applied several data augmentations including linear normalization, random crop, random clip, random intensity shift, and so on. Each image was preprocessed by cropping to a size of $128 \times 128 \times 128$ before being fed into the segmentation model. The network was trained from scratch using four NVIDIA A100 GPUs (40 GB VRAM) for 1000 epochs, with a batch size of 24. The same environment was employed for both federated and centralized training, which were carried out on the same machine. PyTorch Distributed Data Parallel was used for centralized training. The entire training process took approximately 25 h for 1000 epochs. Moreover, we applied Test-Time Augmentation (TTA) for the challenge.

4.3   Federated Validation Result

The performance of different training methods on FeTS 2022 validation data is reported as Table 1. The centralized method yielded a better performance than the two Federated Learning frameworks. Among these frameworks, NVFLARE had better performance than FedML. We speculated that the reason for this could be related to the data splitting methods. FedML split the data based on institution ID, which is more representative of real-world scenarios. However, the datasets split by FedML were more unbalanced compared to NVFLARE, which evenly split the data into 4 sites. In terms of the aggregation policy, FedOPT performed slightly better than FedAvg. The optimizations and modifications applied resulted in a significant improvement in performance compared to the model that was submitted to the challenge.

Table 1. Dice score and Hausdorff distance on FeTS 2022 validation dataset. ET, TC, WT present enhancing tumor, tumor core, and whole tumor respectively.

Validation dataset	Dice			Hausdorff95 (mm)		
	ET	TC	WT	ET	TC	WT
Unet baseline	0.7335	0.7633	0.8266	32.6349	25.3428	17.4926
FedML(FedAvg)	0.7267	0.6772	0.7492	34.6926	40.0021	26.0513
FedML(FedOPT)	0.7235	0.7012	0.7597	33.5342	37.9832	25.7833
NVFLARE	0.7245	0.7231	0.7847	32.8643	34.1002	17.9282
Challenge	0.8113	0.8482	0.9101	18.0867	11.4861	4.39933

4.4 Validation Phase Result for Competition

In terms of challenge, we have this section specially listed for the competition result. The performance of our model on FedTS 2022 validation data is reported as Table 2. Our model reached the mean dice scores of 0.81, 0.84, and 0.91 on ET, TC, and WT respectively. From the deviation, it is evident that the enhancing tumor and tumor core have high variation. By analyzing the median and 25th quantile results, we can see that our model is stable across the entire validation dataset. Upon reviewing the complete validation score table, we found that our model had a score of 0 for enhancing tumor on some validation cases, which also had lower dice scores such as cases 1689, 1797, and so on. We will investigate further the reasons for the differences in performance on these cases.

Table 2. Dice score and Hausdorff distance on FeTS 2022 validation dataset. ET, TC, and WT present enhancing tumor, tumor core, and whole tumor respectively.

Validation dataset	Dice			Hausdorff95 (mm)		
	ET	TC	WT	ET	TC	WT
mean	0.8113	0.8482	0.9101	18.0867	11.4861	4.3993
stdev	0.2477	0.2265	0.0870	73.6223	50.1051	7.0679
median	0.8922	0.9326	0.9357	1.4142	2.2361	2.4495
25th quantile	0.8266	0.8534	0.8935	1.0000	1.0000	1.7321
75th quantile	0.9416	0.9629	0.9586	2.8284	4.3298	4.2426

4.5 Qualitative Results

We selected some validation cases that were close to the dice scores we presented in the last section for visualization. These validation cases were chosen as the best, worst, median, and 75th and 25th percentiles based on their Dice scores. As shown in Fig. 4, the overall segmentation quality is high. The best case is FeTS2022_00153 with dice scores of 0.983, 0.992, 0.988 on ET, TC, and WT. The

75th percentile case is FeTS2022_00129 with dice scores of 0.942, 0.960, 0.953 on ET, TC, and WT. The median case is FeTS2022_00256 with dice scores of 0.869, 0.882, 0.895 on ET, TC, and WT. The 25th percentile case is FeTS2022_00129 with dice scores of 0.824, 0.866, 0.905 on ET, TC, and WT. The worst case is FeTS2022_00213 with dice scores of 0.081, 0.081, 0.506 on ET, TC, and WT.

4.6   Test Phase Result for Competition

The performance of our model on FedTS 2022 test data is reported as Table 3. In the test phase, our model was evaluated on 30 different sites, representing 30 different medical institutions. Each site has an unknown number of test cases with undisclosed ground truth. The performance that we listed in Table 3 is the mean value of all test cases for each site including mean value, the standard deviation, the median value, the best, worst, 25th quantile, and 75th quantile. The total test cases on each local site are still unknown to us. Compared to validation datasets, our model had better performance in terms of mean value among the real test cases. Our model also reached the mean dice scores of 0.854, 0.869, and 0.913 on ET, TC, and WT respectively. From the standard deviation perspective, the values indicate that the performance is stable across all 30 sites, with standard deviations of only 0.06, 0.08, and 0.04 for ET, TC, and WT, respectively. By analyzing the median, worst site, and 25th percentile results, we can see that our model is stable in most medical institutions. However, the values of the worst sites decrease the overall performance of the global model. In the future, we will work to optimize the performance of the worst sites.

Table 3. Dice score and Hausdorff distance on FeTS 2022 test dataset. ET, TC, and WT present enhancing tumor, tumor core, and whole tumor respectively.

Test dataset	Dice			Hausdorff95 (mm)		
	ET	TC	WT	ET	TC	WT
mean	0.8543	0.8688	0.9133	11.7867	12.2827	6.3178
stdev	0.0683	0.0806	0.0470	12.8352	14.5118	5.3278
median	0.8677	0.8931	0.9253	4.7401	5.9342	4.4666
min	0.7151	0.6416	0.7822	47.5965	58.6337	25.0028
max	0.9477	0.9626	0.9650	1.2649	1.8225	1.6413
25th quantile	0.8016	0.8288	0.9053	21.3416	16.4353	7.8095
75th quantile	0.9075	0.9268	0.9460	2.2018	2.9832	3.3202

5   Discussion

In this work, we presented an optimized and modified UNet model for improved segmentation on multi-modality 3D MRI. Our results in the validation phase

T1   T2   FLAIR   Predict

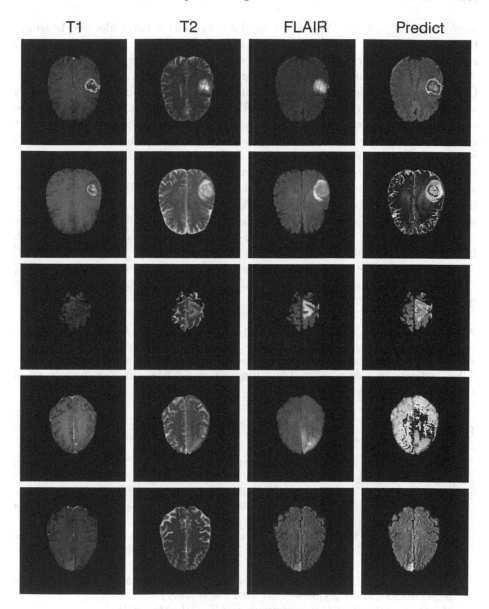

Fig. 4. The visualization of qualitative results is presented as follows: For each row, the raw T1 image is shown in the first left column. The second column to the left is the raw T2 image. The T2 Flair image is next to the T2 image. The predicted outcome is in the last right column. Edema is shown in green, enhancing tumor in red, and necrosis/non-enhancing tumor in blue. From the first row to the last row, we have displayed the best, 75th percentile, median, 25th percentile, and worst validation cases, respectively. (Color figure online)

were generally positive. We also adapted our method to two Federated Learning frameworks, FedML and NVFLARE, and both frameworks performed well and showed potential for federated training on the FeTS challenge data.

In the future, there are several improvements we can make to our method. One aspect we can focus on is implementing a post-processing method for cases where the enhancing tumor is empty. These cases can result in undefined dice scores due to division by 0. To address this, we can apply an algorithm that replaces all empty enhancing tumor predictions with tumor core labels. By removing the empty enhancing tumor and replacing it with necrosis, we can ensure that these voxels are still considered part of the tumor core. This will not affect the performance of the tumor core and improve our Rank score by removing those true positive predictions. Additionally, we can improve our method by using batch dice instead of mini-batch dice. By using batch dice, we can consider the entire dataset as one large sample that is trained in one batch. This approach balances the trade-off between bias and variation.

In conclusion, we achieved mean dice scores of 0.854, 0.869, and 0.913 on ET, TC, and WT, respectively. We will address the proposed improvements in the next challenge.

Acknowledgment. We acknowledge support from the National Science Foundation under Grant 2015254, from the University of Southern California, and from the University of Texas at Anderson Cancer Center, Texas Advanced Computing Center, and Oden Institute for Computational and Engineering Sciences initiative in Oncological Data and Computational Science.

References

1. Antonelli, M., et al.: The medical segmentation decathlon. Nat. Commun. **13**(1), 1–13 (2022)
2. Baid, U., et al.: The RSNA-ASNR-MICCAI brats 2021 benchmark on brain tumor segmentation and radiogenomic classification. arXiv preprint arXiv:2107.02314 (2021)
3. Bakas, S., et al.: Segmentation labels and radiomic features for the pre-operative scans of the TCGA-GBM collection. The cancer imaging archive. Nat. Sci. Data **4**, 170117 (2017)
4. Chen, J., et al.: Transunet: transformers make strong encoders for medical image segmentation. arXiv preprint arXiv:2102.04306 (2021)
5. He, C.: FedML (2022). https://github.com/FedML-AI/FedML
6. He, C., et al.: FedML: a research library and benchmark for federated machine learning. In: Advances in Neural Information Processing Systems, Best Paper Award at Federate Learning Workshop (2020)
7. Huang, G., Liu, Z., Van Der Maaten, L., Weinberger, K.Q.: Densely connected convolutional networks. In: Proceedings of the IEEE Conference on Computer Vision and Pattern Recognition, pp. 4700–4708 (2017)
8. Isensee, F., Jaeger, P.F., Kohl, S.A., Petersen, J., Maier-Hein, K.H.: nnU-net: a self-configuring method for deep learning-based biomedical image segmentation. Nat. Methods **18**(2), 203–211 (2021)

9. Isensee, F., Jäger, P.F., Full, P.M., Vollmuth, P., Maier-Hein, K.H.: nnU-net for brain tumor segmentation. In: Crimi, A., Bakas, S. (eds.) BrainLes 2020. LNCS, vol. 12659, pp. 118–132. Springer, Cham (2021). https://doi.org/10.1007/978-3-030-72087-2_11

10. Kamnitsas, K., Bai, W., Ferrante, E., McDonagh, S., Sinclair, M., Pawlowski, N., Rajchl, M., Lee, M., Kainz, B., Rueckert, D., Glocker, B.: Ensembles of multiple models and architectures for robust brain tumour segmentation. In: Crimi, A., Bakas, S., Kuijf, H., Menze, B., Reyes, M. (eds.) BrainLes 2017. LNCS, vol. 10670, pp. 450–462. Springer, Cham (2018). https://doi.org/10.1007/978-3-319-75238-9_38

11. Langlotz, C.P., et al.: A roadmap for foundational research on artificial intelligence in medical imaging: from the 2018 NIH/RSNA/ACR/the academy workshop. Radiology 291(3), 781 (2019)

12. McMahan, B., Moore, E., Ramage, D., Hampson, S., Arcas, B.A.: Communication-efficient learning of deep networks from decentralized data. In: Artificial Intelligence and Statistics, pp. 1273–1282. PMLR (2017)

13. Milletari, F., Navab, N., Ahmadi, S.A.: V-net: fully convolutional neural networks for volumetric medical image segmentation. In: 2016 Fourth International Conference on 3D Vision (3DV), pp. 565–571. IEEE (2016)

14. Myronenko, A.: 3D MRI brain tumor segmentation using autoencoder regularization. In: Crimi, A., Bakas, S., Kuijf, H., Keyvan, F., Reyes, M., van Walsum, T. (eds.) BrainLes 2018. LNCS, vol. 11384, pp. 311–320. Springer, Cham (2019). https://doi.org/10.1007/978-3-030-11726-9_28

15. NVIDIA: Nvidia federated learning application runtime environment (2022). https://github.com/NVIDIA/NVFlare

16. Pati, S., et al.: The federated tumor segmentation (Fets) challenge. arXiv preprint arXiv:2105.05874 (2021)

17. Price, W.N., Cohen, I.G.: Privacy in the age of medical big data. Nat. Med. 25(1), 37–43 (2019)

18. Reddi, S., et al.: Adaptive federated optimization. arXiv preprint arXiv:2003.00295 (2020)

19. Reina, G.A., et al.: OpenFL: an open-source framework for federated learning. arXiv preprint arXiv:2105.06413 (2021)

20. Ronneberger, O., Fischer, P., Brox, T.: U-net: convolutional networks for biomedical image segmentation. In: Navab, N., Hornegger, J., Wells, W.M., Frangi, A.F. (eds.) MICCAI 2015. LNCS, vol. 9351, pp. 234–241. Springer, Cham (2015). https://doi.org/10.1007/978-3-319-24574-4_28

21. Schmidhuber, J.: Deep learning in neural networks: an overview. Neural Netw. 61, 85–117 (2015)

22. Sheller, M.J., et al.: Federated learning in medicine: facilitating multi-institutional collaborations without sharing patient data. Sci. Rep. 10(1), 1–12 (2020)

23. Shi, Y., Micklisch, C., Mushtaq, E., Avestimehr, S., Yan, Y., Zhang, X.: An ensemble approach to automatic brain tumor segmentation. In: Crimi, A., Bakas, S. (eds.) Brainlesion: Glioma, Multiple Sclerosis, Stroke and Traumatic Brain Injuries. BrainLes 2021. LNCS, vol. 12963, pp. 138–148. Springer, Cham (2022). https://doi.org/10.1007/978-3-031-09002-8_13

24. Wang, G., Li, W., Ourselin, S., Vercauteren, T.: Automatic brain tumor segmentation using cascaded anisotropic convolutional neural networks. In: Crimi, A., Bakas, S., Kuijf, H., Menze, B., Reyes, M. (eds.) BrainLes 2017. LNCS, vol. 10670, pp. 178–190. Springer, Cham (2018). https://doi.org/10.1007/978-3-319-75238-9_16

25. Wang, W., Chen, C., Ding, M., Li, J., Yu, H., Zha, S.: Transbts: multimodal brain tumor segmentation using transformer. arXiv preprint arXiv:2103.04430 (2021)
26. Wolny, A., et al.: Accurate and versatile 3d segmentation of plant tissues at cellular resolution. eLife **9**, 57613 (2020). https://doi.org/10.7554/elife.57613
27. Zerka, F., et al.: Systematic review of privacy-preserving distributed machine learning from federated databases in health care. JCO Clin. Cancer Inform. **4**, 184–200 (2020)
28. Zhang, Z., Liu, Q., Wang, Y.: Road extraction by deep residual u-net. IEEE Geosci. Remote Sens. Lett. **15**(5), 749–753 (2018)
29. Zhou, Z., Rahman Siddiquee, M.M., Tajbakhsh, N., Liang, J.: UNet++: a nested u-net architecture for medical image segmentation. In: Stoyanov, D., et al. (eds.) DLMIA/ML-CDS -2018. LNCS, vol. 11045, pp. 3–11. Springer, Cham (2018). https://doi.org/10.1007/978-3-030-00889-5_1

Author Index

A

Abderezaei, Javid II-35
Adamski, Szymon I-186, II-218
Alasmawi, Hussain II-90
Albarqouni, Shadi I-25
Aldahdooh, Ahmed I-25
Alhoniemi, Esa II-121
Almahfouz Nasser, Sahar II-15
An, Ning II-142
Atzori, Manfredo I-241
Avestimehr, Salman II-228
Azeem, Mohammad Ayyaz II-121

B

Baheti, Bhakti I-68
Bakas, Spyridon I-3, I-68
Berger, Derek I-57
Bi, Lei I-273
Bossa, Matías I-80
Bouchet, Philippe I-149
Boutry, Nicolas I-149
Braghin, Stefano II-183
Burgert, Oliver I-127, II-25

C

Canalini, Luca I-262
Canton-Bacara, Hugo I-149
Cetinkaya, Coskun II-79
Chen, Zhaolin II-173
Cho, Jihoon I-138
Chopra, Agamdeep II-35
Christensen, Søren I-45
Chung, Albert C. S. I-231
Colman, Jordan I-102

D

Dawant, Benoit M. II-109
de la Rosa, Ezequiel I-3
De Sutter, Selene I-80
Deloges, Jean-Baptiste I-149
Dou, Qi II-161

Duan, Wenting I-102
Duerinck, Johnny I-80

E

Egan, Gary II-173
Elbaz, Othman I-149
Epperlein, Jonathan P. II-183
Ezhov, Ivan I-3, II-209

F

Fan, Yubo II-109
Farzana, W. I-205
Feng, Dagan I-273
Fidon, Lucas I-3
Finck, Tom I-3
Fischi-Gomez, Elda I-45
Futrega, Michał I-162

G

Gao, Hongjian II-228
Geens, Wietse I-80
Gerken, Annika I-262
Ghorbel, Ahmed I-25
Großbröhmer, Christoph I-252
Guan, Cuntai II-68
Gulli, Giosue I-102

H

Hahn, Horst K. I-262
Hakim, Arsany I-45
Hamghalam, Mohammad I-195
Hamidouche, Wassim I-25
Han, Ji-Wung II-100
Han, Luyi II-49
Hansen, Lasse I-252
Harandi, Mehrtash II-173
Hardan, Shahad II-90
Hayat, Munawar II-173
Heinrich, Mattias P. I-252
Heldmann, Stefan I-262

Heo, Keun-Soo   II-100
Hering, Alessa   I-262
Horvath, Izabela   I-3
Hou, Qingfan   I-174
Hou, Xiangjian   II-90
Hu, Qingyu   II-142
Huang, Tsung-Ming   I-216
Huang, Yunzhi   II-49
Hung, Chih-Cheng   II-79

I
Iftekharuddin, K. M.   I-205

J
Jafaritadi, Mojtaba   II-121
Jiang, Jian   I-174
Jiang, Meirui   II-161
Jurgas, Artur   I-241

K
Kadhe, Swanand   II-183
Kaissis, Georgios   I-14
Kam, Tae-Eui   II-100
Kanagavelu, Renuga   II-196
Kang, Bogyeong   II-100
Karar, Mohamed E.   I-127, II-25
Khan, Muhammad Irfan   II-121
Khan, Suleiman A.   II-121
Kim, Jinman   I-273
Kirschke, Jan   I-3
Klein, Jan   I-262
Kober, Tobias   I-45
Kofler, Florian   I-3
Kontio, Elina   II-121
Kotowski, Krzysztof   I-90, I-186, II-218
Kurian, Nikhil Cherian   II-15
Kurt, Mehmet   II-35

L
LaMaster, John   I-3
Levman, Jacob   I-57
Li, Hongwei   I-3
Li, Tiexiang   I-216
Liao, Jia-Wei   I-216
Lin, Wen-Wei   I-216
Liu, Han   II-109
Liu, Hong   II-79
Liu, Yong   II-196
Lu, Shiyu   I-115

M
Mächler, Leon   II-209
Machura, Bartosz   I-90, I-186, II-218
Madrona, Antoine   I-45
Malara, Wojciech   II-218
Mann, Ritse   II-49
Marcinkiewicz, Michał   I-162
Marini, Niccolò   I-241
Mathis-Ullrich, Franziska   I-127, II-25
Mazerolle, Erin   I-57
McKinley, Richard   I-45
Meena, Mohit   II-15
Meissen, Felix   I-14
Meng, Mingyuan   I-273
Menze, Bjoern   I-3, I-68
Mojtahedi, Ramtin   I-195
Mok, Tony C. W.   I-231
Müller, Henning   I-241

N
Nalepa, Jakub   I-90, I-186, II-218
Nam, Hyeonyeong   II-100

O
Oguz, Ipek   II-109
Otálora, Sebastian   I-45

P
Paetzold, Johannes   I-3, I-14
Paetzold, Johannes C.   II-209
Park, Jinah   I-138
Passerrat-Palmbach, Jonathan   II-154
Pati, Sarthak   I-68
Peiris, Himashi   II-173
Peng, Yanjun   I-174
Pinot, Lucas   I-149
Pionteck, Aymeric   II-35
Piraud, Marie   I-3
Pusel, Gaëtan   I-149

R
Rafael-Patiño, Jonathan   I-45
Rahman, M. M.   I-205
Ravano, Veronica   I-45
Rawat, Ambrish   II-183
Ren, Jianxun   II-142
Ribalta, Pablo   I-162
Richiardi, Jonas   I-45
Rueckert, Daniel   I-14

S

Sadique, M. S.   I-205
Sethi, Amit   II-15
Shamsi, Saqib   II-15
Shi, Yaying   II-228
Shit, Suprosanna   I-3, II-209
Siebert, Hanna   I-252
Simpson, Amber L.   I-195
Singh, Gaurav   II-133
Siomos, Vasilis   II-154
Song, Enmin   II-79
Soufan, Othman   I-57

T

Tan, Tao   II-49
Tarroni, Giacomo   II-154
Temtam, A.   I-205

V

Vanbinst, Anne-Marie   I-80
Vandemeulebroucke, Jef   I-80
Vercauteren, Tom   I-3

W

Wang, Han   I-216
Wang, Hao   I-115
Wang, Jiao   I-174
Wang, Jueqi   I-57
Wang, Lisheng   II-59
Wang, Yuan   II-196
Wang, Zhuofei   I-174
Wei, Qingsong   II-196
Wiest, Roland   I-45

W

Wiestler, Benedikt   I-3
Wodzinski, Marek   I-241

X

Xu, Kaixin   II-68

Y

Yan, Kewei   II-3
Yan, Yonghong   II-3, II-228
Yang, Hongzheng   II-161
Yang, Tao   II-59
Yang, Xulei   II-68
Yang, Yechao   II-196
Yaqub, Mohammad   II-90
Yau, Shing-Tung   I-216
Ye, Chuyang   I-115
Ye, Xujiong   I-102
Yeo, Huai Zhe   II-68

Z

Zarudzki, Lukasz   I-186, II-218
Zeineldin, Ramy A.   I-127, II-25
Zhang, Lei   I-102
Zhang, Shaoting   II-161
Zhang, Wei   II-142
Zhang, Xiaofan   II-161
Zhang, Youjia   II-142
Zhao, Ziyuan   II-68
Zhou, Ying   II-142
Zhuang, Yuzhou   II-79
Zimmer, Claus   I-3
Zizzo, Giulio   II-183

Printed in the United States
by Baker & Taylor Publisher Services